PSYCHOTHERAPY IN CHEMICAL DEPENDENCE TREATMENT

A Practical and Integrative Approach

D0059170

BOOKS OF RELATED INTEREST

Concepts of Chemical Dependency, Third Edition
Harold E. Doweiko (1996)
ISBN 0-534-33904-2

Exploring Psychological Disorders, Version 3.0
Douglas L. Chute and Margaret E. Bliss (1995)
ISBN 0-534-23179-9

Substance Abuse Counseling: An Individualized Approach, Second Edition
Judith A. Lewis, Robert Q. Dana, and Gregory Blevins (1994)
ISBN 0-534-20053-2

Under the Influence: Alcohol and Human Behavior
John Jung (1994)
ISBN 0-534-20448-1

PSYCHOTHERAPY IN CHEMICAL DEPENDENCE TREATMENT

A PRACTICAL AND INTEGRATIVE APPROACH

GEORGE D. BUELOW
University of Southern Mississippi

SIDNE A. BUELOW
Clearview Chemical Dependence Treatment Center

Brooks/Cole Publishing Company

I(T)P® An International Thomson Publishing Company

Pacific Grove ◆ Albany ◆ Belmont ◆ Bonn ◆ Boston ◆ Cincinnati ◆ Detroit
Johannesburg ◆ London ◆ Madrid ◆ Melbourne ◆ Mexico City
New York ◆ Paris ◆ Singapore ◆ Tokyo ◆ Toronto ◆ Washington

TO JOE STEINER, SR., AND THE TREATMENT STAFF AT SERENITY LANE AND CLEARVIEW CHEMICAL DEPENDENCE TREATMENT CENTERS

Sponsoring Editor: *Eileen Murphy*
Marketing Team: *Romy Taormina,*
 Jean Vevers Thompson, and Deanne Brown
Editorial Assistant: *Susan Carlson*
Production Coordinator: *Laurel Jackson*
Production Service: *Scratchgravel Publishing*
 Services

Manuscript Editor: *Catherine Cambron*
Permissions Editor: *Cathleen Collins Morrison*
Interior Design: *Anne Draus*
Cover Design: *Laurie Albrecht*
Typesetting: *Scratchgravel Publishing Services*
Cover Printing: *Phoenix Color Corporation*
Printing and Binding: *R. R. Donnelly & Sons, Inc.*

For more information, contact:

BROOKS/COLE PUBLISHING COMPANY
511 Forest Lodge Road
Pacific Grove, CA 93950
USA

International Thomson Editores
Seneca 53
Col. Polanco
11560 México, D. F., México

International Thomson Publishing Europe
Berkshire House 168-173
High Holborn
London WC1V 7AA
England

International Thomson Publishing Japan
Hirakawacho Kyowa Building, 3F
2-2-1 Hirakawacho
Chiyoda-ku, Tokyo 102
Japan

Thomas Nelson Australia
102 Dodds Street
South Melbourne, 3205
Victoria, Australia

International Thomson Publishing Asia
221 Henderson Road
#05-10 Henderson Building
Singapore 0315

Nelson Canada
1120 Birchmount Road
Scarborough, Ontario
Canada M1K 5G4

International Thomson Publishing GmbH
Königswinterer Strasse 418
53227 Bonn
Germany

Printed in the United States of America

10   9   8   7   6   5   4   3   2   1

Library of Congress Cataloging-in-Publication Data
Buelow, George, [date]–
    Psychotherapy in chemical dependence treatment : a practical and
 integrative approach / George D. Buelow, Sidne A. Buelow
     p.   cm.
    Includes bibliographical references and index.
    ISBN 0-534-26118-3 (alk. paper)
    1. Substance abuse—Treatment.   2. Psychotherapy.   I. Buelow,
 Sidne A.   II. Title.
 RA564.B84   1998
 616.86'0651—dc21   97-23147
                                                          CIP

CONTENTS

◆ PART ONE ◆
A MODEL FOR CHANGE

3 CASE CONCEPTUALIZATION, TREATMENT PLANNING, AND TREATMENT   93

4 MAINTENANCE, RELAPSE, AND RELAPSE PREVENTION   124

◆ PART TWO ◆
CHEMICAL DEPENDENCE PRACTICE CONCERNS

5 INDIVIDUAL TREATMENT   145

6 FAMILY DYNAMICS AND TREATMENT   172

PREFACE

This book provides a concise, practical guide to the assessment, case conceptualization, treatment planning, treatment, and aftercare of substance abuse and dependence. It fills a relative vacuum between substance abuse education texts on the one hand and psychopharmacology texts that stress the structure of abused and psychiatric drugs on the other. The book is written for students and practitioners who are or plan to be in the trenches working on treatment and relapse issues with substance abusers. In particular, the book provides a transtheoretical model of how change takes place in chemical dependence treatment—a model that utilizes Prochaska, DiClemente, and Norcross's work on common stages and processes of personal change. Most counseling and psychotherapy techniques can be used effectively at some time in chemical dependence treatment. Knowing when, how, and why to use particular techniques distinguishes the well-trained clinician, whether he or she is a psychologist, counselor, certified alcohol and drug counselor (CADC), psychiatric nurse, or social worker.

This text is a nuts-and-bolts approach to the domains of chemical dependence treatment. It emphasizes the consultative nature of relationships between therapists and clients and between therapists and other therapists, common in concurrent psychotherapy and structured chemical dependence treatment. The book focuses on issues often confronted by therapists working with dual-diagnosis clients. The introduction, which describes a transtheoretical model of chemical dependence self-change and psychotherapy intervention, uses a structured approach to decision making about diagnosis, referral, dual diagnosis, inpatient versus outpatient treatment, and choosing specific treatment strategies. This structured approach offers a framework within which critical decision points can be made more explicit for both client and therapist. For example, whether a practitioner decides to refer a client to an inpatient or outpatient treatment setting will have important ramifications for the client for the duration of treatment and lifelong aftercare.

We believe that psychotherapists and CADC practitioners already in the field will find important ideas in this text to enhance their present work. Issues relevant to CADCs—especially concurrent treatment and dual-diagnosis issues—are addressed throughout the book in a variety of important intervention, assessment, treatment, and aftercare domains.

Acknowledgments

We would like to thank the following reviewers of this book for their valuable insights and suggestions: Robert Q. Dana, University of Maine; Stephen R. Kahoe, El Paso Community College; John C. Lewton, University of Toledo; and Clayton T. Shorkey, University of Texas–Austin.

We also want to thank the staff at Brooks/Cole—especially Eileen Murphy, Laurie Albrecht, Deanne Brown, Susan Carlson, Laurie Jackson, Cat Collins Morrison, Kelly Shoemaker, Romy Taormina, and Jean Thompson—for their hard work on this book. In addition, special thanks go to Anne and Greg Draus, Catherine Cambron, and James Minkin for their valuable contributions to the production process.

INTRODUCTION

THE CHEMICAL DEPENDENCE TREATMENT FIELD

Our field is fragmented by forces that affect all segments of public life. Political, economic, social, religious, and technical forces have directly influenced, and in many cases determined, the goals, structure, and clinical application of treatment. Treatment specialists cannot easily leave aside the biases of society where chemically dependent clients are often held in low esteem despite their best efforts at sobriety. Clinicians' beliefs, knowledge, and treatments are focused through their ethnic and cultural values, which are in turn directly influenced by forces of moral and social control. Even though clinical judgments in the chemical dependence field may themselves be clouded by negative stereotypes, clinicians must work toward the objectivity necessary to provide the highest level of client-patient care in this developing field. In addition, we must be constantly aware of the social, legal, and political pressures that influence the funding and publication of research in our growing discipline. We must also be realistic about nonpractitioners' overly simplistic views of the substance abuse and dependence "problem." In reality, substance abuse and dependence consist of a collection of diverse problems, only some of which are the result of drugs themselves.

This book is about treatment for individuals and small groups of substance abusers; it is *not* about reforming society. Few believe that individual treatment specialists are going to solve the chemical dependence problem by treating individuals and small groups; to do so would be to imagine that a physician who worked hard enough could vanquish disease. Unfortunately, only about one out of ten who need treatment for chemical dependence receive it. The drug war, a multitude of complex geopolitical problems, will expand and contract due to forces for which clinicians, as individuals, have important responsibility, but over which they have only modest control. Fortunately, clinicians *are* in control of their own level of expertise in individual and group treatment. This book, then, is aimed at helping clinicians gain more practical insight into the chemical dependence treatment field—not at winning a war on drugs.

An old joke in the chemical dependence war game has our hero and a friend picnicking near a river when he hears the cries of people floating downstream. He and his friend rush out into the water and begin dragging people to shore. The longer they are in the water, though, the more struggling victims come downstream, and they are soon exhausted. Our tired hero thrashes to shore and begins to walk upstream. "Wait," cries his friend, "I'm wearing out. I can't handle all these people alone!" "Right. Me either," our hero yells back. "So I thought I'd go upstream and suggest that they stop jumping in!" The moral of the story is, simply, that chemical dependence treatment, important as it is, is far downstream. If you pace yourself, working downstream is feasible. If and when you decide to work farther upstream, having worked downstream will definitely give you a clearer perspective with which to accomplish your work. We advise working both ends of the stream concurrently when that is possible.

Although social forces are always important to our actions, each of us makes individual decisions about our behavior around drugs. No one makes those decisions for us. High-risk drugs will probably always be for sale just around the corner. They will always be a part of modern life. They will not go away. Denial will not armor us against their effects. Therefore, we must have both a broad knowledge of drugs themselves and a deep understanding of the social forces that determine treatment funding, goals, and clinical activities.

Due to myriad political, social, and academic pressures, some would have us believe that treatment approaches are mutually exclusive. For example, individualized treatment approaches are often juxtaposed to 12-step approaches modeled on the recovery process in Alcoholics Anonymous (AA). Scientific psychology is often described in opposition to self-help. Fortunately, these seemingly contradictory perspectives can be integrated. In some cases individualized approaches are called for. Other cases call for stepwise approaches, like AA, that stress group affiliation and spirituality. Whether or not we share the religious views typical of AA, many of our clients are desperately hanging on to every support they can find. We need not sit in judgment of other people's belief systems, but rather help them integrate their beliefs into a more drug-resistant whole that includes a more complete armamentarium.

In a majority of cases, a variety of assessment and treatment perspectives are called for. Even psychodynamic approaches of "working through" (much vilified because psychoanalytic psychotherapists misattributed addictions almost exclusively to early psychic injuries and minimized the influence of the drugs themselves) may serve some practitioners very well later in therapy if (mis)attributions of etiology are carefully examined. Chemical dependence and abuse are not a uniform class of actions and cannot be fully understood from any one perspective. An important key to chemical dependence treatment, therefore, is knowing when, how, and why to take a particular perspective or to use a particular technique.

Treatment personnel often have practical insight that researchers who are new to the field lack. Fortunately, research has generally verified and helped us refine what practitioners have learned through clinical experience. Although treatment strategies forged in the trenches and verified by treatment success must ultimately be validated by broader clinical research, innovation based on treatment experience is usually the basis for treatment change. Thus, we should not be wedded forever to particular techniques of dubious value or be afraid to innovate. After all, we are asking clients to change, and we must be willing to do so as well. Executed correctly, each treatment is an example of a single-subject research experiment, the outcome of which must be evaluated on its own terms.

In the absence of strong research support for the efficacy of techniques that have proved useful in individual cases, we must have the courage to continue to innovate. We should follow research when it is rational and well done, but not be afraid to follow our clinical instincts. Our understanding must be informed by both the richness of data provided by our clients and by our understanding of and intuition about the course of the addiction process. Techniques that cannot be clearly shown to be effective with specific individuals or subgroups should be abandoned.

Reasons for Optimism

Viewed overall, modern alcohol and drug treatment has shown good success. Research gives us many reasons for optimism. Although we will present data supporting our conclusions, we first provide a nontechnical overview. When clients and counseling strategies are matched on the basis of the difficulty of the problem and client and counselor expectations, success rates have been very high—in some limited cases, as high as 70%. This rate is certainly as high as those found in many other treatment areas such as pain management. Chemical dependence therapy is most successful when it provides both width—as in the integration of individual, group, and family counseling—and depth of experience, which includes the counselor's concern for the client as a complex and dynamic organism, as well as the client's education and supervised practice in refusal skills and other behaviors.

Like many therapy concerns, drug use problems are multifaceted and intercorrelated. Emotional and behavioral problems and drug use are certainly correlated. This correlation, however, does not mean that emotional problems usually cause alcohol or other drug problems. The cause-and-effect relationship is as or more likely to be the other way around.

For most of us, problems come in bunches: The greater the number of economic, social, emotional, behavioral, and drug problems one has (and the more different kinds of drugs one takes), the poorer the prognosis for reduction of use, for length of abstinence, and for length of time until retreatment. Regardless of race or sex, there is a linear relationship between the stresses of social and economic status (SES) and both short-term and long-term drug treatment success. In particular, employed people do drugs less and have better luck with treatment if they have jobs (and family) they are worried about losing.

As a treatment specialist, if you worry excessively about clients who relapse, you will either have many relapse dynamics yourself or you will not stay in the treatment field very long. *Both lapses and relapses are part of the often lengthy process of treatment, not necessarily failures of treatment.* Interestingly, and unlike our expectations for the chemically dependent, our expectations for clients with schizophrenia include both lapse and relapse; moreover, we usually do not view their relapses as failures. Most of us are aware that clients with schizophrenia would relapse even if we could control every psychosocial factor that affects them. We are not expected to feel as if we have failed when these clients' illnesses are exacerbated. Overly perfectionistic expectations for the chemically dependent are particularly unrealistic since the chemically dependent are, perhaps, more sensitive to relapse stresses than any other psychiatric group. From our point of view, relapses are not losses. They are part and parcel of a syndrome that we treat with varying levels of success. Remember, physicians do not discontinue treatment with cancer patients who have relapsed after treatment. Not every physician, however, is capable of working in oncology, where patients die so often. In order to learn to live and prosper in the face of significant losses, you must have reasonable expectations and enjoy what you are accomplishing on a day-to-day basis.

Fortunately, you don't need to be a "recovering" chemically dependent person to work successfully in this field. Long experience with drugs is not, in and of itself, a good social skills teacher; many die of their addiction or related problems before they learn very much. A primary contributor to social skills and insight is empathy, a trait that usually develops long before people discover drugs. If you haven't walked the walk, don't try to talk the talk—speak in your own voice about what you do know. That knowledge will be sufficient. A few drug abusers do rediscover how important they are as people and, therefore, how important others are. That rediscovery process, not the drug experience itself, leads them to overcome their drug-acquired narcissism and devote themselves effectively to becoming treatment personnel. Hats off to this hardy group. However, research has not found that recovering chemical dependence counselors have an easier time, are better liked by recovering clients, or do a better job than counselors who have not used drugs.

Academically trained and occupationally trained chemical dependence counselors perform at similar levels as treatment specialists. This equivalence indicates that success as a chemical dependence treatment specialist may be as much due to counselor's courage to support, confront, and be authentic with clients as it is due to specific experience with drugs. Experience matters, but so does honesty, personality, and courage. Our advice is to get as much direct, hands-on experience in an inpatient treatment facility as you can. A good rule for counselors who cannot work in an inpatient setting is to start by acting as cocounselors in an aftercare group that meets in the evening at a local inpatient or outpatient setting. Then, work back into the treatment cycle toward early intervention as your time allows. A wide experience with all forms of psychotherapy is important now in the chemical dependence treatment field and will become more of a prerequisite for employment in the future.

Finally, medications that reduce craving and withdrawal are also valuable. The view that chemically dependent individuals should not use psychiatric medications that aid them in breaking the abuse cycle is unreasonable and perfectionistic. Drug abusers, who are often more expert on their drug of choice than most counselors will ever be, usually know very well which drugs feed their addictions and which do not. Since we cannot go back to an idyllic period prior to the discovery of alcohol and other drugs, we must forge ahead using ethically reasonable technology when it comes our way. It is not unlikely that long-term drug agonists and antagonists with few side effects will be developed that negate the reinforcing properties of entire classes of abusable drugs. Those drugs will be powerful tools indeed, even though new illicit drugs will always be discovered to offset them.

Counselors and psychotherapists are the linchpins of drug therapy. By *counselor* we mean someone who has been trained to give good counsel and to help normative individuals solve problems of living (Hershenson & Power, 1987). Counselors come in a surprising variety of flavors. Each group (alcohol and drug counselors, marriage and family counselors, and psychiatric social workers, for example) usually gains certification through an accrediting body such as the American Counseling Association. Each is usually also licensed by the state and may perform tasks that are specifically described by the licensing legislation. Counselors who work for the state or federal government do not need to maintain a license because they are presumed to have knowledge and supervision within their area of expertise by virtue of the jobs they hold. Also, religious practitioners are exempted from licensure as counselors, because religious counseling is viewed as an ordinary ongoing component of pastoral care.

We define a *psychotherapist* as a therapist who addresses the psyche. From a historical perspective, the psyche is the life principle or inner world, a world composed of the mind, the emotions, and the self. Practitioners who consider themselves psychotherapists come from a variety of disciplines, including psychology, psychiatry, psychoanalysis, and also counseling. Most psychotherapists work toward both structural and functional changes in the client's internal existential world. Only some of these changes will be reflected in noticeable changes in behavior. According to their inclination and training, some counselors become psychotherapists; many do not. Counselors with a facility for working at deeper levels often do. We draw attention to this distinction because counseling is rooted in psychotherapy. Although chemical dependence counselors, like other counselors, can give good advice, education, and counsel without a deeper understanding of the client's internal world or psyche, they often fail to make progress with the many dual-diagnosis clients who are disturbed at the biological or characterological level. These failures are reflected in the growing rigidity and programmatic character of their work, leading to stress and burnout. Education, closely guided practice, and self-exploration are essential to development as a psychotherapist. We encourage all counselors, regardless of their training, continually to deepen not only their work but, necessarily, themselves.

Before exploring some of the important myths about chemical dependence treatment and treatment specialists, we should state several assumptions. First, we assume you are, or are becoming, a counselor or psychotherapist and that your training is taking place in either an academic, continuing education, or treatment facility setting. Second, we assume that you have supervision and know how to make use of it and that you have exposure to the consultation literature. Third, we assume that you have coherent theories of multicultural counseling, of personality development, and of psychological development over the life span, that are well grounded in both the theoretical and empirical literature. Without these training essentials, you cannot develop your own theory of change or understand how psychotherapy and chemical dependence counseling fit into the change process.

COMMON MYTHS ABOUT CHEMICAL DEPENDENCE TREATMENT

A number of myths about chemical dependence counselors and treatment should be briefly explored at the outset. They include the following:

Myth 1: One can become an excellent chemical dependence counselor without simultaneously becoming a psychotherapist. *Reality:* Counselors who do not deepen and enrich their own inner lives rarely enrich the field. Chemical dependence treatment cannot be provided by technicians and is rarely successful over the long run unless clients develop insight and responsibility. Chemical dependence counseling involves not just counseling, case management, and problem solving, but psychotherapy as well.

Myth 2: Generalist counselors can or should leave drug problems to chemical dependence counselors. *Reality:* In fact, *all* counselors are chemical dependence counselors, either by design or accident, whether they like it or not. In our experience one-third of all counseling clients (individual, couple, family, and group) have significant chemical abuse or dependence problems. Therefore, many of your clients are having drug problems of which you may be unaware and that will affect therapy in important ways. In some cases, drug use exacerbates an existing emotional problem that must be dealt with if psychotherapy is to be successful. In many cases, however, emotional problems are simply camouflaging the real problem: drug abuse or dependence. Can you diagnose the difference? Do you routinely attempt to assess the etiological significance of drugs in your clients' well-being? How do you diagnose such a difference and how do you handle ambiguous cases? This text will attempt to answer these questions.

Myth 3: Chemical dependence counseling is like other kinds of counseling and doesn't require special training. *Reality:* Although many counseling skills are directly transferable into chemical dependence settings, there are critical points at which strategic decisions must be made if clients are to receive adequate care for chemical dependence. In an important sense, chemical dependence counselors are defined by their ability to help clients make these decisions. Making decisions such as whether to refer the client to an alcohol diversion program (intervention for driving under the influence, for example) rather than treatment, or whether to begin a structured inpatient rather than outpatient treatment program, is drug counseling. Unlike other forms of counseling, where critical concerns have been addressed from the beginning of counselors' training, critical decisions in drug counseling are less well understood, and counselors' chemical dependence training is often neglected. When working with chemically dependent or substance abusing clients, generalist therapists often face decisions that do not at first appear important, but later turn out to be critical. Understanding how we make—sometimes, mismake—these critical decisions is crucial to providing better care for chemically dependent clients. Drug problems may be distorted or masked completely by the client's presentation of problems and social facade. Also, counselors who are inexperienced or naive often find themselves enabling their addicted clients, perhaps because they do not feel comfortable intervening with the goals and objectives that clients set for their therapy. Client problems may also be complicated or enabled by experienced recovering counselors who believe that their personal experience with drugs will give them special immunity from being "sucked in" to their clients' relapse dynamics. Our advice is: Trust but verify. Enabling behaviors may include not asking sensitive questions, not noticing and not asking about physical symptoms, missing signs of treatment impasse, using supportive techniques but not also authentically confronting the client about drug use behavior.

Remember also that confidentiality, which is meant to protect the client, can at times act against the client's self-interest. Privacy concerns may stop us from obtaining necessary releases and caveats on confidentiality that keep us from collecting much-needed information from cocounselors, spouses, and family members. Each counselor must decide whether he or she is willing to work with chemically dependent clients (or any clients) in a virtual vacuum of collaborative information. Also, enmeshment with clients (sometimes disguised as "building the relationship") can increase counselors' vulnerability to drug-related manipulations.

Myth 4: Chemically dependent clients prefer recovering counselors and have fewer relapses when treated by clinicians who are in recovery themselves. *Reality:* On the contrary (and in keeping with research on counseling in general) the counselor's gender, race, and recovering status have only minor influence on treatment satisfaction, perception of counselor empathy, and clients' risk of relapse after treatment (Johnson & Prentice, 1990; Machell, 1991; Shipko & Stout, 1992). Like clients in other therapy domains, chemically dependent clients respond most to the expertise, personal attractiveness, and trustworthiness of their therapists. Chapman (1988), for example, found cultural encapsulation and bias to contribute significantly more to poor counseling outcomes than race. Although it does not appear necessary that clients and counselors share a wide range of social and political values, they do need to share values about personal conduct, particularly as it applies to behaviors that may enable a return to drug use (Tyler, Clark, & Wittenstrom, 1989).

Myth 5: Recovering males with little postsecondary formal education make up the great majority of counselors in chemical dependence settings. *Reality:* The numbers differ greatly from state to state, but in Massachusetts, a survey of more than 1300 chemical dependence counselors found, first, that the number of women roughly equaled the number of men; second, that the number of recovering counselors roughly equaled those who were not; and, third, that the number of counselors with graduate training roughly equaled those with less than a bachelor's degree (Mulligan et al., 1989). Recovering counselors apparently are more likely to work in inpatient than outpatient settings (65% versus 35%, respectively), a difference that may stem from their being less intimidated by the more complex cases that are typical of inpatient settings. Inpatient therapists also tend to receive higher pay.

Myth 6: Recovering counselors are more difficult to train than counselors with degrees. *Reality:* Even though recovering counselors generally have less education, research has found that they learned as much from state-sponsored chemical dependence certification training as those with advanced degrees (Gideon, Littell, & Martin, 1980). Therefore, even though less formally trained in psychology and therefore less able to provide psychotherapy for dual-diagnosis clients, for example, non-degreed counselors can be expected to perform as well in many areas, to profit from training and experience equally, and ultimately to contribute as greatly to the field, if perhaps in a different way.

Myth 7: Chemically dependent clients want and need emotional (or religious) conversion in order to benefit from counseling. *Reality:* Research indicates that, like other clients with a variety of psychological concerns, chemically dependent clients consider understanding, concern, caring, experience, honesty, listening, directness, openmindedness, street smarts, and professional certification the most important qualities in a counselor (Rohrer, Thomas, & Yasenchak, 1992). Rationally designed intervention approaches are more convincing than purely emotional or religious appeals.

Myth 8: Chemical dependence clients require aggressive, "in-your-face" confrontation about their problems in order to change. *Reality:* Excessive argument and confrontation are directly associated with client resistance and, therefore, poorer outcomes (Miller, Benefield, & Tonigan, 1993). The therapy clients need is face to face, not in their face. When confrontation is construed to imply directness, openness, and honesty of appraisal, then we agree that it is not only worthwhile, but crucial. Like all counselors, chemical dependence personnel need to be flexible, self-actualized, and reasonably self-disclosing, traits furthered by broad, multimodal training (Gideon, Littell, & Martin, 1980).

Myth 9: Recovering counselors work harder than nonrecovering counselors. *Reality:* No productivity differences between sober recovering alcoholics and people who have never habitually abused drugs have been identified in any work setting (Blum & Roman, 1985). There is no reason to believe that significant differences in work-related performance would be found between recovering and other treatment staff. The treatment field is particularly attractive to those who come from dysfunctional family backgrounds, however (Buelow, Bass, & Ackerman, 1994); as you might expect, counselors often themselves seek treatment. A dysfunctional and, often, substance-abusing family background can be a double-edged sword. On the one hand, treatment personnel are used to assessing and working with family and substance abuse dysfunction. On the other hand, they are vulnerable to being sucked in to the client's problem, becoming for all practical purposes a part of the client's larger dysfunctional family. Even though a dysfunctional family background can provide some inoculation effects for some counselors, all chemical dependence counselors, as all counselors in general, require close supervision by an experienced psychotherapist.

Myth 10: Chemical dependence psychotherapy differs from other forms of psychotherapy because alcohol and drugs are the problem regardless of clients' culture, race, sex, gender, age, physical limitations, and ethnicity. *Reality:* As we find for psychological intervention in general, the many issues confronted daily by special populations present concerns for optimum chemical dependence treatment. For a practical guide to confronting and resolving many of these issues, refer to *Overcoming Unintentional Racism in Counseling and Therapy* by Ridley (1995) and *Counseling American Minorities* by Atkinson, Morten, and Wing Sue (1989). Chemical dependence counselors should keep in mind the following guidelines:

1. Watch for the fundamental attribution error (my problems are circumstantial whereas others' problems are dispositional). Remember to pay equal attention to both environmental factors (such as drug use) and dispositional (or internal) factors while working with the chemically dependent.
2. Continue to assess contemporary client behavior (that is, provide evaluation) rather than simply confirm original diagnostic and theoretical biases.
3. Ask clients to explain their views and values about chemical dependence treatment and to describe difficulties they experience fitting into their own culture or special population that may influence their utilization of treatment.

4. Read broadly and keep current on cross-cultural, ethnicity, gender, sexuality, and disability issues through continuing education.
5. Rather than remaining satisfied with the status quo, continue to question how prejudices and stereotypes influence chemical dependence among special populations.
6. Whenever possible, help the client remove obstacles to receiving treatment (by helping to find day care for a woman's young children, for example), and always provide a bridge back into the work force by addressing career and work concerns as a normal part of therapy.
7. Pay special attention to treatment centers' dependence on tests and test results, many of which are subject to significant loss of reliability and validity across culture, age and disability.
8. Help move exploited clients away from victimization toward survivorship.
9. Keep daily case notes and behavioral summaries rather than relying on memory to reconstruct client interactions. Memory is notoriously biased by immediate actions, salient events, and underlying emotional and cultural preferences.
10. Attend closely to ways in which clients differ from both majority and minority stereotypes, and explore how clients expect differences to affect treatment.

Myth 11: Recovering chemical dependence counselors have special immunity from relapse dynamics or active relapse. *Reality:* Most recovering counselors do appear to show some inoculation effects. These effects are apparent, however, only so long as overall stress levels are moderate and of short duration. Like recovering people generally, when stress levels spiral out of control, counselors should use their internal and external resources and interpersonal support to reduce stress to manageable levels. If stress cannot be reduced, relapse, illness, or psychiatric problems often result.

Unfortunately, we know much less about the problems drug treatment personnel face than we know about drugs, clients, and treatment outcomes. Too little is known about counselors' relapse rates, specific relapse dynamics, transference-countertransference issues, and private practice concerns. Although many treatment center staff maintain that working in the field keeps them aware of their relapse dynamics and thus reinforces their sobriety, we need a much better understanding of how these factors influence one another. Do recovering therapists handle stress differently than nonrecovering treatment personnel do? Are recovering treatment personnel vulnerable to specific triggers of which we are unaware and which exist specifically in treatment centers? Knowing the answers would certainly help us reduce staff burnout and relapse.

Chemical dependence counselors appear to be subject to most of the same problems that produce burnout in other treatment personnel. Whether burnout is actually higher under particular center conditions is unclear. It certainly results from unreasonable and unmet expectations for client recovery. Unclear and unrealistic personal and professional goals also contribute to burnout. Helping others as a way to postpone helping oneself almost invariably leads recovering counselors back into their dependence on others for emotional regulation and, ultimately, back into a relapse dynamic.

Large substance abuse treatment centers, especially those with inpatient, residential, outpatient, diversion, and intervention divisions, have extensive paperwork demands; large numbers of very ill, dual-diagnosis clients; limited time; and tight budgetary constraints. These centers often produce enough stress that they negatively influence recovering counselors and contribute to their relapse dynamics. Such centers must constantly guard against making excessive demands on their staff and work to relieve stress, rather than assuming it is natural product of the setting. Settings where stress levels are high generate low morale, high turnover, and constant relapse dynamics in staff that will ultimately be transferred to clients. Busy is good; stressed-out is not.

All treatment centers, whether for chemical dependence problems or other kinds, should have clear personnel guidelines concerning therapists who may be lapsing or relapsing. These guidelines should explicitly spell out the center's and the staff's responsibilities for interaction concerning suspected lapses. These personnel guidelines should be discussed in detail at hiring and at periodic workshops and retreats. The center's written policies and procedures should cover each phase of the relapse intervention plan. Positive reinforcements for counselors' owning up to their relapses should be included, as should clear consequences for not taking that responsibility. Personnel guidelines should be very specific about how treatment is conducted, how follow-up drug screens are handled, how leave is arranged, and what due process rights employees have concerning advancement, demotion, and termination.

Whether a single-episode lapse or a full-scale relapse has taken place, written intervention, counseling, or treatment plans must be accepted (signed) by both employer and employee. Treatment should not take place at the employee's center. The center director should have signed permission to discuss the employee's progress with the treatment director of the cooperating treatment center. If the lapse or relapse involves a return to drug use, interruption of the therapist's services to clients should ensue: The therapist's clients should be informed about the relapse in a straightforward manner (Kinney, 1983). The counselor's relapse should be discussed openly by the counselor's group and with individual clients. If the counselor is available to debrief the group, a cocounselor who will continue with the group should be present. As Kinney (1983) indicated, special supervision and support will be necessary to facilitate counselors' return to work and help them deal with clients' concerns about their own possible relapse dynamic.

Treatment personnel who are actively using either legal or illegal drugs present special problems whether or not they are recovering. It is our experience that counselors who can and do drink without abusing alcohol often underestimate clients' drinking, because such counselors are unused to focusing on drinking as a problem that requires special attention. Counselors who are abusing alcohol have a clear reason to avoid scrutinizing their clients' alcohol or other drug use. Counselors who are smoking marijuana are likely to sweep the client's ashes under the rug along with their own. Finally, we might ask how many therapists who smoke cigarettes feel free to talk with addicted clients about getting help when these counselors know that tobacco kills more than 400,000 people each year.

It is reasonable to assume that approximately the same percentage of counselors use drugs as do professional people in general. Given the greater numbers of counselors who come from dysfunctional family backgrounds, however, when it does occur their drug use may have more extreme consequences for a larger percentage of the group and certainly for their clients. The nonresilient are particularly vulnerable to the effects of family dysfunction, low self-esteem, social role distortion, and close relationship dysfunction. Without being hypervigilant about our coworkers, we must learn to provide the kind of supportive work and interpersonal environments within which not only clients but therapists will develop greater resistance to the dynamics of burnout and relapse.

PART ONE

A MODEL FOR CHANGE

1

AN INTEGRATIVE MODEL OF CHEMICAL DEPENDENCE TREATMENT

An integrative model of chemical dependence treatment successfully blends a variety of specific theories into a more meaningful, useful, and empirically justifiable whole than can be found in any particular theory or group of techniques. Such a meta-theoretical model should be empirically based and congruent with testable theories of behavior and personality; the model must provide an accurate picture of clients' psychological change processes. A successful model should focus first, and in great depth, on people and their successes and failures in overcoming chemical dependence. The broad range of myths and political concerns surrounding chemical dependence as a syndrome is interesting but of secondary importance. Chemical dependence treatment is about people who have problems; a successful metatheoretical model cannot be divorced from those people's intrapersonal change processes.

During the often complex progression of chemical dependence intervention and treatment, every microskill, psychotherapy technique, and explanatory paradigm traditionally used by psychotherapists will be of use to the chemical dependence counselor. Counselors need not reject personal practice theories that are congruent with their experience. Rather, they should work to integrate their personal and psychological theories into the general framework presented in this book. Practitioners do need to suspend the belief that only one theory is practicable and defensible in chemical dependence treatment—whether that theory is cognitive, behavioral, interpersonal, spiritual, or psychodynamic.

Even though chemical dependence counseling and psychotherapy may differ in specific ways from other kinds of psychological interventions, psychotherapists treat people, not problems. Thus, we must always be aware of our clients' individual, cultural, and gender differences, however much their problems may resemble those we have encountered before in others. Problems can be separated from the individuals who evidence those problems only on a theoretical level; therapy must proceed first and foremost from a detailed assessment of the person-in-culture.

As psychotherapists we are participant-observers with our clients. Not only will our views of treatment reality directly influence the client, but clients' views also will (and should) significantly affect us. Therefore, we will also discuss counselor issues as they are affected by client issues. Finally, although the present work represents 30 cumulative years of psychotherapy and health care experience, it is neither perfect nor finished. Our advice should be put into practice only after it is tempered by the reader's specific experience and creativity.

THE TRANSTHEORETICAL MODEL

Although we intend to work toward an independent integration of prior theory and empirical findings as we explore the assessment, conceptualization, and treatment of chemical dependence, we readily accept and gratefully acknowledge that a transtheoretical model like that described by Prochaska, DiClemente, and their colleagues (McConnaughy, DiClemente, Prochaska, & Velicer, 1989; McConnaughy, Prochaska, & Velicer, 1983; Prochaska, 1991; Prochaska & DiClemente, 1992; Prochaska, Norcross, & DiClemente, 1994) provides important structure for understanding many of the successes and failures of chemical dependence treatment. We have borrowed liberally from these authors' research findings and theory of change. Based on our own chemical dependence treatment experience, we will try to show where and how a therapist can enter chemical dependence intervention and treatment with a client, whatever the counselor's or the client's theoretical persuasion. Like Prochaska and DiClemente's, our views are metatheoretical and integrative, as opposed to nontheoretical and purely eclectic. In other words, our views do not depend on any particular counseling or behavioral theory, but rather on clinical experience and research findings, organized from a developmental perspective, about common, successful self-help and formal pathways people use to quit drugs, develop more creative coping mechanisms, and rebuild their lives.

In joining our specific approaches to chemical dependence case conceptualization and psychotherapy with the transtheoretical model, we will show how common decisions that counselors and clients must make in relapse prevention can be viewed as features of an integrative process. While the transtheoretical approach provides a useful model for change, we will also focus on the specific critical decisions that are so often of great practical concern to chemical dependence counselors, particularly those common to assessment, case conceptualization, referral, and treatment planning. In particular, we will focus on concurrent psychotherapy and the many complexities of working with dual-diagnosis clients.

Prochaska and DiClemente's transtheoretical model evolved from Prochaska's (1979) comparative analysis of the therapeutically unifying processes of change of 18 leading therapy systems. Prochaska looked specifically at preconditions for therapy, content to be changed, processes of change, and the therapeutic relationship concerns common to the therapies. He found that a majority of the approaches employed similar processes in attempting to effect change in a variety of problems, including consciousness raising, self-liberation, catharsis, counter-conditioning and stimulus control, and contingency management. Table 1.1 outlines the processes of change, and Table 1.2 the stages of change. Inventories used to ascertain stages and processes of change may be found in Worksheets 1.1 and 1.2 at the end of this chapter.

Over many years, Prochaska and his colleagues empirically verified that these processes are typical both to self-change and to formal therapy, and that intervention is most successful when the personal and environmental change processes take place at appropriate developmental problem-solving stages (Prochaska, DiClemente, &

TABLE 1.1   Titles, Definitions, and Representative Interventions
of the Processes of Change

Process	Definitions: Interventions
Consciousness raising	Increasing information about self and problem: observations, confrontations, interpretations, bibliotherapy
Self-reevaluation	Assessing how one feels and thinks about oneself with respect to a problem: value clarification, imagery, corrective emotional experience
Self-liberation	Choosing and commitment to act or belief in ability to change: decision-making therapy, New Year's resolutions, logotherapy techniques, commitment enhancing techniques
Counterconditioning	Substituting alternatives for problem behaviors: relaxation, desensitization, assertion, positive self-statements
Stimulus control	Avoiding or countering stimuli that elicit problem behaviors: restructuring one's environment (e.g., removing alcohol or fattening foods), avoiding high-risk cues, fading techniques
Reinforcement management	Rewarding oneself or being rewarded by others for making changes: contingency contracts, overt and covert reinforcement, self-reward
Helping relationships	Being open and trusting about problems with someone who cares: therapueutic alliance, social support, self-help groups
Dramatic relief	Experiencing and expressing feelings about one's problems and solutions: psychodrama, grieving losses, role playing
Environmental reevaluation	Assessing how one's problem affects physical environment: empathy training, documentaries
Social liberation	Increasing alternatives for nonproblem behaviors available in society: advocating for rights of repressed, empowering, policy interventions

From "In Search of How People Change," by J. O. Prochaska, C. C. DiClemente, and J. C. Norcross, 1992, *American Psychologist, 47,* p. 1108. Copyright © 1992 by the American Psychological Association. Reprinted with permission.

Norcross, 1992). Our research and clinical experience validates this view: People change when they are ready. Their readiness to change, and their continuation and maintenance of change, are contingent on a variety of interpersonal factors (job and family, for example) and intrapersonally, existentially meaningful states—including, insight, commitment, and courage.

Stages and processes of change common to both self-changers and psychotherapy clients have been found in a wide variety of change situations, including (1) quitting alcohol, cigarette, and other drug use; (2) weight control; and (3) pain and illness management (Prochaska et al., 1994). The stages observed by Prochaska include precontemplation (inactivity or stasis), contemplation of action (increasing convergence of the forces pushing away from substance dependence and pulling toward sobriety), preparation for action (interventions showing positive effects), action to change, and maintenance of change or relapse prevention (Prochaska, DiClemente, &

TABLE 1.2 Stages of Change in Which Particular Processes of Change Are Emphasized

Precontemplation	Contemplation	Preparation	Action	Maintenance
Consciousness raising Dramatic relief Environmental reevaluation				
	Self-reevaluation			
		Self-liberation		
			Reinforcement management Helping relationships Counterconditioning Stimulus control	

From "In Search of How People Change," by J. O. Prochaska, C. C. DiClemente, and J. C. Norcross, 1992, *American Psychologist, 47*, p. 1109. Copyright © 1992 by the American Psychological Association. Reprinted with permission.

Norcross, 1992). From Prochaska's perspective, "the underlying structure of change is neither technique-oriented nor problem specific. The evidence supports a trans-theoretical model entailing (1) a cyclical pattern of movement through specific stages of change which often includes regression back to prior stages and continued re-working, (2) a common set of processes of change, and (3) a systematic integration of the stages and processes of change" (Prochaska, DiClemente, & Norcross, 1992, p. 1110). To understand these processes and stages, and to link them meaningfully to treatment, requires a coherent conceptualization of each client's chemical dependence concerns as they affect his or her social and psychological world.

Prochaska and his colleagues also impressively documented that clients, family, and therapists must be involved in intervention processes integral to appropriate stages before constructive long-term change is likely. In fact, their research showed that change processes predicted progress through stages better than demographics, problem history or severity, health history, withdrawal symptoms, or reasons (Prochaska, DiClemente, Velicer, Ginpil, & Norcross, 1985). These are very important findings indeed. Therefore, let us look closely at a mapping of the change processes typical to developmental stages within chemical dependence treatment.

STAGES AND PROCESSES OF CHANGE

A stage of change represents both a time period and a set of functional tasks (processes, activities, and interventions) that must be completed to enable a person to move to the next stage. Unless motive forces—interpersonal, intrapersonal, or environmental—are at work, individuals do not perceive the need to change. Further, unless change forces are appropriate to the stage in which people live their immediate lives, people will quite reasonably resist change. Therefore, chemical dependence interventions and treatment must be executed and supported in a systematic way, one that takes the client's stage of change into close consideration.

Clients who are in stasis or precontemplation are often unaware of the immediate and long-term dangers of their behavior; they resist change and may actively deny that a problem exists. They invest little energy in examining the ramifications of their problems, are not generally open to discussions, and may actively resist heroic interventions to the great frustration of those around them who are concerned about these problems. We have observed that the chemically dependent are moved from precontemplation toward contemplation by a combination of growing and pressuring circumstances. Such circumstances may include referrals to employment assistance programs by employers, gathering family and health crises, doctors' advice, legal complications, and public education. One perfectly contented alcoholic client was moved into contemplation of her problem after she idly filled out an alcohol problems questionnaire in a women's magazine in her doctor's office.

Clients who have been moved by either internal or external circumstances into the contemplation stage are usually open to consciousness-raising activities, including feedback from others, supportive dialogue, and explicit education. During contemplation of action, clients may use a wide variety of self-evaluation and self-assessment strategies as they attempt to diagnose the extent and ramifications of their chemical dependence problems. Integral to this self-assessment process are bibliotherapy, discussions with close friends and clergy, values clarification, and observation of the usefulness of self-help actions clients are trying. During the contemplation stage, clients begin to assess their expectancies for change and to weigh the pros and cons of quitting use. As clients prepare for change, the decisional balance begins to shift from the pro side to the con side. Negative expectancies can then play a greater and greater role in tipping the balance against sobriety, unless modified by well-planned psychoeducational counseling and consultation.

During the stage of preparation for change, clients are more willing to undergo formal assessment, including discussions with professionals. Clients also assess their family and employment social support systems, including their family's willingness and ability to give clients emotional support, to endure slips along the way, and to deal firmly with family members' own enabling behaviors. Many clients come to psychotherapists during this stage to investigate the roots of their problems. They often minimize, or simply underestimate, the extent of their alcohol and other drug use. Therapists are often misled about the importance of clients' chemical dependence by a lack of assessment training and a willingness to begin psychotherapy immediately for the many problems clients present. Thorough assessment, client problem conceptualization, and treatment planning are necessary to help move clients who need formal treatment from the stage of preparation to responsible action.

During the action stage, a wide variety of cognitive, affective, and behavioral change processes are used. These include existential processes like self-liberation and behavioral processes like reinforcement management, counterconditioning, and stimulus control.

Understanding the level of the client's chemical dependence and the stage of change in which the client is usually cycling requires a detailed clinical interview, which will be outlined in subsequent chapters. Unless the therapist understands the client's readiness and position within the present stage of change, change is often thwarted by ill-timed or misdirected interventions. Before we explore the concepts of addictionology and look at definitional dilemmas that occur in the field, we will present five brief case histories describing clients who have entered or are moving into each stage of change.*

◆ PRECONTEMPLATION ◆

An example of someone coming out of denial of his substance abuse, Howard, a 21-year-old German-American student, was brought to the university counseling center by Jeffrey, a friend and fellow student, who played with him in a string quartet. Each term of the last four, Howard had dropped one or two courses, citing stress, fatigue, and depression as his reasons for falling behind his classmates.

With Howard's consent, his friend Jeffrey attended the initial counseling interview. Jeffrey reported that Howard had become increasingly reclusive and, after preparing to move in with Jeffrey, had said he just was not ready to have other people around him all the time and needed space. Jeffrey informed the counselor that Howard smoked marijuana almost daily and had complained of experiencing LSD flashbacks when fatigued. Several times over the past couple of months, Jeffrey had been asked to give excuses for why Howard missed rehearsals. Two weeks prior to counseling, Howard called Jeffrey and said he needed help because he could not breathe. At the emergency room, Howard was di-

---

*All the case studies in this book use fictitious names for the clients and the counselors.

agnosed as having had a panic attack. Since then Jeffrey had taken the liberty of reading a few pages of Howard's diary and believed Howard had come to view his use of marijuana and LSD as religious experiences and that talking with anyone about his drug experiences would interfere with his spiritual development because no one could understand what he was experiencing. Also, Jeffrey recalled that Howard had written a paper on mind-altering drugs for a biology class and had become intrigued by the idea of heightened states of consciousness. When Howard asked if Jeffrey would cancel a performance, Jeffrey realized Howard needed professional help.

During the sessions, Howard characterized himself as a little down and as going through an identity crisis. He was unable to identify any precipitating factors for his depressive symptoms. He described recently staying alone in the dark for hours in his apartment and doing mystic exercises to transport himself to a higher dimension of consciousness. He initially denied significant drug use problems. When pressed in Jeffrey's presence, however, he acknowledged using marijuana daily for two years and LSD one to three times per week for the past ten months. He identified feeling more anxious and having trouble concentrating when reading or rehearsing when not smoking marijuana.

Prior to the initial interview, Howard was in a state of precontemplation with respect to his chemical dependence. He felt that his friends just did not understand his spirituality and his special relationship with drugs, and he came to treatment only to appease his friend and to seek advice on coping with his feelings of fatigue and depression, which he considered unrelated to his drug use. His friend's intervention in bringing Howard to counseling and describing Howard's drug use, along with the counselor's initial supportive exploration with Howard of his drug-related behaviors and consequences (particularly embarrassment and loss of credibility in his work), began the process of moving Howard from precontemplation to contemplation: a willingness to consider that his drug use contributed to his dysphoria and a growing inability to follow through on commitments. Most critical to working with a client who presents for counseling in the precontemplation stage is forming a therapeutic alliance. Clients who do not yet recognize a need for self-change—instead either not seeing a problem or seeing change as something others need to make happen, not the clients themselves—are at greatest risk for prematurely dropping out of therapy and continuing unhealthy patterns of coping.

◆ CONTEMPLATION ◆

Charlene, a 35-year-old African American legal secretary and single mother of three, represents the stage of contemplation. She began therapy as a concerned parent. Her 16-year-old daughter had started an intensive outpatient treatment program for cocaine and alcohol abuse, and Charlene attended family therapy sessions with her. During the first session, Charlene found herself disclosing a great deal about herself, including her inability to sleep without prescription medication and her frequent need for nerve pills to cope with financial stress and the responsibilities of being a single mother and the daughter of aging parents. She reported that—following in her mother's footsteps—she had first begun taking benzodiazepines (like Valium), prescribed by her family physician when Charlene was a teenager, to help her cope with PMS. Her use of sleeping pills began when she was 25, following the birth of her first child. She remembered being unable to get back to sleep after nursing the baby and sharing pills out of her aunt's prescription. Charlene considered herself a nervous person and had viewed her use of benzodiazepines and muscle relaxants as entirely normal until watching a television talk show on people with addictions to prescription pain medication. Also, a character on her favorite soap opera had been required to enter a chemical dependence treatment facility after being arrested for a traffic violation and found with prescriptions for codeine from three different doctors. Charlene wondered for the first time whether something more than convenience was involved in her obtaining prescriptions from her gynecologist, her orthopedist, and her family doctor. When her daughter was arrested and given the option of juvenile detention or treatment, Charlene first blamed her daughter's boyfriend for corrupting her daughter. During the first family session, as Charlene related her own history and how she had modeled medication abuse, she began to understand both her own need for change and the impact of her behavior on her daughter.

To help Charlene move from contemplation to preparation for change, the therapist should work with Charlene on the processes of social and self-reevaluation. Charlene should be encouraged to explore in a concrete and detailed way the impact of her drug-using behavior on her own development and on her relationships with her children. She should also be encouraged to write a list of the pros and cons of her continuing drug use for discussion with the therapist and to begin the process of better understanding why her drugs of choice are addictive and what long-term consequences might be expected from their use.

◆ PREPARATION FOR CHANGE ◆

Lincoln, a 35-year-old Native American veteran with a history of combat-related PTSD, began preparation for change while hospitalized for three months with pneumonia and a broken leg. While hospitalized he went through heroin and alcohol withdrawal. Three months earlier, after hitting his wife for the first time in their 12-year marriage, Lincoln had left his wife and three daughters to live in a shelter because he believed his family would be better off without him. While in the VA hospital, he became actively suicidal. The psychologist who evaluated him supported Lincoln's interest in contacting his wife, with whom he had not spoken since leaving home. Lincoln's roommate on the medical ward talked him into going with him to an in-hospital AA meeting.

Previously, Lincoln had actively resisted the concept of chemical dependence, believing that he had full control over his behavior. He was moved toward contemplation during a family therapy session with his wife and their three children. His 7-year-old son told his father how scared of him the son felt when Lincoln was drinking, but also how much the son loved his father. Lincoln's family was supportive but also confronted him about the problems of having him at home without treatment. By the time he began family therapy, Lincoln had been sober and drug-free long enough to begin to examine his life and his situation more realistically. He came to recognize the impact of growing up in a family in which more than half the men of the three preceding generations were alcoholic. Lincoln also saw that he had felt doomed to fail in treatment because of his genetic vulnerability to alcohol as a Native American. His 7-year-old son reminded Lincoln of himself at that age and the sobriety he had wished for his own father. Through psychoeducational reading and AA, Lincoln began to better understand the concepts of chemical dependence. During following sessions, Lincoln struggled with the possibility of relapse on release from the hospital, claiming that he would kill himself if he began drinking or using drugs again because that would mean his situation was hopeless. He also struggled with his deeply held view that attending AA or NA meetings was a sign of weakness. He did continue to attend AA/NA meetings with his roommate, however. Over several weeks, Lincoln came to understand the disease concept of addiction and to appreciate the support of other patients. Lincoln liked listening to newer members and began to talk about the importance of support in staying clean and sober. In therapy sessions, he wrote out and discussed the pros and cons of sobriety versus continued chemical dependence. By the time he was discharged from medical treatment, he had begun to make preparations for change. He decided to move back home and had taken the initiative to find an NA sponsor who lived in the same community. His sponsor would be able to take him to three meetings a week until he could afford his own vehicle. He had an appointment at the local community mental health center for evaluation for intensive outpatient chemical dependence therapy, which offered four group and two individual sessions per week. He also had requested applications from two junior colleges in the area and found out what school financial aid was available through the Veterans Administration. He became more realistic about sobriety, and though developing a comprehensive relapse contingency contract was difficult for him, he promised his counselor that, rather than harm himself, he would call one of three 24-hour emergency numbers if he did relapse.

◆ ACTION STAGE ◆

Brandon exemplifies the action stage of change. On his 16th birthday, Brandon completed one month of inpatient treatment for major depression related to having been sexually abused by his uncle, and his therapist referred him to outpatient substance abuse treatment to go on concurrently with the continuing therapy. Since age 12, Brandon had become increasingly involved with marijuana, ecstacy, volatile solvents (such as glue), and cocaine. In the hospital, he had experienced strong drug cravings and early on he viewed drug-using friends as the only people who truly liked and accepted him. He indicated that everyone else hated him, especially his family. The teenagers he became close to during his hospitalization also had significant drug abuse histories. As the relationship with his therapist developed, Brandon was able to talk about the relationship between his depression and his using, and it became clear to him that rather than decreasing his dysphoria, the drugs were contributing significantly to it. He also began to recognize that his relationships with others who were using lacked depth and meaningful intimacy and were focused on using drugs rather than relating. People he had considered friends became irritable and demanding or unavailable after he talked with them about his considering not using. When his therapist recommended that he be discharged to an outpatient adolescent substance abuse program, he felt strong enough to continue his sobriety. He left the hospital armed with basic substance abuse knowledge and skills for coping with depression, which would help him as he entered outpatient treatment for polysubstance abuse. During his first session with his outpatient alcohol and drug counselor, he said that in the hospital he worked on self-esteem issues by challenging negative self-statements. He had begun to practice progressive muscle relaxation to help him sleep and had become more comfortable identifying and talking about the emotional impact of his drug use in group therapy.

◆ MAINTENANCE STAGE/RELAPSE PREVENTION ◆

Andrea, a 28-year-old Italian American nurse with a history of bipolar disorder and alcohol dependence entered couples therapy with her partner, Jane. Andrea had three years of sobriety. Following multiple failed attempts to stop drinking, which commenced at age 20 and included inpatient detoxification and treatment at ages 21 and 24, Andrea stopped drinking, began attending AA meetings, and obtained a sponsor at age 25, three months after her father died of cirrhosis. She had been hospitalized at ages 18 and 23 for manic episodes, which may have been related to amphetamine abuse. She had not been under the regular care of a psychiatrist since her trust fund ended when she was 26, and she had stopped taking lithium 18 months prior to couples therapy. Andrea had remained drug-free for several years.

Andrea and Jane began attending couples counseling to improve communication and adapt to differences in personality and lifestyle. Their longer term goals were to make a decision about whether to formalize their relationship through a legal contract about common property and to address their conflict about whether to have children. Other than the increased complexity of questions around becoming parents, they presented no issues specific to having a lesbian orientation and reported having a supportive community of friends. Two sessions into counseling, at Andrea's suggestion, Jane abruptly moved in to Andrea's small apartment to escape her parents' nagging and criticism. Andrea had always lived by herself, and the level of conflict between them predictably escalated. Additionally, Andrea's mother was in increasingly poor health and called on Andrea almost daily to run errands and help at home. Finally, Andrea had just learned that the home health company she worked for was in financial trouble and, though she earned a good salary, she could not yet afford to return to school.

About six sessions into couples counseling, Andrea volunteered that she was becoming more aware of her chronic irritability, hypersensitivity, and negative expectations about the future. She described herself as experiencing "dry drunk" syndrome or "white-knuckled sobriety." She said, "I've stopped working my program." She reported that about a year earlier she had stopped attending AA meetings because she had begun running into former patients and felt uncomfortable. Further, she reported not having spoken with her sponsor in several months: "She's always busy and I just felt I should be able to do it on my own." She also wondered aloud whether she was putting in increasing amounts of overtime at work with patients in crisis in order to forestall her own emotional needs. As Andrea continued to talk, she became aware that she had erected other roadblocks to attending AA meetings. For example, she had maintained that other meetings (where she was less likely to see patients) were always too far away or were held at the wrong times, even though she had several possible choices. She had also turned down Jane's offers to go with her to more distant meetings. Finally, although Andrea now had adequate medical coverage, she reported postponing seeing a psychiatrist because she was sure she would be expected to go back on lithium. With further discussion, Andrea became more clear about how not working her program not only affected herself but was having a negative impact on her relationship with Jane and their work together in couples therapy. Andrea agreed to resume attending two AA meetings weekly, supported Jane's interest in going to weekly open AA meetings with her, and made an appointment for a psychiatric evaluation in order to evaluate her status with respect to her bipolar disorder and to begin to establish a relationship with a psychiatrist who could work with her to manage medically any future manic or depressive episodes.

Change appears to be cyclical rather than linear. Like many chemical dependence counselors, Prochaska and his colleagues have found that people often relapse into their old behavior and thinking patterns and then cycle back to the contemplation and preparation stages before taking further action. This cycling process results in critical junctures during which therapists can intervene through further assessment, reconceptualization of the client's problems, and encouragement to begin preparing for the action phase once more. Interestingly, research indicates that although 15% cycle back to stasis, fully 85% cycle back to contemplation and preparation for action (Prochaska, DiClemente, & Norcross, 1992). Prochaska also found that, even though many smokers in the contemplation stage said they would use a self-help smoking program, only 4% of the study group actually signed up when a program was offered. But although intensive action-oriented counseling failed to change smoking behaviors among cardiac patients who were in the precontemplation and contemplation stages, interventions were successful for more than 90% of patients judged to be in the action phase, who were also found to have continued abstinence from smoking as much as six months later.

Prochaska and his colleagues suggested that clients in the precontemplation and contemplation stages need consciousness-raising techniques instead of action-oriented counseling. Counselors may, for instance, use motivational interviewing to engage these clients. Without well-designed interventions that take their stage of change into consideration, people often remain in contemplation for many years without instigating preparation for new behavior, even when apparently appropriate programs are offered. Therefore, chemical dependence assessment must entail a close understanding of not only the client's chemical dependence problems (using chemical dependence assessment instruments and clinical interviews), but also the client's history of self-supported and externally supported change. Case conceptualization requires understanding the client's unique processes and resources for change. Treatment planning must be justified on the basis of that conceptualization and extend from it both structurally and functionally.

Drug Abuse, Dependence, and Addiction

Addictionology, the modern study of the addiction process, began for practical purposes with the pioneering work of E. M. Jellinek in the 1940s. Even today Jellinek's work provides us an insightful assessment and treatment perspective based on close observation, empirical research, and clinical work with individuals suffering from alcoholism (Jellinek, 1952a, 1952b, 1960). Although Alcoholics Anonymous is usually associated with helping addicts through a social and spiritual model of change, the disease model of alcoholism actually arose primarily from early writings of AA's founders and Jellinek's extensive writings.

Jellinek was one of the first to conclude that people suffering from alcoholism had physiological problems with the drug itself. He believed that the drug, not moral depravity, produced profound psychiatric consequences, including a withdrawal syndrome, craving, physical deterioration, and loss of control over both the drug and social functioning. He concluded that most of the physical, cognitive, and emotional problems alcoholics suffered were the aftermath of a diseaselike syndrome and, therefore, that alcoholics could more usefully be considered as suffering from or recovering from an illness.

Jellinek was aware that the defect in an addict's so-called will—the addict's inability to stop, even while feeling motivated and willing to change—was caused by a physiological process peculiar to addiction. Jellinek also saw that moral condemnation or punishment only further exacerbated the client's problem by further lowering the client's self-esteem. Although Jellinek certainly considered an individual's use pattern and adaptation to alcohol (and to other drugs) important, he chose instead to study *the addiction's effects on the individual.* This approach does not seem very novel now, but it was almost revolutionary in the 1940s, shifting emphasis from individual variables (level of willpower) to aspects of the drugs themselves (addiction potential) and their effects on the total human system. This breakthrough set the stage for modern education and treatment.

By disease process we mean the progressive biopsychological deterioration fundamental to addictions, which results in an erosion of control and judgment and a multiplicity of insults to various organ systems. While an addiction is not a disease in a traditional sense—because the pathogen is not bacterial, but rather is like some parasite that mimics a necessary constituent of the brain—an addiction is sufficiently like a disease process to make the designation a useful one. Our field is not facilitated by constant self-serving arguments over whether and how closely addictions mimic disease processes. From a semantic point of view, all definitions tend to break down under rigorous philosophical analysis. In the end, research must focus on the essential facts and their relationships—not the precision of a definition. We consider addiction a disease process because it rapidly erodes our control, however strong our will. In other words, the addiction has a life of its own, as Jellinek made clear, though it does depend on the individuals who manifest it.

The acceptance of alcoholism, and by association other drug addiction, as a disease by the American Medical Association in the 1950s put medical and psychological treatments for addictions on a footing with other health care and psychiatric concerns. Although treatment outcome data prior to the 1960s are sketchy, it is doubtful that non-AA, religious exhortations and psychiatric interventions for addiction were successful more than 5% of the time (George, 1990). In fact, these treatments often did more harm than good! In comparison, then, contemporary treatment is an outstanding success.

Definitions and classifications in and of themselves cannot provide empirical answers, but they can help us delimit our study and clarify our theorizing. Therefore, we will look at some of our definitions and psychiatric assessment classifications.

DEFINITION AND CLASSIFICATION

The word *drug*, once used synonymously for *medication*, is now commonly used to refer to illicitly obtained psychoactive substances, whether or not the substance is (or was) also a medication. Today, alcohol and tobacco—which are clearly psychoactive and addictive—are also more frequently referred to as drugs, even though they are used legally. The public is slowly accepting the fact that alcohol and tobacco are addictive psychoactive substances; in the media, they are often referred to as drugs. Despite the historic overlap between the terms *drug* and *medication*, we will use the term *drug* to refer to a psychoactive substance used for nonmedical purposes, whether it is legal or not.

Psychoactive medications are those prescribed by licensed health care providers to produce therapeutic changes in affect (antidepressants, for example), cognition (antipsychotics, for instance), and behavior (for example, mood stabilizers like Tegretol or Lithium (Buelow & Hebert, 1995). We will define psychoactive drugs, both licit and illicit, as those that are misused to produce these changes for personal, nonmedical reasons. These personal reasons are rarely therapeutic in nature, unless the definition of self-medication is distorted to include feeding one's drug dependence to avoid withdrawal (Gold, 1994).

It is also difficult to define terms like *alcoholism* and *drug* or *alcohol abuse, addiction,* and *dependence* so that they describe only discrete scientific categories. A term like *alcoholism* demonstrates this problem clearly because it developed in a common lexicon that has no particular allegiance to science. Common usage of the term has changed over time and will probably continue to change. While change is reasonable, it does cause difficulties for scientists who want a more stable and precise vocabulary.

The following substantive concerns, for example, arise through definitional imprecision. Should specialists use the term *alcoholism* to include only alcohol addiction or dependence? That course might be wise, but the definition seems to ebb and flow on the basis of a variety of important states and traits. Are there multiple pathways into alcoholism? There probably are, and people may confuse these different pathways into alcoholism for different types of alcoholism. Is physical dependence on alcohol only one sign of addiction? Must dependence on a drug include emotional, cognitive, and behavioral components before it can be considered an addiction? That depends, of course, on one's definition of dependence and addiction; some equate the two, some see them as separable concerns. Is gambling an addiction or an obsession? Is an addiction the same as a compulsion? We will offer answers to these questions in the following sections.

Given the definitional imprecision and research complexities, it is small wonder that social and biological scientists of good will often find themselves in heated arguments comparing apples and oranges when they thought they were comparing different species of grape. Not infrequently, researchers also reach very different conclusions from the same data source (for example, compare Vaillant & Milofsky, 1982 with Zucker & Gomberg, 1986). Understandably, the public and the client often want simple answers to very complex questions. The realities of our field, however, often dictate very complex answers even to relatively simple questions.

We will define a drug addiction as a dependence process marked by increasing levels of tolerance and withdrawal, craving or preoccupation, and loss of control over the drug and ordinary social behavior. According to Jellinek (1960) and a variety of subsequent researchers, it is specifically the risky use of a drug in the face of severe harm, loss of control, and periodic relapse back into use, even in the face of a strong desire to abstain, that indelibly marks an addiction process. Remember that no one symptom is ultimately conclusive; what matters instead is how each symptom fits into an evolving process of physical, psychological, behavioral, and emotional deterioration.

Addictive processes also lead to the deterioration of personal, individual consciousness. Through time, the phenomenological representation of the self is ultimately degraded or destroyed. Although some writers use the term *spiritual* to indicate that the inner self is being destroyed, we will limit our use of that term here because of its religious connotations and the sectarian battles that its use often occasions. In working with clients who are religious, however, we often use the concepts interchangeably.

As we have indicated, then, drug dependence is traditionally defined to include preoccupation with the drug, long periods of high-level use of the drug, loss of control over drug use, increasing use in the face of negative consequences, drug cravings, and abstinence withdrawal. The roots, causes, or etiology of drug dependence, which we will define as functionally equivalent to addiction, are multifactorial (the product of multiple biological and social factors) and polygenic (the expression of more than one gene with varying levels of penetrance) (Gold, 1994; Schuckit, 1994). The roots are also evolutionary in the sense that dependence adapts to circumstances through time and through the host's life stages. Drugs are usefully viewed as parasitic: They extend and consolidate their influence through changes wrought in the victim, and gradually they kill.

Although the physical and psychological components of addictions are primarily dictated by the drug itself, premorbid (preaddiction) personality characteristics or social conditions may directly influence many individuals to continue their experimentation with drugs into an abusive phase. Alcohol use is an excellent example of this process, because it is selectively addictive. In other words, unlike morphine—a drug on which an overwhelming majority of individuals are capable of rapidly forming a dependence—only a minority of individuals seem capable of developing the neurochemistry necessary for an addiction to alcohol (Blum, 1982; Milam & Ketcham, 1983; Schuckit, 1994). Alcohol is, therefore, a very sneaky drug. About 10% of men and 5% of women will develop an unnoticed but growing tolerance for and dependence on alcohol even though they began its use in socially approved situations. This tolerance and dependence is primarily independent of social factors, but social factors (social stress, for example) accelerate use. As Milam and Ketcham (1983) pointed out, although the descent from social use to abuse of alcohol may be only a moderate slope, it is an extraordinarily slippery one for vulnerable people, especially considering that the drug is advertised as healthful, harmless, and, of course, fun.

Addiction can be roughly equated with the American Psychiatric Association (APA) *Diagnostic and Statistical Manual of Mental Disorders, Fourth Edition* (DSM-IV, 1994) criteria for drug dependence, which includes the following characteristics:*

Substance Abuse
A. A maladaptive pattern of substance use leading to clinically significant impairment or distress, as manifested by one or more of the following occurring at any time during the same 12-month period:
   (1) recurrent substance use resulting in a failure to fulfill major role obligations at work, school, or home (e.g., repeated absences or poor work performance related to substance use; substance-related absences, suspensions, or expulsions from school; neglect of children or household)
   (2) recurrent substance use in situations in which it is physically hazardous (e.g., driving an automobile or operating a machine when impaired by substance use)
   (3) recurrent substance-related legal problems (e.g., arrests for substance-related disorderly conduct)
   (4) continued substance use despite having persistent or recurrent social or interpersonal problems caused or exacerbated by the effects of the substance (e.g., arguments with spouse about consequences of intoxication, physical fights)
B. Has never met the criteria for Substance Dependence for this class of substance.

*Reprinted with permission from the *Diagnostic and Statistical Manual of Mental Disorders, Fourth Edition*, pp. 181–183. Copyright © 1994 American Psychiatric Association.

Substance Dependence

A maladaptive pattern of substance use, leading to clinically significant impairment or distress, as manifested by three or more of the following occurring at any time in the same 12-month period:

- (1) tolerance, as defined by either of the following:
  - (a) need for markedly increased amounts of the substance to achieve intoxication or desired effect
  - (b) markedly diminished effect with continued use of the same amount of the substance
- (2) withdrawal, as manifested by either of the following:
  - (a) the characteristic withdrawal syndrome for the substance (refer to criteria A and B of the criteria sets for withdrawal from the specific substances)
  - (b) the same (or closely related) substance is taken to relieve or avoid withdrawal symptoms
- (3) the substance is often taken in larger amounts or over a longer period than was intended
- (4) a persistent desire or unsuccessful efforts to cut down or control substance use
- (5) a great deal of time is spent in activities necessary to obtain the substance (e.g., visiting multiple doctors or driving long distances), use of the substance (e.g., chain smoking), or recovering from its effects
- (6) important social, occupational, or recreational activities given up or reduced because of substance use
- (7) continued substance use despite knowledge of having had a persistent or recurrent physical or psychological problem that was likely to have been caused or exacerbated by the substance (e.g., current cocaine use despite recognition of cocaine-induced depression, or continued drinking despite recognition that an ulcer was made worse by alcohol consumption)

The criteria for substance abuse are subsumed within those of substance dependence. They include preoccupation with getting and using the drug, risky use, and recurrent behavioral problems. Diagnosis of dependence hinges on both the absolute number and severity of behavioral problems that are arising and on the existence of tolerance or withdrawal symptoms. Diagnostically, no single threshold defines addiction: Addiction is a syndrome made up of many parts, some of which are less and some more significant for particular clients.

Drugs alter drive states and deposit hidden markers in the memory and the pleasure centers to continue use and to achieve a new baseline for homeostasis. These altered drives are effective in sabotaging sobriety. In a competing fashion, treatment lays down both conscious and unconscious markers designed to reactivate prosocial drives. These drives are reinforced as the client learns new coping skills, social reinvolvement subroutines, and help-seeking strategies. We will discuss the drive components of addiction further in our discussion of treatment and relapse prevention.

COMMON PATHWAYS AND REWARDS IN ADDICTION

Abusable drugs act along common neural pathways to produce similar pharmacodynamic effects in the pleasure centers of the brain, particularly the medial forebrain bundle (MFB). It is principally through the MFB, and other reward centers as yet undiscovered, that drugs produce their most important cognitive and affective reinforcements. As Gold (1994) and Miller, Dackis, and Gold (1987) pointed out, people generally use drugs to feel good (proactive), rather than not feel bad (reactive). The view that people principally use drugs to avoid feeling bad—the self-medication theory—has received only partial support (Schinka, Curtiss, & Mulloy, 1994). Research has shown, first, that when people indicate they use drugs because they feel bad, the usual reason for their feeling bad is that they don't have the drug in their system. Prior to using drugs, these people didn't feel any worse than others in their social set who didn't use drugs. Second, treated individuals relapse about as often during good times (and presumably because they want to feel even better) as during bad times! Gold (1994, p.93) stated, "It is my belief that these [addictive] 'feeling states' can be seen as a new drive state, similar to drives for food and sex, that has developed in response to the powerful reward associated with all drugs of abuse. Furthermore, it is my contention that the self-medication hypothesis for drug abuse addiction may be in reality an attempt by the user to satisfy the drive for drug reward."

Gold's view is entirely reasonable and supportable for the general population of alcohol and other drug-dependent individuals, most of whom were relatively normal prior to addiction. A clear overview of this population is distorted by two problems. First, individuals with more severe psychopathology, particularly street people, are likely to use drugs whenever they are available. Because drugs are endemic to this group, the strength of the relationship between their earlier psychopathology and their present drug use can tilt the overall picture, even in large samples, toward one that shows a significant relationship between drug use and underlying psychopathology (Alterman, 1985). In opposition to the self-medication hypothesis, however, many street people will use mood- and mind-altering drugs even when they are aware that use will exacerbate their mental illnesses. Even the chronically mentally ill make upside (pro) and downside (con) choices about drugs. Second, studies linking drug use and psychopathology are usually biased because they compare treatment groups with normal controls. Treatment groups are much more likely to be composed of the most difficult cases, many of whom do have a dual-diagnosis component.

Other findings have emerged that diminish support for the self-medication hypothesis (Gold, 1994; Miller & Gold, 1991; Vaillant, 1983; Vaillant & Milofsky, 1982). First, evidence shows that drugs rarely cause irrevocable changes in basic personality, even though they cause a variety of emotional problems. Therefore, as we would expect, longitudinal studies have shown that many recovering clients, particularly alcoholics, do not have any underlying psychopathology that might have needed medicating in the first place. Second, research has not found that respondents who are experiencing more severe bouts of preexisting anxiety and depression prefer to drink more than anyone else. In other words, preexisting mood dysregulation is not predictive of increased substance abuse or dependence in a majority of cases. Third, we usually find that depressed alcoholics improve very little with antidepressants; their depression improves dramatically, however, when they have sobered up. After reaching a high-quality sobriety, clients who continue to suffer from depression may get good results with antidepressant medications if they are concurrently learning new coping skills through psychological treatment.

Clearly, any chronically mentally ill population characterized by impulse control problems, lowered reaction to risk, or antisocial leanings is more likely to engage in risky behavior of all kinds, including drug use. Thus this group will show a greater than average association with drugs, but these higher levels of drug use do not support the self-medication hypothesis. Additionally, clients with antisocial personality traits or disorders are more likely to use drugs because they lead the clients to feel even more disinhibited, not because the drugs medicate or inhibit their already antisocial leanings (Alterman, 1985; Vaillant & Milofsky, 1982).

Even though the self-medication hypothesis has not received wide empirical support over the broad spectrum of clients, some people do attempt to self-medicate underlying psychiatric problems (Schinka, Curtiss, & Mulloy, 1994). Whether the client is medicating an underlying disorder or inhibiting his or her withdrawal syndrome, however, can be determined only after the client has been sober for a significant period of time and after a complete psychological assessment has been conducted.

Research has consistently implicated the excitatory neurotransmitter dopamine (DA) as the principal stimulant in the brain's pleasure centers (Gold, 1994; Miller, Dackis, & Gold, 1987). Drugs like cocaine and amphetamine that closely mimic and enhance the availability of dopamine have the same basic effects. A variety of animals, including humans, will self-administer some addictive drugs (such as cocaine) that stimulate the medial forebrain bundle until they are starving in the presence of food (Julien, 1995). Researchers have found a variety of abusable drugs, even those not classed as stimulants, to cause DA-induced MFB reinforcement, including marijuana (tetrahydrocannabinol, THC), alcohol, opiates, tobacco (nicotine), and cocaine. This common pathway finding is particularly important given that abusable drugs act on the body with a variety of pharmacodynamic outcomes, and they have been divided into drug classes based on their differences. For example, cocaine is considered a stimulant, whereas alcohol and other sedative hypnotics are considered depressants. Thus, even though they may produce varying levels of neural excitation or inhibition, their common pathway is one which increases dopamine concentrations and, therefore, rewards in the pleasure centers, particularly the nucleus accumbens (NAc) (Gold, 1994).

Because we have no litmus test or biological assay for addictions, dependence is best defined through a set of affective, cognitive, and behavioral characteristics, which includes preoccupation with, compulsive use of, and persistent relapse to drugs. Tolerance, in which increasing doses produce the same effect as earlier doses, and withdrawal syndromes develop with the use of a majority of drugs, including cocaine, amphetamine, marijuana, and LSD. The ability of a drug to produce tolerance and withdrawal cannot be equated with addiction, however, because tolerance can develop without producing preoccupation, compulsive use, or relapse (as in some pain sufferers who take morphine, for example).

Further, we should remember that some behaviors that become habitual, satisfying, and highly reinforcing may also produce neurochemical changes in the brain that subsequently alter more fundamental drive states. Gambling and sexual acting out are primary examples. Clearly, multiple physiological and behavioral pathways influence drive states positively or negatively. If this were not the case, talk treatments for addictions would have no effect, because changes in cognition and affect would not combat addictive drive states in any significant way. Fortunately, underlying and mediating drive states can be influenced by persistent use of behavioral-emotional therapy techniques as well as by medication. In fact, talk treatments and medications may act on the same areas of the brain. For example, treatment of obsessive compulsive syndrome with either fluoxetine or cognitive behavioral therapy decreases local metabolism of glucose in the same areas of the brain (Baxter et al., 1992).

THE INHERITANCE OF DRUG ADDICTION

To thoroughly understand how chemical dependence is passed from generation to generation, one must consider the multifactorial nature of social and genetic transmissibility, and how these factors interact. Inheritance of heightened risk for drug dependence includes the passing from generation to generation of specific genetic material. First, people may inherit genes that act alone to produce drives that specific drugs reduce. So far, no such single gene has been found. The fact that identical twins who drink show only an 80% concordance rate for alcoholism, rather than a 100% concordance rate, indicates that no single gene with complete penetrance exists. Therefore, a triggering mechanism involving at least several genes must also be necessary (and activated) for a behavioral phenotype to emerge. Second, individuals may inherit a number of interactive genes that produce predispositions toward a general class of behaviors under given conditions, rather than strong drives toward specific acts. Third, we might inherit psychophysiological vulnerabilities to particular drug effects that increase our likelihood of addiction; an example can be found in Blum's 1982 research on the importance of morphinelike compounds (tetrahydroisoquinolones, THIQs) in alcoholism. Fourth, high-risk individuals may inherit low emotional cognitive resilience in the face of environmental challenges like family dysfunction or peer pressure and internal challenges like depression. Finally, and quite likely, we may inherit a combination of these processes and a vulnerability to their synergistic effects.

The inheritance of alcoholism has been more fully researched than any other drug, probably because the social costs of alcoholism have been evident for several thousand years. Due to these costs, some Scandinavian countries have collected family and individual data on community efforts to constrain alcoholism for many generations. With the exception of the prohibition period in the United States, alcohol, like tobacco, has long been freely available over much of the Western world. Limits on its penetration into society have been minor. While around 90% of adults drink, only a minority appear to drink addictively. It is relatively easy, therefore, for people to accept the traditional folklore, supported by the alcohol industry, that vulnerability to dependence is not inherited but caused by personal problems or overindulgence.

In an overview of genetic influences in alcohol dependence, Schuckit (1994, p. 5) made the following comments:

> Alcoholism or alcohol dependence, as defined by repetitive severe life problems with alcohol (American Psychiatric Association, 1987), runs strongly in families, without a remarkable familial rate of most other psychiatric disorders such as schizophrenia and manic-depressive disease (Cotton, 1979; Schuckit, 1992). A genetic contribution to this familial pattern for alcoholism is best supported by the half-sibling (Schuckit et al., 1987) and adoption studies (Bohman, 1978; Cadoret, 1980; Goodwin et al., 1974), all of which demonstrate an increased risk for severe alcohol-related problems in children of alcoholics who were adopted out, even if they had been raised without knowledge of their

biological parents' problems. Further solidifying the relationship between alcohol dependence and genetic influences are most, but not all, of the comparisons of concordance rates of monozygotic and dizygotic twins (Gurling et al., 1984; Kai, 1960)

Schuckit (1994) described several parameters that help make the study of transmissibility of addictions more effective. We need to look, first, at those who are truly addicted. Individuals who may be abusing a drug are not necessarily becoming addicted to it; therefore, including them in our samples may potentially dilute our findings. Effectively separating abuse from addiction requires that we have an accurate definition of addiction and effective, easily available threshold tests. Also, because addictions are defined by progressive levels of dependence, we should compare individuals whose dependence is at roughly the same level. If we do not, we may be comparing important but qualitatively different processes at work. For example, different inheritable processes may well influence initial use (low impulse control) as opposed to late (deteriorative) stage addiction.

Second, our research samples should include individuals whose addiction is not complicated by other social or genetic factors (schizophrenia, for example) to which the addiction might be secondary. As Schuckit (1994) pointed out, it is not hard to understand why someone who learns poorly from experience, who has poor impulse control, or who lives hand-to-mouth on the street would have drug problems, independently of any underlying predisposing genetic factors.

As Goodwin (1986) noted, it is no secret that alcoholism runs in families. That fact has been obvious since the time of the Greek city states or earlier. Reviews of the literature several decades ago (Cotton, 1978) showed that families with alcohol histories produced alcoholics at abnormally high rates, whereas those without such histories produced them at very low rates. It continued to be unclear, however, how much of the inheritance was due to nature and how much to nurture.

An important way to help establish the causal contribution of social and genetic transmission was to study alcoholism longitudinally in a large cohort of people. In the early 1980s Vaillant reported on the results of a 30-year longitudinal study in which he found that having an alcoholic parent was a much better predictor of the development of alcoholism in adult children of alcoholics (ACOAs) than any combination of other factors, including family functioning. Families with an alcoholic parent (including those without high levels of family dysfunction) were five times more likely to produce offspring with alcoholism than those with a variety of severe family dysfunctions but without an alcoholic parent. Controlling for intervening social variables is difficult, however.

The best way so far devised to capture the relative contribution of nature and nurture in addiction has been through research on adopted-out children of alcoholics (Anthenelli & Schuckit, 1993; Cloninger, Sigvardsson, von Knorring, & Bohman, 1988; Goodwin, 1986; Schuckit, 1994). Research found that sons of alcoholic mothers or fathers were between three and four times more likely to become alcoholic as men with nonalcoholic parents (30–40% of samples versus 10%) (Goodwin, 1986, 1989; Schuckit, 1994). Sex-linked factors (whether mother or father was alcoholic) do not appear to influence the level of inheritance. Daughters do seem to inherit alcoholism less often, however. Why this sex-linked difference exists among male and female offspring is not clear, but ACOA daughters are about half as likely to become alcoholic as ACOA sons. In a majority of studies, the factor of whether the ACOA was raised by an alcoholic parent, was adopted out at birth, or lost the alcoholic parent to death or abandonment during infancy has not been found to significantly affect ACOA alcoholism rates. Also, alcoholism may skip generations (with phenotypic expression absent), but still be passed to subsequent generations. Alcoholism may also appear to skip a generation only because a parent was a teetotaler. Having an alcoholic grandparent or other close relative who is alcoholic is also associated with a higher than expected risk of inheriting the problem.

Monozygotic twins possess identical genetic makeups. If one is alcoholic, the twin is also alcoholic in around 80% of cases (Anthenelli & Schuckit, 1993; Cloninger et al., 1988). This high rate of concordance occurred even when the twins were adopted out at birth and therefore not raised by either of their biological parents; it also occurred when only one twin was adopted out and raised by a nonalcoholic family, while the other was raised by the natural parents. These are the strongest proofs available that alcoholism, complex though it may be, has a fundamental and powerful genetic determinant. Fraternal (dizygotic) twins have an approximately 30 to 40% concordance rate for alcoholism whether or not they were raised together. These high concordance and inheritance rates have led to predictions that between 60 and 80% of the variance in alcoholism is explained by genetics, while 10 to 30% is explained by sociological variables (Cloninger et al., 1988). Although some revisions have been made as empirical research has accumulated, the basic implication of inheritability from the twin studies has held firm. Finally, although Cloninger believes that different discrete forms of alcoholism exist, this view has not been confirmed. Correlations between alcoholism types and psychosocial variables are inconclusive.

Unfortunately, we know much less about the genetic factors predisposing clients to addictions to drugs other than alcohol. It is likely, however, that other addictions share many genetic mechanisms in common with alcoholism. Because much drug use tends to occur in fads, use rates may vary greatly compared to an old legal standby like alcohol. Also, because use of multiple drugs is so common, it is difficult to study the transmission of vulnerability to a single drug independently. We do know, for example, that opiate dependency runs higher in the members of particular families than would be expected in the general population and also that identical twins show high concordance rates not only for alcohol but for a variety of drugs, including the opiates (Anthenelli & Schuckit, 1993).

A number of mechanisms that may serve as markers of genetic susceptibility have been advanced. They include the following:

1. Inherited low excitability: Those who are less excitable take more stimulation to reach satisfaction and satiation. Decreased changes in cortisol, prolactin, and EEG reaction may make susceptible people less able to recognize when they should discontinue drinking.
2. A highly sensitive DA excitation system: High sensitivity, especially in the pleasure centers, might encourage chronic small doses of drugs to trigger the system. Chronicity might encourage dependence.
3. A highly successful DA-dominated drive system, with concurrent low activity of other drives (such as food and sex): In this scenario, the artificial drive system comes to restrict or supplant other drive systems.

4. High overall system excitability: Such excitability might lead to self-medication using sedative hypnotics.
5. High tolerance for alcohol due to heightened ethanol breakdown (liver efficiency) without concurrent acetaldehyde breakdown: This explanation rests on the assumption that chronic high levels of acetaldehyde either initiate or induce aversive effects, and therefore lower than average drug use, or else trigger the expression of a system in the brain that uses acetaldehyde to produce other more reinforcing biochemicals (THIQs) (Blum, 1982; Milam & Ketcham, 1983).
6. Lowered perception of degree of intoxication found in ACOAs: This research finding, together with findings that ACOAs produce lower sway following drinking measured amounts, indicates that ACOAs might simply be less able to tell how much to drink based on what they feel from drinking, and this insensitivity leads to higher tolerance (Anthenelli & Schuckit, 1993).

As we have seen, genetic influences are very important in the transmission of alcoholism. Genetics may be less important in the transmission of other addictions, but it continues to be of major influence. We began with the biological model because the contribution of genetics has been underrepresented in psychology for a variety of reasons. First, the moral model of addiction—that individuals use drugs because they are spiritually depraved—held sway for many centuries and remains very strong. The involvement of inherited stress reactivity as a triggering mechanism (the stress-diathesis model) in the transmissibility of complex biopsychological problems like schizophrenia that clearly contradict moral models have not existed until recently. Second, overly simplistic behavioral theory dominated academic psychology until very recently. The irrational belief that alcoholism and other addictions are simply overlearned behaviors with limited genetic bases has remained an important tenet in behavioral dogma. Third, academic researchers found it easier, less time consuming, and less expensive to study social correlates of addictions than to delve into genetic components of transmissibility. Also, confirmatory cross-cultural and longitudinal studies are costly and complex.

Finally, we will direct our attention to the social correlates of addictions. Even if only 30% of the variance in transmission of addictions is of a social, interpersonal origin, talk therapy may be most effective on this 30%. Only 30% may be under social control, but that 30% is an area for action by counselor and client.

PSYCHOSOCIAL FACTORS IN THE ETIOLOGY AND TRANSMISSION OF ADDICTIONS

Addiction is clearly a biosocial reinforcement process. Although biology may account for much of a person's vulnerability to drugs, social processes interact with biological processes (the stress-diathesis model) and often determine the course of treatment. Nonbiological components include social and ethnic reinforcers and their interactions. Ethnic reinforcers include actual interaction with peers, family, self, and partners. Cultural reinforcers include cultural rules, symbols, facts, history, cognitive schemas, roles, shared values, and worldview that are contingent upon the wider culture for their existence, transmission, and resistance to change.

Addictions foster characteristic dysfunctions that are passed on to subsequent generations in a variety of ways. All family dysfunction cannot be attributed to drugs, and all individual psychopathology, even among ACOAs, cannot be attributed to addictions in prior generations (Hadley, Holloway, & Mallinckrodt, 1993). Left untreated over generations, however, addictions produce not only typical family dysfunctions but typical patterns of dysfunction. For example, familial addiction dysfunction tends to grow from generation to generation, with each subsequent generation becoming more disorganized, fragmented, and rigid. Not only do individuals within families become symptomatic, the social and economic standing of entire family groups may collapse. Fortunately, many treated individuals and families have been shown to have better than average functioning (Buelow, 1994b).

Although it is important to understand individual and family characteristics that are passed from generation to generation, it is equally important to understand the processes through which these factors arise. We must ask not just what specific characteristic was passed, but also by what process and to whom, with what specific individual and family result. All chemically dependent families are made up of both dysfunctional and resilient members. Some family groups are resilient even in the face of severe dysfunction. How is it that dysfunctional families produce some very resilient offspring? Is there an inoculation effect? Is dysfunction more persistent than resilience, so that resilience will be overcome over several generations? We will attempt to answer some of these questions and to provide a preliminary biosocial model.

Before we begin, it is important to restate an important caveat: Even though particular traits are found to be common across the entire group of children from chemically dependent homes (CDs), any particular individual may have none of the traits. Appraisal of the client's potential problems may be informed by group data but must be verified by clinical assessment.

Individuals from homes that were not dysfunctional and not drug abusive have been found to differ from CDs and ACOAs in their frequency of substance abuse and in levels of psychiatric problems, social skills deficits, and educational attrition (Barnard & Spoentgen, 1986; Claydon, 1987; Kinney, 1991; West & Prinz, 1987; Woodside, 1982/1984). Children from dysfunctional families where alcohol or other drug use is typical appear to be worse off psychologically than children from otherwise dysfunctional families. These differences are often the product of distortions of family roles and rules (Nardi, 1981; Potter & Williams, 1991). For example, research has found that students from alcoholic and chemically dependent homes are significantly higher in overall family dysfunction, family role dysfunction, and alcoholism scores, and significantly lower in social and emotional components of college adjustment (Buelow, 1995).

Many family-induced dysfunctions appear more fully virulent and destructive of relationships as children age (Black, Buckey, & Wilder-Padilla, 1986; Jacob & Leonard, 1986). It is clear from observing the attachment styles of very young children, however, that dysfunctional parenting causes difficulty in the development of effective relationship styles even in infancy (Ainsworth & Bowlby, 1991). Research among adults from alcoholic and chemically dependent families indicates that adult attachment patterns are often seriously disrupted by early experiences with caregivers. These disruptions cause high levels of social anxiety, avoidance, ambivalence, and interpersonal disorganization (Brennan, Shaver, & Tobey, 1991; Buelow, McClain, & McIntosh, 1996). These attachment failures are not easily remediated because they negatively affect personality formation, especially identity development and individuation, which in turn affects children's and young adults' ability to create necessary psychological separation from their parents. Therefore, ACOAs often do not achieve effective adult relationships (Buelow & Hebert, 1995; Quintana & Kerr, 1993; Quintana & Lapsley, 1990; Rice, 1992). In severely addictive and dysfunctional families, particularly those where physical and sexual abuse are typical, disordered personality traits and fully developed personality disorders frequently arise.

In conclusion, a variety of other factors also appear to have a significant social transmission component. They include propensities toward antisocial traits, low academic and professional achievement, higher levels of relationship conflict, and emotional problems (Zucker & Gomberg, 1986). Intergenerational transmission of alcohol and other drug dysfunction occurs through the agencies of neglect of social interaction and isolation from the general community (Black, 1981), poor role modeling and the development of compensatory but dysfunctional family roles (Buelow, 1995; Nardi, 1981; Potter & Williams, 1991; Thorton & Nardi, 1980), and disruptions to the development of important family rituals or ceremonies through which both family and general culture is passed from generation to generation (Wolin, Bennett, Noonan, & Teitelbaum, 1980).

Study and Discussion Questions

1. What is the transtheoretical model developed by Prochaska and DiClemente?
2. What is the relationship between the stages and processes of change in the transtheoretical model, and why is this relationship particularly useful in understanding chemical dependence treatment?
3. What is the meaning of "decisional balance" as it applies to the transtheoretical model?
4. How is decisional balance important to our understanding of chemical dependence case conceptualization?
5. What is addictionology?
6. Describe the strengths and weaknesses of the disease model of addictions.
7. Explain what we mean when we say that the etiology of addictions is multifactorial and polygenic.
8. Outline the differences between the DSM-IV criteria for substance abuse and for substance dependence.
9. What are the common pathways and rewards in addictions?
10. Outline the case for the genetic and social transmissibility of alcoholism, including an overview of the data and mechanisms.

STAGES OF CHANGE INVENTORY

Stages of Change Assessment

Name or ID # _____   Date _____

Please read the following instructions carefully:

Each statement below describes how a person might feel when they are in therapy and approaching problems in their lives. Please indicate the extent to which you tend to agree or disagree with each statement. In each case, make your choice in terms of how you feel right now.

For questions that refer to your "problem," please answer in reference to the difficulties you are dealing with in therapy. Any questions that use "here" or "this place" are referring to the treatment center.

Circle the number that best describes how much you agree or disagree with each statement.

There are five possible responses to each statement:

1 = strongly disagree
2 = disagree
3 = undecided
4 = agree
5 = strongly agree

1. As far as I'm concerned, I don't have any problems that need changing.   1 2 3 4 5

2. I think I might be ready for some self-improvement.   1 2 3 4 5

3. I am doing something about the problems that had been bothering me.   1 2 3 4 5

4. It might be worthwhile to work on my problems.   1 2 3 4 5

5. I'm not the problem one. It doesn't make much sense for me to be here.   1 2 3 4 5

6. It worries me that I might slip back on problems I have already changed, so I am ready to work on my problems.   1 2 3 4 5

7. I am finally doing some work on my problems.   1 2 3 4 5

8. I've been thinking that I might want to change something about myself.   1 2 3 4 5

9. I have been successful in working on my problem but I'm not sure I can keep up the effort on my own.   1 2 3 4 5

10. At times my problem is difficult, but I'm working on it.   1 2 3 4 5

11. Working on my problems is pretty much a waste of time for me because the problems don't have to do with me.   1 2 3 4 5

Source: From "Measuring Processes of Change," by J. O. Prochaska et al., 1988, *Journal of Consulting and Clinical Psychology*, 520–528. Copyright © 1988 by the American Pyschological Association. Reprinted with permission.

1 = strongly disagree
2 = disagree
3 = undecided
4 = agree
5 = strongly agree

12. I'm hoping this place will help me to better understand myself. 1 2 3 4 5

13. I guess I have faults, but there's nothing that I need to change. 1 2 3 4 5

14. I am really working hard to change. 1 2 3 4 5

15. I have problems and I really think I should work on them. 1 2 3 4 5

16. I'm not following through with what I had already changed as well as I had hoped, and I'm here to prevent a relapse of the problem. 1 2 3 4 5

17. Even though I'm not always successful in changing, I am at least working on my problem. 1 2 3 4 5

18. I thought once I had resolved my problems I would be free of them, but sometimes I find myself still struggling with them. 1 2 3 4 5

19. I wish I had more ideas on how to solve my problem. 1 2 3 4 5

20. I have started working on my problems but I would like help. 1 2 3 4 5

21. Maybe this place will be able to help me. 1 2 3 4 5

22. I need a boost right now to help me maintain the changes that I have already made. 1 2 3 4 5

23. I may be part of the problem, but I don't really think I am. 1 2 3 4 5

24. I hope that someone here will have some good advice for me. 1 2 3 4 5

25. Anyone can talk about changing; I'm actually doing something about it. 1 2 3 4 5

26. All this talk about psychology is boring. Why can't people just forget about their problems? 1 2 3 4 5

27. I am working to prevent myself from having a relapse. 1 2 3 4 5

28. It is frustrating, but I feel I might be having a recurrence of a problem I thought I had resolved. 1 2 3 4 5

29. I have worries but so does the next guy. Why spend time thinking about them? 1 2 3 4 5

30. I am actively working on my problems. 1 2 3 4 5

31. I would rather cope with my faults than try to change them. 1 2 3 4 5

32. After all I had done to try and change my problems, every now and then they come back to haunt me.

URICA Scale Profile–Psychotherapy Sample

T-scores are based on an outpatient psychotherapy sample using all 8 items per scale.

Name or ID # _____ Date _____

	Precontemplation	*Contemplation*	*Action*	*Maintenance*
Item # 1._____	2._____	3._____	6._____
5._____	4._____	7._____	9._____
11._____	8._____	10._____	16._____
13._____	12._____	14._____	18._____
23._____	15._____	17._____	22._____
26._____	19._____	20._____	27._____
29._____	21._____	25._____	28._____
31._____	24._____	30._____	32._____
TOTALS _____	_____	_____	_____

Please circle the number in each column corresponding to the total scale score and connect with lines for Stage of Change profile.

Scores	Precontemplation	Contemplation	Action	Maintenance
100				
95				
90	38–39–40			
85	36–37			
80	33–34–35			
75	30–31–32			
70	27–28–29			40
65	24–25–26	40	39–40	37–38–39
60	22–23	38–39	37–38	34–35–36
55	19–20–21	36–37	34–35–36	30–31–32–33
50	16–17–18	34–35	32–33	27–28–29
45	14–15	32–33	29–30–31	24–25–26
40	11–12–13	30–31	26–27–28	20–21–22–23
35	08–09–10	28–29	24–25	17–18–19
30		26–27	21–22–23	14–15–16
25		24–25	19–20	11–12–13
20		22–23	16–17–18	08–09–10
15		20–21	14–15	
10		18–19	11–12–13	
05		16–17	09–10	
00		14–15	08	
–05		12–13		
–10		10–11		
–15		08–09		

PROCESSES OF CHANGE INVENTORY

Processes of Change Scale
Psychic Distress Form (Current)

We would appreciate your perspective on how you are dealing with psychological distress. Please indicate how frequently you use each of the following procedures in helping yourself overcome psychic distress. Circle the appropriate number on the right-hand side of the page.

1 = never
2 = seldom
3 = occasionally
4 = often
5 = repeatedly

1. I relate less often to people who add to my distress.	1	2	3	4	5
2. I see signs in some public places trying to help people cope with distress.	1	2	3	4	5
3. I read about people who have successfully changed.	1	2	3	4	5
4. I can be open with at least one special person about my distressing experiences.	1	2	3	4	5
5. I tell myself I can choose to change or not.	1	2	3	4	5
6. I engage in some physical activity when I am beginning to feel distressed.	1	2	3	4	5
7. I seek out people who support my changing.	1	2	3	4	5
8. I try to understand the historical causes of my distress.	1	2	3	4	5
9. I notice that some public places are designed to help reduce stress.	1	2	3	4	5
10. I struggle to alter my view of myself as a distressed person.	1	2	3	4	5
11. I use willpower to keep from getting distressed.	1	2	3	4	5
12. I recall information people have personally given me on the benefits of overcoming my distress.	1	2	3	4	5
13. I have someone who understands my problems with psychic distress.	1	2	3	4	5
14. I am considering the belief that people overcoming distress will make the world a better place.	1	2	3	4	5
15. I think about information from articles and advertisements on how to overcome distress.	1	2	3	4	5
16. I take some type of medication for my distress.	1	2	3	4	5
17. Remembering studies about illnesses caused by distress upsets me.	1	2	3	4	5

Source: From "Measuring Processes of Change," by J. O. Prochaska et al., 1988, *Journal of Consulting and Clinical Psychology*, 520–528. Copyright © 1988 by the American Pyschological Association. Reprinted with permission.

1 = never
2 = seldom
3 = occasionally
4 = often
5 = repeatedly

18. Other people in my daily life try to make me feel good when I overcome my distress.   1   2   3   4   5

19. I have someone who cares about my distress.   1   2   3   4   5

20. I try to express feelings related to distress.   1   2   3   4   5

21. I tell myself I am able to overcome my distress if I want to.   1   2   3   4   5

22. I have someone who listens when I need to talk about my distress.   1   2   3   4   5

23. When I am becoming distressed, I try to relax myself.   1   2   3   4   5

24. I do something nice for myself in return for not giving in to my distress.   1   2   3   4   5

25. I try to change personal relationships that are distressing.   1   2   3   4   5

26. I leave places where other people are adding to my distress.   1   2   3   4   5

27. I tell myself that if I try hard enough I can keep from being distressed.   1   2   3   4   5

28. I read books that help me release my distressing feelings.   1   2   3   4   5

29. I make commitments not to become distressed.   1   2   3   4   5

30. I reward myself when I don't give in to distress.   1   2   3   4   5

31. I notice that distressed people are asserting their rights.   1   2   3   4   5

32. I take some type of drugs for my distress.   1   2   3   4   5

33. I stop to think that my distress is hurting my environment.   1   2   3   4   5

34. I can expect to be rewarded by others if I don't act distressed.   1   2   3   4   5

35. I keep things around my place of work that remind me not to get distressed.   1   2   3   4   5

36. I find society changing in ways that make it easier for distressed people.   1   2   3   4   5

37. I get upset when I think about my giving in to my distress.   1   2   3   4   5

38. I remove things from my home that remind me of distress.   1   2   3   4   5

39. When I am beginning to feel distressed, I think about something else.   1   2   3   4   5

40. I am considering the view that my friends and family deserve a distress-free environment in which to live.   1   2   3   4   5

41. I do something else instead of worrying when I need to deal with tension.   1   2   3   4   5

42. I remove things from my place of work that remind me of distress.   1   2   3   4   5

1 = never
2 = seldom
3 = occasionally
4 = often
5 = repeatedly

43. I find that doing things is a good substitute for feeling distressed.   1   2   3   4   5

44. Dramatic portrayals about distress affect me emotionally.   1   2   3   4   5

45. I have someone whom I can count on when I'm having problems with distress.   1   2   3   4   5

46. I am rewarded by others if I don't act distressed.   1   2   3   4   5

47. I look for information related to distress.   1   2   3   4   5

48. I consider the view that distress can be harmful to an interpersonal environment.   1   2   3   4   5

49. I realize the fact that being content with myself includes changing my distress.   1   2   3   4   5

50. I encounter social situations designed to reduce the distress of people.   1   2   3   4   5

51. I consciously struggle with the issue that being distressed contradicts my view of myself as a caring and responsible person.   1   2   3   4   5

52. I put things around my home that remind me not to get distressed.   1   2   3   4   5

53. My tendency to get distressed makes me feel disappointed in myself.   1   2   3   4   5

54. I am considering the idea that the world would be a better place without my being distressed.   1   2   3   4   5

55. I react emotionally to warnings about distress.   1   2   3   4   5

56. Warnings about health hazards of distress move me emotionally.   1   2   3   4   5

57. I try to understand why I get distressed.   1   2   3   4   5

58. I use tranquilizers to relax.   1   2   3   4   5

59. I alter my diet in order to feel better.   1   2   3   4   5

60. I take a drink of alcohol to feel better.   1   2   3   4   5

Scoring Key for 60-Item Processes of Change Scale
for Psychic Distress

Process

I.	Consciousness raising	3, 8, 12, 15, 28, 47, 57
II.	Self-reevaluation	10, 37, 49, 51, 53
III.	Environmental reevaluation	14, 33, 40, 48, 54
IV.	Self-liberation	5, 11, 21, 27, 29
V.	Social liberation	9, 31, 26, 50
VI.	Counterconditioning	6, 23, 39, 41, 43
VII.	Stimulus control	2, 35, 38, 42, 52
VIII.	Contingency management	18, 24, 30, 34, 46
IX.	Helping relationship	4, 13, 19, 22, 45
X.	Dramatic relief	17, 20, 44, 55, 56
XI.	Interpersonal control	1, 7, 25, 26
XII.	Substance use	16, 32, 58, 59, 60

2

PRACTICAL DECISIONS IN ASSESSMENT AND REFERRAL

Assessment instruments such as the Michigan Alcoholism Screening Test (MAST; Selzer, 1971) are important aids to diagnosis and may be useful for other care providers and for insurance purposes. But the essence of assessment is a thorough clinical interview. Assessment instruments should be used to further confirm hypotheses strongly supported in the clinical interview, not as stand-alone predictors of alcoholism or other drug dependence.

THE CLINICAL INTERVIEW

Treatment is most effective when therapist and client are working together at the same stage of change. For that reason, the clinical interview should allow the therapist to formulate a clear conceptualization and treatment plan, correctly identifying the client's present stage of change and movement within that stage, as well as what self-help processes the client has used or is now using. Stages of change involve setting meaningful goals. Therapy is impeded when client and therapist are working toward different goals (on different levels, or with different purposes). The interview must also frame the client's concerns with ethnographic clarity—clarity about culture, family, and environmental setting.

Prochaska and DiClemente (1992) described assessment priorities as follows. Therapists need to learn the client's attitude and actions regarding a problem behavior. Therapists also need to evaluate the time and energy clients may have used in accomplishing the tasks of any prior stage of change. Also important is the extent to which the problem has been brought under intentional control in the past, as are the problem's symptomatic expression (such as the client's history of use and nonuse) and situational (family, environmental) determinants. Respect for the client's relative (and changing) position in the change process is perhaps the most important first step toward forming a therapeutic alliance between therapist and client. The Addiction Severity Index (ASI; McLellan, Luborsky, O'Brien, & Woody, 1988; McLellan, Kushner, Metzger, Peters, et al., 1992), a structured interview that should form the basis for the clinical interview, is presented in Worksheet 2.1, at the end of this chapter.

Although we will discuss the general features of such a clinical interview, we encourage therapists to design their own interview schedules taking their particular practices into consideration.

The clinical interview is designed to help the therapist understand how best to utilize the client's change processes and coping resources in developing a structured approach to self-focused treatment. In a very real sense, therapists do not act on clients in an independent way. More accurately, clients themselves learn, through a variety of cognitive and affective interactions, to use therapists' knowledge about and resources for change, and therapists' structured, supportive, and interpersonal involvement, to make changes in the clients' own lives. The first task for the therapist in this process is to determine why an individual is in the intake and assessment process. This understanding involves not only learning the client's explicit reasons but assessing the internal and external process underneath the surface. Second, the therapist needs to determine the current stage of change. Third, the therapist must determine what processes the client has used in the past to make changes in his or her life. Fourth, the therapist should outline the client's history of drug use, health concerns, use of prior therapy, and level of chemical dependence dysfunction. In addition to the DSM-IV Axis I diagnosis of chemical dependence and concurrent Axis II concerns, equally important are Axis III (medical problems), Axis IV (impact of environmental stressors), and Axis V (global functioning)—all of which will dramatically affect treatment response.

In determining the client's stage of change it is important to discuss each stage and not reach hasty conclusions. Clients' readiness to change may seem evident, but all stages should be explored. The initial intake interview may, therefore, take several hours during one session or several sessions spread over several days. Explore with the clients what their life was like before they made a decision to be interviewed. Were they or are they now basically satisfying someone else's demands? Do they clearly understand the problem, or are they considering treatment because they were coached or coerced? What issues of potential dependence do clients deny reasonably? Unreasonably? If a client is actually in stasis, and not committed to contemplate future action, a psychoeducational approach respectful of the client's indecision can help the client begin the contemplation process.

If the client appears to be contemplating change, the therapist must discover what events actually brought the client into the present interview—both in general and at this very moment. Other indicators of the client's movement into contemplation include, for example, self-estimates of the pros and cons of use, views about other successful and unsuccessful previous attempts to change, desires to be different (you might ask what the client would do with a magic wand), and thoughts about how life would be different during and after treatment. The therapist can also expect periods during which the client regresses from contemplation of change back into stasis.

Clients who are in the preparation stage have often made small structural and personal changes to facilitate action to stop drug use; even if these changes have been brief. Clients may have tried, with many lapses, to limit their use rather than quit altogether. Before beginning direct action, clients may be marshaling time, money, and emotional support. You the therapist play an important role in providing that emotional support. Clients in the preparation stage may also be in therapy for related problems, as preparation for action on their drug use. Do not, however, assume that because a client is in the midst of an interview with you, the client is actually preparing for change. Clients may be stuck long-term in an information-gathering cycle. You will rarely be able to lead them into action until they feel prepared on cognitive, emotional, behavioral, and situational fronts. Both client and therapist must fully discuss and understand each of these fields of action.

The action stage is assessed by a thorough examination of the change processes and coping resources clients have used in prior and present situations. Therapists should assess the extent to which clients have used consciousness raising, self-evaluation (and self-assessment), self-liberation and catharsis, helping relationships, reinforcement management, stimulus control, and counter-conditioning, on their own or with others' help. Has the client sustained action in the past but lapsed or relapsed? Clearly, relapse failures make an independent contribution to undermining the client's sense of self-efficacy and must be addressed as challenges, not as failures of past work and moral collapse.

Finally, clients who are presently in the maintenance stage often seek help because they are caught in a relapse dynamic. As we will discuss in more detail in Chapter 4, relapse is not an act but a process, one that must be redirected in a structured, developmental way. Assessment of relapse requires a thorough understanding not only of techniques or therapies that the client may see in retrospect as failures, but of current interpersonal and intrapersonal conditions that may be blocking the positive effects of prior treatment and self-help.

CRITICAL DECISIONS IN INTAKE AND ASSESSMENT

In perhaps his best-known poem, Robert Frost took us on a walk down a winter path, one that divided in a snowy wood. Of the two, he took the path less traveled, and explained in the poem the significant influences on his critical decision—his past, his desires for the future. Critical decisions like this one define the subsequent course of events not only for oneself, but for others. In counseling, a critical decision is one that defines a new path for therapy and, often, a strategic intervention for a client. For example, when you as counselor drop your social and professional mask and confront your client as an important person in your life, a defining moment takes place for both you and the client. This confrontation with reality is viewed as pivotal in interpersonal approaches to counseling, because an authentic relationship between counselor and client is necessary for a therapeutic alliance to develop. That alliance is the cornerstone of therapeutic communication generally (Teyber, 1992), and especially in chemical dependence psychotherapy. In an important sense, the counselor's effectiveness depends on whether this critical interaction takes place.

Added to their role as psychotherapists, chemical dependence counselors are further defined by the critical assessment, conceptualization, and treatment decisions that they make. In each of these areas are critical points—forks in the path, if you like—at which decisions have to be made if clients are to receive exemplary care. Examples include whether to begin therapy immediately or refer the client, and whether or not to refer the client to a structured inpatient or outpatient program.

In other forms of counseling, critical decision points are better understood because they have more historical depth. In contrast, turning points in chemical dependence counseling are less well understood. Chemical dependence often misrepresents itself as a psychological or physical problem. The actual drug use—often minimized and defended if not denied outright—is the tip of an iceberg, the dimensions of which are often lost in clients' historical and emotional depths. Because counselors in training are often less sure of themselves, they may consider some questions about drug use intrusive and therefore not ask those questions, or not pursue them in enough depth. The client's drug use may therefore be minimized or attributed to psychological problems. For this reason chemical dependence assessment and case conceptualization require a highly structured approach. We will look more closely at turning points—alternative paths in our snowy wood.

Intake, assessment, and case conceptualization are the three main activities that make treatment planning and, therefore, successful treatment possible. Of these, the most often underutilized activity is intake, and the most misunderstood is conceptualization. The three activities overlap, and because formative evaluation is always occurring as treatment and aftercare take place, assessment and conceptualization are never truly completed.

INTAKE

Assuming that we are not directly involved in the intervention that provides the pressure necessary to guide the client toward therapy, intake is the period between the client's decision to submit to an assessment and active treatment. Intake involves answering questions about treatment, about the therapist, and about the program that come over the telephone, in person, or through family emissaries. Intake's purpose is to include, to bring in—even if referral is the ultimate decision. In an important sense, intake is the first real step in assessment; the client provides not only verbal information, but also clinically important nonverbal data.

Treatment centers make routine use of standard intake forms, which inexperienced staff can quickly be taught to administer. But intakes, and the clinical interviews that give them meaning and substance, should be either performed by the most highly trained staff available or guided by close supervision. The reasons are several. First, a few clients leave against medical advice (AMA) during a lull in the intake. More expert staff can sometimes see what is coming and defuse the situation. Second, even though formal intake instruments and questionnaires used as part of a structured interview can be administered by less well-trained personnel, instruments cannot substitute for expert clinical investigation of the problems that arise during the clinical interview. Often, it is the information gleaned during the intake from sources other than a written instrument that is crucial to treatment planning. Of central importance are whether the client means to stay in treatment or not and whether the client intends to be successful in treatment or is "sandbagging" (waiting, with a hidden agenda). Sometimes clients answer honestly about their hidden agendas if the right questions are asked before clients are more sober and have their defenses securely erected. Moreover, during intake, clients often make decisions that will affect not only treatment but relapse prevention.

What questions should be asked early in the assessment process as the basis for immediate critical decisions? For starters, find out whether your client is sober now. Is he or she high? Can you tell? If you are in private practice and your client does not appear sober, will you continue to assess and work with the client on an intervention while the client is under the influence? If you are in a treatment center and your client is drunk, will you refer the client to a coworker who has more experience, or ask the client to return when she or he is sober? All these decisions speak to the training, interests, and expertise of the counselor. They also speak to the issue of how intakes are best done with chemically dependent clients.

If you decide to continue with the client, what signs, signals, and traditional wisdoms will help you decide whether you or someone else will work with the client? Are there ethical issues involved in your working with this particular client? For example, have you considered your own alcohol and drug experience, expertise, current use, family use, and dependency, or codependency?

How will you determine your client's mental status? Is the client's reality testing intact? If not, is the difficulty recent drug use, mental illness, or both? Does the client have a dual diagnosis, so that mental problems may complicate or interfere with evaluation and treatment planning? Does the constellation of symptoms or their onset indicate a need to refer the client for a medical evaluation?

Finally, it is important to ask, how might any sexual, racial, cultural, or physical status differences between you and this client impinge on your conceptualization of the case? How clear is your conceptualization of the case? How might the client's dual diagnosis interact with his or her cultural differences and your cultural biases?

All these questions are important; but perhaps the most important issue for what must be a cooperative project is whether the counselor has underlying moral views about chemical dependence that may make the client's recovery more difficult. Questions important to this decision are, first, whether you have such powerful religious proscriptions against alcohol and other drug use that you believe that those who use drugs are reprehensible. Treatment specialists need to be objective and nonjudgmental, to take a nonpunitive stance toward drug users. Clearly, our judgmental biases will even more forcefully affect our responses to those who are actively drunk or high.

Second, do you come from an alcoholic or chemically dependent home? A history of living in a family with a parent who abused drugs can distort a therapist's ability to remain objective about clients' drug use. If seasoned through therapy, however, that early experience can become a powerful resource and ally. Further, the role you played in your family of origin will arise in your interactions with your clients. Be aware that alcohol and drug clients have long antennae for searching out individuals in the treatment field with whom the clients can reenact dysfunctional family relationships. If you come from a dysfunctional home and have not worked out your own family role problems in treatment, you may be more vulnerable to being hooked into clients' seductive role playing.

But let us suppose that you are working on your family issues and that you understand the physical actions of drugs in the nervous system—does that mean that you should work with chemically dependent clients? Even if your job description includes them? In our view you should work with the chemically dependent only to the extent that you choose that work. Nothing is more damaging to drug-abusing clients' long-term prospects for sobriety than working with treatment personnel (in any kind of setting) who don't want to work with these clients. Inexperience is much less deadly than the reluctance of a therapist who has been coerced to work with a client. Still, even if the therapist decides not to attempt to provide alcohol and drug follow-up treatment, the therapist must nevertheless make an informed decision about how, when, and where to refer the client. For clients' mental and physical protection, and for counselors' professional and legal protection, counselors need to assess clients' immediate suicide risk, their risk for accident upon leaving the office, and their likelihood of following through on any referral counselors make to alternative or concurrent treatment.

What to Do About a Client Who Appears Drunk or High

In my experience few counselors have much patience with people who initiate an intake or come to treatment drunk or high, even when the client is asking for substance abuse treatment. In these circumstances, counselors routinely feel threatened and frustrated. This lack of patience usually stems more from a moral judgment than from the more rational objection that it is often more difficult to cope with people who are high. Counselors' distress around coping with clients who are drunk or high can often be traced back to negative childhood experiences with an abusing parent or family member. This early distress often engenders a sense of powerlessness and threat. It is important to remember, therefore, that expecting an addict to show up clean, not under the influence of a drug, is somewhat like expecting someone who is bipolar to come for help when their medications are under proper regulation. We usually see clients when there problems are worsening, not when they are coping well.

Because a typical dose of a drug of choice usually has a normalizing effect on someone who is dependent on it, stable addicts usually appear out of control in the following three circumstances. First, a particularly stressful event has caused the client to use a larger than routine dose of the drug. Second, the client's physical condition has deteriorated to an extent that a typical amount of the drug causes a growing cascade of adverse side effects. Many of us have come into contact with late-stage alcoholics, for example, whose livers can no longer effectively process alcohol or other drugs and who, as a result, are easily disoriented by relatively small amounts of alcohol. Also, because alcohol cannot find its usual escape route from the body, more of the drug may be excreted through the skin and exhaled from the lungs, causing the person to smell strongly of alcohol, even though he or she may have imbibed no more than usual. Third, by design or circumstance, the client is in a state of withdrawal resulting from lack of drug intake.

We must be cautious about sending individuals who need medical attention and supervised detoxification onto the street. This admonition is especially true for late-stage alcoholics who have experienced prior withdrawal hallucinosis or detoxification seizure disorders like delirium tremens (DTs), because many die during unsupervised withdrawal. As difficult as it is to follow through on the lengthy and often frustrating hospitalization process, alcoholics who live on the street often need to be mandated into protective treatment.

If the client is high but cooperative, you may have the client call a friend or relative to provide transportation to a detox center. Or, if you have an emergency mental health system in your area, and your client is becoming uncooperative, let them provide transport. If the client is clearly becoming aggressive or threatening, the police will provide transportation to supervised detoxification or to jail if they judge that the client is a risk to self or others. Unless you are a trained expert who is being paid to do so, do not offer to convey clients who are drunk or high anywhere at any time for any purpose, no matter how humanitarian it may seem at the time, and no matter how long you have known them or how well you think you know them. Let the emergency system come to you and the client. More than a few therapists have been injured by clients, or have had clients injure themselves by stepping out of moving vehicles into the middle of traffic.

Worksheet 2.2 provides physical and psychological indicators for behavior that is related to recent intake of alcohol and other drugs, and some pointers for rational self and client management (such as reducing stimulus for some and increasing awareness of breathing lapses for others).

Your first critical decision as a counselor in training may be to decide whether and how you will work with someone who comes into your office or center high. Have you thought out your options?

Practical Concerns

You do not need to be a chemical dependence treatment specialist to properly refer a client to structured inpatient or outpatient treatment. Counselors are trained to conduct both psychological and psychosocial assessments—therefore, half the assessment battle is already won. Remember that you are not starting from scratch; most of your prior learning can be brought to bear on future chemical dependence assessments and interventions.

From a practical standpoint, and in conjunction with the clinical interview, chemical dependence intake procedures contain at least five initial critical appraisal activities. The first, as we have indicated, is appraising the client's present sobriety. Second, we must determine the extent to which the client is in touch with reality, through a mental status examination; the contribution of present drug intoxication, of course, is an integral part of the client's mental status. Third, we must assess the client's dual-diagnosis status—that is, the relationship between their drug dependence and possible concurrent psychiatric conditions. Fourth, we must carefully consider the cultural, ethnic, and gender components of the client's present behavior and potential psychiatric acting out. And, fifth, we must consider special issues that may arise from the client's specific drug of choice (for example, paranoia in crack cocaine users).

Even though chemical dependence assessment extends beyond ordinary psychological assessment, many important aspects are the same for both. And although the focus should be on the immediate behavioral, emotional, cognitive, and developmental effects of the drugs on the individual and his or her social network, therapists must first establish an effective working relationship. Without a developing therapeutic alliance, the client will neither accept your proposals about referring them for structured treatment, nor return to you for continued psychological care or aftercare.

While working to develop a relationship based on reality, we must work to keep the client focused on the contribution of the drugs to their current problems. It is important to feel comfortable gently confronting a compliant client about digressions and leading the client away from war stories. It is equally important to remain objective and direct without being punitive with a less compliant client. With chemically dependent clients, who usually are high on the paranoia scale and do not trust others easily, the working alliance must be based on shared commitment to reality testing and to tasks agreed on as important for clients' immediate safety. This working alliance does not prosper in an atmosphere of threats, aggressive confrontation, or judgment.

THE MENTAL STATUS EXAMINATION

The mental status exam should be integrated into the clinical interview to the fullest extent possible. Carrying out a mental status exam is not an exotic task, even for the novice counselor in training. We all update mental status reports on ourselves and others constantly: "How am I acting?" "Am I doing OK?" "Is my friend being weird, or what?" Empathy for others necessitates psychological awareness; social competence demands it.

Mental status generally indicates the level of clients' arousal, orientation, intellectual functioning, and cooperativeness. In assessing arousal we look at clients' affect and mood, behavior and mannerisms. Is the client depressed or manic, anxious or overconfident? Throughout the assessment process we must be especially sensitive to cultural differences that could bias our interpretations, and we must try to make our limitations explicit in our reports. In assessing orientation we look at whether the client is disoriented about one or more domains of time, place, or person on the one hand, or obsessed with the minutiae of unfolding events on the other. Is the client able to move cooperatively and flexibly between a focus on his or her immediate issues and the counselor's frame of reference without losing track of the stream of interaction?

The purpose of the mental status exam is to better understand your clients' level of functioning. This cannot take place if clients feel they are being interrogated rather than accepted and dealt with as people. Nothing will cause a client who is high on a drug to shut down more quickly than to feel that he or she is involved in a power struggle over information. Unfortunately, emergency room staff, and often emergency mental health staff, react in an angry or judgmental way when they suspect that a chronically mentally ill (CMI) patient is using drugs. Being judgmental in this way interferes with assessment.

The following section outlines the data that should be collected during a mental status examination. Although all centers should provide a structured form for mental status examinations somewhere among the clinical interview forms, you should work with this kind of examination until it is your own, independent of the forms.

Areas of Mental Functioning

The following areas of the client's functioning should be examined.

1. *General appearance:* Describe the client's observed characteristics, including sex, age, ethnic group, gender considerations, dress, grooming, and obvious health markers, including needle marks, nasal discharge, cleanliness, body and breath odor. Outline the conditions under which the exam is being completed, including whether treatment is outpatient or inpatient, voluntary or involuntary. An inventory of the physical contents of pockets and baggage should be made when ap-

propriate and possible, even if only a verbal check with the client. This inventory should include a check on drugs, drug paraphernalia, and, especially important, weapons. The client should be strongly encouraged to leave any weapons with center security or return them to the client's locked vehicle. If the client refuses, leave the area and call security. You as a clinician are obviously not encouraged to disarm clients, but you do need to ask them to disarm themselves.

2. *Sensorium:* Determine the client's orientation to time, date, place, and person. For example, ask whether the client can tell you what time it is, and the date. Ask whether the client can tell you where the two of you are now. Get specific answers: If the client responds that you are in the hospital, ask what part. Ask whether the client can tell you who he or she is. Determine whether the client's orientation is clear or clouded, precise or vague.

3. *Behavior and mannerisms:* Look at whether the client appears active or passive.

4. *Stream of talk:* Look for pressure of speech, poverty of speech and mutism, compulsive talking, halting speech, rhythmic or melodic patterns. Also determine the client's coherence, including loosening of association, tangential ideas, digressions, clanging, or rhyming.

5. *Cooperativeness:* Examine the client's attitude toward interviewer and situation—whether the client is compliant, overly compliant, resistant, seductive, manipulative, combative.

6. *Mood and affect:* These are analogous to climate and weather, with affect being more transitory than mood. Look at the client's inner feelings—surface and deeper feelings. Is the client stable or labile? Aroused or depressed?

7. *Perception:* Look for illusions, which involve a misperception of reality; hallucinations, which involve seeing, hearing, smelling, tasting, or feeling things not present in reality; depersonalization, which is the feeling that one's reality or self is lost; and delusions, which may concern persecution, grandeur, health, guilt, or other aspects of the client's reality (see DSM-IV).

8. *Thought processes:* Is the client's thinking logical and reasonable? Or is it strange or bizarre, perhaps including ideas of reference, mind control, and automatism or robotism.

9. *Intellectual functions:* Look at the client's general knowledge, memory, and ability to reason and interpret. Memory includes recall of remote past experiences, recent recall, immediate impressions, general grasp and recall of materials, and digit span and serial subtraction, both of which speak not only to short-term memory impairment, but to immediate attention and concentration.

10. *Insight and judgment:* Insight includes insight into one's problems and what brought one into the present setting, as well as insight into abstract phenomena.

Principles Governing the Mental Status Examination

Although the structured mental status examination can help us distinguish between drug-induced and non-drug-induced mental symptoms and can help us rule out dual diagnosis, the mental status examination should be considered an ongoing evaluative process, involving the assessment of data that will be collected over a period of hours, days, weeks, or sometimes months. These data should be viewed diagnostically using standardized, objective inventories. Remember, however, that the predictive power of psychiatric instruments like the Minnesota Multiphasic Personality Inventory (MMPI) may be especially low early in alcohol and drug treatment. The following general rules apply to mental status examinations.

Distinguishing the Primary Diagnosis   Distinguishing which component of a dual diagnosis is the primary diagnosis, and which the secondary one, is not usually possible without follow-up assessment. Some diagnostic schemes simply base their priority on which process began first—alcoholism or schizophrenia, for example. Many counselors might reasonably contend that attribution of primary or secondary status to a diagnosis contributes little to the outcome of therapy. But accurately assessing, for example, whether depression is primary (began prior to alcoholism) or secondary (began after depressant drug use) often makes a substantial difference in long-term treatment planning. The distinction frequently makes an important practical difference early in treatment as well. For example, a client who sobers up from extensive sedative use expects to be less depressed, but is unlikely to if primary depression underlies drug use and goes untreated. For this reason antidepressants may be a necessary adjunct to chemical dependence treatment for some clients.

Building a Relationship with the Client   Mental status information should be developed within the framework of a relationship with the client. That relationship, to the extent possible, should be built upon the client's free consent. The client's level of cooperation with the examination and with intake workers should be clearly noted. It is important to remember that angry clients have the right to be resistant, whether we like it or not. As difficult as it is, we must remember during stressful moments that, as Fritz Perls (1971) reminded us, other people were not born into the world to live up to our expectations.

Assessing the Client's Physical Symptoms   Throughout the process of the mental status exam, the counselor must take into consideration the client's level of drug intoxication or withdrawal, anxiety, depression, physical pain, abstraction, or outright psychosis. Direct observations should be recorded. Make as complete a list as possible of prescription and over-the-counter (OTC) drugs that the client is using on medical advice. Also make a list of drugs that the client may be abusing. Find out whether the client has any medications or drugs with him or her now, and if so whether the client will allow you to look up their characteristic effects in the best source available. If the client has been prescribed psychiatric medications, you can consult the *Physicians Desk Reference* (PDR), the *Counselor's Resource on Psychiatric Medications* (Buelow & Hebert, 1995), or a similar resource. Find out when the client last took the prescribed amount. Also assess when the client last used any other drug and determine the client's present level of craving for or withdrawal from the drug. The client may feel the need to drink or use to forestall withdrawal. Help the client plan for detoxification as immediately as possible and contact an on-staff expert in detoxification.

Is the client sweating in a cool room, or feeling cold even though it is warm? Failure to regulate body temperature properly is often a sign of drug withdrawal. Note the size of pupillary dilation. Are the pupils pinpoint (mydriasis) in a moderately lit room (narcotics and hallucinogens, perhaps), or fully dilated (miosis) in a brightly lit room (marijuana or cocaine, perhaps)? It is our experience that drug users and abusers are very likely to be open about their immediate use, even though they may deny the long-term effects the drug is having. Honesty about their drug use is not foreign to the chronically mentally ill either. They are often, however, unable to concentrate meaningfully or for long on the question. They are also more likely to become belligerent if they think you are threatening them about their use of drugs. These issues must be approached in a forthright, nonantagonistic manner.

Paying Attention to Context   Mental status must be interpreted within the cultural, racial, sexual, and educational context within which clients live out their lives and emotional problems. To interpret mental status you must know in some detail what those cultural, ethnic, sexual, and educational differences are. Simply asking people for their ethnic affiliation does not help you define how they or their cultural peer group view their behavior. Ask clients how people in their own family and social group view their current problem and behavior. Whether we like their values or not, a member of the Dying Demons motorcycle gang may be unlikely to ask for help using the same language you might, but may need help just as much. Psychological and sociological jargon should be left out of the exam and the write-up. Describe behaviors and what the client says, leaving interpretation to a minimum. Interpretation should generally be limited to the written summary and diagnosis.

Assessing the Client's Neurological Symptoms   All indications of neurological dysfunction among children and adolescents suspected of drug use should be taken very seriously. Both the child and the child's guardians should be questioned closely about prior head injury, history of neurological signs or diagnoses (epilepsy, for example), and prior drug use, especially solvents. Adolescent dementia may be caused by the toxic effects of inhaling evaporants—glue, gasoline, and paint thinners in particular. Chronic as well as episodic subacute use of evaporants may produce toxic brain syndromes that are signaled by significant declines in school and social performance; standardized intelligence test performance may be affected as well. Review the characteristics of solvent inhalation provided in Worksheet 2.2. Remember that amotivational syndromes and malaise can be caused by inhalants as well as by marijuana.

Angry, elderly clients are likely to produce "positive" but ambiguous (soft) neurological signs on mental status examination. Remember that elderly and adolescent clients are often coerced into treatment and that their anger may be justified, regardless of the views of their families (Yesavage, 1992).

Repeating the Examination   Drug-induced brain syndromes and psychoses are usually reversible. Thus, the longer clients are observed, the less likely they are to display signal symptoms. There should be a relatively steady improvement in depth and stability of affect, irrational or contradictory behavior, pressure or poverty of speech, uncooperativeness, perceptual distortions, and bizarre thought patterns. If the mental status examination is taking place in an emergency mental health setting, for example, and you believe that the patient is becoming more normalized because the effects of a drug are wearing off, the full examination or parts of the examination that showed pathological functioning should be repeated after a reasonable interval, two hours, for example. Client should be discouraged from leaving the facility until hard evidence has been collected demonstrating how partial detoxification may affect them. Time is also necessary to rule out delirium or dementia resulting from other (disease) sources.

Evaluating Dual Diagnosis   Finally, dual diagnosis, which indicates a client who suffers from a combination of drug abuse or dependence and mental illness, cannot be ruled present or absent on the basis of a mental status examination alone. We can always be in error as clinicians about the degree to which a drug or withdrawal from a drug may be contributing to the exacerbation or production of a mental disorder. The relative contribution of substance abuse to any mental disorder must be examined over time and contact with the client. We will look more fully at dual diagnosis concerns in Chapter 5.

REFERRAL TO STRUCTURED TREATMENT

Structured chemical dependence treatment settings offer a wide range of services that are designed to provide integrated treatment for clients at each stage in the addiction process. Structure implies repeated timed sets of social and behavioral activities built upon the completed learning patterns of prior steps. Treatment steps, whether cognitively derived or modeled on Alcoholic Anonymous–type 12-step programs, should be clearly defined in behavioral terms and graduated in difficulty. In structured settings, clients are not only encouraged but shown how to make each step toward their sobriety goal; for example, clients role-play a variety of the negative thinking traps that lead them away from a rational appraisal of their current situation. Structured treatment also provides a wide range of intervention services, from short-term alcohol diversion and education for the episodic drinker who drives drunk, to daily supervised treatment for the drug dependent. Rarely do structured community-supported programs that focus primarily on the drug dependent help clients work toward controlled drinking outcomes. The history of research on using controlled drinking options among clients with extensive backgrounds of drug use has inspired little confidence among active treatment specialists (Beck et al., 1993).

Reasons for referring clients to residential rather than outpatient treatment are varied, such as the client lives in an environment not conducive to sobriety, or the client has personality or behavior problems amenable to positive peer pressure in a structured living situation. Inpatient treatment or partial hospitalization may be indicated for a client with a coexisting psychiatric disorder that needs to be stabilized with medication, or for a client with a serious medical condition that requires frequent monitoring with detox or chemical dependence treatment. (For full criteria on client placement, see American Society of Addiction Medicine, 1996.) Clients with strongly antisocial or borderline tendencies present major challenges in any treatment setting. Therefore, they should always be in concurrent individual therapy.

In a structured program, the treatment team talks with the client in advance about each individual, group, and family concern in the client's treatment. Each critical point in the patient's therapy is signaled by behavioral milestones documented by treatment personnel. For example, how well did the client move from semi-isolation in detox into greater contact with other clients? Has the client made the transition from completely self-focused attention to other-focused so that group treatment can begin?

In structured community programs that are modeled on 12-step concepts, milestones are viewed as points of progress toward more deeply considered personal responsibility and spiritual development. Step- or phase-designed programs that do not encourage notions of a higher spiritual power are structured on milestones of insight and personal responsibility and are usually based on existential, humanistic writings. Here, the emphasis is on development of responsibility to the self, to society at large, and to the family in particular (Ellis & Velten, 1992; Ellis et al., 1988).

Unstructured programs usually provide short-term intervention or detoxification, emergency mental health treatment, and client-focused and client-led self-help groups that may not be supervised by a formally trained treatment specialist. Alcoholics Anonymous might best be considered a semi-structured self-help group; it is certainly the most effective of its kind in the world. Also, marriage and family counselors often work with families affected by an abusing, dependent, or recovering member. Unfortunately, many formal systems therapists tend to focus too exclusively on family interaction and neglect the dependence cycle as it applies to addicted individuals, especially intrapersonal dynamics and neuropsychological correlates.

Structured programs may be inpatient, residential (so that clients are housed for treatment but continuous medical care is not provided on-site), or outpatient. Many facilities provide a variety of options. Structured, intensive, outpatient programs focus directly on the addiction and dependence cycle and provide facilities and staff for evening treatment if the client works during the day or daylong outpatient treatment if the client is not employed during the day. Many programs provide structured settings and staff for either inpatient or outpatient detoxification. Programs vary greatly in duration—usually one month for inpatient and two to several months for residential and outpatient. In a structured program—whether it is inpatient, residential, or outpatient—clients are expected to commit themselves to the change process, to follow the rules of the program, and to make behavioral, cognitive, and emotional changes at a rate consistent with clients' individual functioning. If clients do not make consistent progress, the treatment team needs to initiate a formal reassessment, focusing especially on present sobriety (for example, through drug screening) and dual diagnosis status. For those who are not able to make steady progress in a short-term (one month) inpatient or residential setting, halfway houses and therapeutic communities are available that can house recovering individuals for extended periods of time (occasionally more than a year), enabling them to continue to build social skills and to establish employment.

Inpatient Treatment Versus Outpatient Treatment

Outpatient treatment is less expensive than residential and inpatient treatment (perhaps $1,500–$3,000 as opposed to $9,000–$15,000) and has generally been shown to be as therapeutic for its clientele as inpatient treatment (Miller & Hester, 1986). So why not refer all clients exclusively to outpatient treatment? Unfortunately, uncertainty in evaluating outcomes precludes a definitive answer.

Residential treatment outcomes have been underresearched. Much of the research compares inpatient success rates with outpatient success rates based on self-selected samples rather than randomly assigned ones; this is like comparing apples and oranges. It is not clear whether outpatient treatment would be as successful with typical inpatient populations, where the typical client is traditionally conceived to be more deeply embedded in the addiction cycle. It is difficult to find comparable inpatient and outpatient programs in which patients reflect similar use characteristics, including, for example, drug enculturation factors and addiction history. Studies involving random assignment of clients seeking treatment have been few, due to the ethical and legal ramifications of assigning drug-addicted individuals and especially alcoholics, who may clearly need inpatient detoxification and intervention, to less supervised outpatient treatment. In the few, relatively small-scale random assignment studies that exist (Miller & Hester, 1986), it is not clear that the treatment groups, methodologies, or actual therapy applications found in the inpatient versus outpatient research settings were directly comparable.

Unfortunately, many insurance programs continue to pay only for inpatient treatment, assuming (shortsightedly) that if a person really needs treatment (is addicted), the person needs inpatient services with a physician on staff. Those insurance companies and health maintenance organizations that do pay for outpatient treatment virtually never pay for residential programs. Residential treatment, such as group therapy, can sometimes be billed to outpatient coverage. Those rigid views are changing in the face of better research and escalating costs, but earlier beliefs about chemical dependence and its treatment failures die hard. In the final analysis, a large number of individuals who could probably have been as well served by outpatient treatment have gone through inpatient treatment. Of course, this treatment was better than none at all.

Miller (1992) described several further important reasons that outcome research has failed to document the success of chemical dependence treatment adequately. First, treatment programs have failed to keep up with research and have relied exclusively on older methods (heavy confrontation, less sophisticated 12-step approaches, for example), when newer ones (behavioral contracting, for example) might work better for a particular client population (such as juveniles). Second, in many cases effective treatments are ineffectively administered through lack of training, care, and ongoing assessment of clients' progress. Third, short-term effectiveness of interventions has been overshadowed by posttreatment lapses or relapses. In other words, relapse may color a treatment as ineffective that may have been very effective, but which may have needed a specific reinforcement or required application in a different setting; for example, a client may have been likely to relapse regardless of the treatment type because specific follow-up was needed but not provided. Fourth, for-profit providers have provided "overly sufficient" forms of treatment (usually inpatient) in order to maximize profits. That over-treatment has complicated evaluation by masking the efficacy of particular treatments for those for whom these methods were specifically designed. Finally, treatment has not been responsive enough to individual client differences. Miller (1992, p. 99) usefully pointed out that "the impact and cost-effectiveness of the treatment system are diminished when treatment is standardized rather than individualized." Some standardization, however—especially movement through structured developmental steps as we find in most forms of cognitive and interpersonal therapy—is crucial.

In brief, alcohol and drug therapy has reached a stage comparable to that of psychotherapy as a whole. Given that our treatments have been shown to be generally effective, we now need to know which treatment will work most effectively over what period of time for which particular clients under what conditions. In many cases, and not only to satisfy insurance providers, we need well-written technical (operational) manuals that take a variety of current technologies into consideration so that outcomes can be compared. Although the research necessary to compare the effectiveness of specific techniques within particular stages of change is now under way (Prochaska et al., 1994), these questions are complex, especially with dual-diagnosis clients and polydrug users. Even tentative answers, however, will make treatment personnel's work more manageable and more meaningful.

Given their many potential similarities, in what significant ways do inpatient and outpatient treatment differ? Perhaps the most important difference is that it is more difficult for the individual to obtain alcohol and other drugs during inpatient and residential treatment—not impossible, certainly, but more difficult. Second, inpatient treatment involves more ongoing interaction between client and peer group, through which social control can be exerted on each individual during group and milieu therapy. Third, in inpatient treatment there are fewer intervening variables that keep clients from utilizing individual and group counseling responsibly and effectively. Fourth, drug-using family members and friends are forced to stay out of the inpatient treatment center until their positive input is sought (and, perhaps, simultaneous treatment is arranged for them). Separation from people who are using drugs can have important buffering effects for many clients.

Unlike many residential settings in which clients must be medically stable, inpatient clients have access to 24-hour-a-day medical supervision, usually through a nursing staff that is in continual communication with a medically trained addictionologist on site. In both inpatient and residential settings, however, the client has regularly planned meals and exercise. Alcoholics Anonymous and other self-help groups are usually available in-house and function every day. Education, treatment, activity, nutrition, counseling, and consultation go on for 16 hours each day, and supervision extends to 24 hours. Unstructured time is held to a minimum. Even though many clients eventually relapse, few come out of such an intensive experience without a good grasp of the importance of their problems. As a rueful client once said, "Treatment may not keep me from drinking forever, but it sure spoiled all the fun!"

The Value of Abstinence from All Drugs

Although we believe that total abstinence from drugs is an important social goal, many of our private clients do not come to us as for help quitting drinking or smoking, and their use of these drugs cannot be said to complicate the therapy for which they did come. Although suspicion is always warranted about whether drugs are causing immediate harm, clients who may not need structured treatment generally include those who are using a drug legally, have been able to cut down or limit drug use without difficulty when they or others feel they need to, do not engage in risky behavior, have no physical problems of any kind, are not pregnant, and are not taking any therapeutic medications.

Clients should clearly be encouraged to move in the direction of total abstinence from alcohol and other drugs under the following conditions:

1. Repeated failure to cut down the amount or limit the frequency of drinking or use of other legal drugs
2. Use of illegal drugs

3. Physical problems that alcohol or other drugs can exacerbate in any way (drugs affect all other physical problems adversely)
4. Pregnancy or risk of pregnancy
5. Prior dependence upon, or addiction to, any drug
6. Concurrent use of medications known to be affected by alcohol or other drugs
7. Prior decision to abstain—why take the risk that some use presents?

Conditions for Referral to a Structured Setting

Although clients' signs and symptoms may differ somewhat from drug to drug, referrals are usually made to a structured inpatient or outpatient program under any of the following general circumstances.

1. The client has failed at attempts to control use of legal drugs or abstain from use of illegal drugs after a reasonable period of time and a reasonable number of trials. The word *reasonable* must be behaviorally defined by the client with the counselor's help; the counselor should not immediately impose his or her own definition as a condition for the client's proceeding with treatment.
2. The client has failed to remain abstinent after agreeing to refrain from drug use during the evaluation and education phase of your work together.
3. The client is having substantial difficulty refraining from drug use and has a genogram (family tree) composed of individuals who could not refrain from use and who needed structured treatment.
4. The client is clearly dependent on a drug as defined by DSM-IV diagnosis, has not been in a structured program, and has repeatedly failed to abstain for more than a short period of time, even where there are no clear signs of work or social impairment.
5. The client's work and social relationships are becoming impaired due to drug use, even though the signs of drug dependence are equivocal.
6. After repeated attempts to educate clients about the nature of addictions, they seem vague or counterrational about what they have learned or become so paradoxically compliant that we question their motives.
7. Even though clients have had structured treatment, they are clearly in relapse: Thinking is distorted, actions are subservient to the drug, relationships are being reordered to enable use, and use is escalating.
8. A psychiatric condition has asserted or reasserted itself, so that drug relapse appears imminent. In this case the client must be referred to a center that is staffed to provide services for those with dual diagnoses.
9. Clients have a history of marked personality changes or inadequacies under the influence of the drug. These personality difficulties can be affective (such as depression), cognitive (such as criminal thinking), or behavioral (such as impulsiveness).

ASSESSMENT

Because of the long-range importance of the decision, time delays, interventions and interference from spouses and other family members, and the many procedural and financial difficulties that often arise in helping clients bridge from individual appraisal and treatment into structured programs, referrals to structured inpatient or outpatient treatment are rarely routine. Each such referral has a life of its own. Let us look closely, then, at some of the important assessment and referral issues that might arise with a new client.

Let us assume that you have a clear idea at this point that you will continue to work with the client and not refer him or her immediately for assessment by a colleague. The client has checked off on an intake form that he wants help for personal problems, and because a partner has suggested he may have an alcohol problem. Do you begin by collecting a history of his personal problems first, or start with drug involvement?

We usually ask clients which area seems most important to their visit at the moment we are talking to them. If they pursue personal issues, we indicate that we will probably pursue issues from one domain to another as we are struck by things they are telling us, so they should not be startled by our changing topics. If they select alcohol and drug issues, we indicate that we will probably want to talk about the effects of the drugs on their emotional and social life, and then we begin to probe their immediate problems with alcohol and other drugs prior to ascertaining their background family abuse and dependence. So that the client is not overly disturbed by our interventions, we also make it clear that we will ask for time-outs to redirect our discussion when we feel it necessary. If the client did not fill out a standard alcoholism assessment inventory like the Michigan Alcoholism Screening Test (MAST) or the Brief MAST (BMAST; see Worksheet 2.3) describing themselves and their parents on intake, we ask the MAST questions from memory in as nonthreatening a way as possible, and in whatever order seems best suited to the particular discussion. You should commit the MAST questions to memory. In addition, other excellent alcoholism and drug screening instruments can be found in Worksheet 2.3. It is important to remember, when working with the MAST or any other screening instrument as part of a structured interview schedule, that our purpose is twofold. Not only are we trying to establish whether the individual's substance problem is abuse or dependence as defined by DSM-IV, but we are also attempting to understand the trajectory and speed with which the client is moving through stages of dependence and stages of change (Milam & Ketcham, 1983; Prochaska & DiClemente, 1992).

Rarely is the use of drugs completely irrelevant to a client's mental and emotional situation. However, a majority of individuals have experimented with legal and illegal drugs at some point in their lives, and, fortunately, most of them abandon drug use before it becomes a significant and chronic problem. How, then, do we know when someone is going through ordinary age-related experimentation, as opposed to being on a high-risk spiral into further drug use? Some of the more obvious indicators are the following.

1. Is the use related to the individual's age and peer group? A majority of teenagers experiment with alcohol and pot before graduating from high school, but most give up all but occasional use of marijuana in late adolescence—has your client?
2. Is the behavior strongly linked to peer group use where there are few options to find new friends? Is the use endemic in the family—do the parents and siblings have problems with alcohol or other drugs? If drug use is closely tied to dysfunctional family dynamics, untying it may be very difficult without family treatment.

3. Is the drug use linked with serious emotional problems? Do drugs act as a form of emotional regulation?
4. Does entrenched alcohol and marijuana use show signs of branching into episodic use of harder drugs, especially cocaine? If so, a major step in escalation toward polydrug dependence may be in process.

Let us assume that you have identified a group of significant emotional problems, some of which seem driven by family dysfunction (the person's father was alcoholic, for example) and some of which appear driven by growing alcohol or drug involvement (for example, the person scores in the alcoholic range on the MAST, has lost a partner because of drinking, or has had blackouts). Now what? Our usual strategy is to focus closely on how willing the client is to commit to continued assessment, education, and counseling concerning their emotional problems and their drug use. This strategy may delay an immediate assessment of the client's likelihood of following through on a referral to structured inpatient or outpatient treatment. Without building a therapeutic alliance that will bear some discord, and without helping the client understand the present risk clearly, however, referrals to further treatment often fail. Also, given the time and expense involved in structured treatment, clients have every reason to want you to help them assess the problem and solve it. Are you willing to do a thorough assessment? If you think you can help, how long will it take, and what guideposts are you going to find along the way to be sure you are heading the client in the right direction?

Deciding About Treatment Options

We believe that it is important to work with a relatively sober client for at least six sessions in order to identify whether he or she needs structured treatment and, if so, what form that treatment should take: partial hospitalization, structured outpatient, structured inpatient, or concurrent psychotherapy. During the course of those six sessions, which may need to be scheduled as two or three sessions each week, we complete our structured interview and, at the same time, begin to educate clients about the many facets of drug abuse and dependence. As we move through an explanation of what chemical dependence therapy and concurrent psychotherapy are, we explore their family history in depth, as well as important facets of their drug use history that supplement the ongoing clinical interview. In our role as consultant-psychotherapists, we help them explore the relationship between their immediate emotional problems and their drug use.

Do not deeply explore clients' internal dynamics at this consultative, educative stage (even though you may be forming hypotheses necessary to your overall conceptualization of a client's problems), but rather focus on helping clients make a connection between their drug use and current emotional states. During this early period, if they are at low risk for withdrawal seizures or delirium tremens (that is, they have routinely maintained abstinence for three weeks each month without serious consequences, for example), we verbally contract with them not to use drugs between sessions. We are not surprised or punitive if they do lapse, however. We also ask clients to undergo routine drug use screening as a part of our mutual commitment to the assessment process. If clients feel unable or unwilling to commit to abstinence during our evaluation, we will continue the evaluation over a fixed and limited number of sessions, but will not continue with them in psychotherapy if we discover that they do, in fact, have an abuse or dependence problem but are unwilling to commit to a concurrent structured abstinence program.

Avoiding Pitfalls in Concurrent Treatment

In general, a counselor without extensive chemical dependence experience working alone in a private practice, or with a large caseload in a community mental health center or college counseling center, needs readily available structured referral support services to provide the high level of continuing care necessary for clients who are actively struggling with drug dependence. In these cases, concurrent psychotherapy may be welcomed once the client is in a structured program. Important legal and professional issues can arise due to standard of care concerns. Let me paint the following scene.

Shouts have drawn you to the edge of the famous La Brea Tar Pit. Because you live close by, you are aware that many people and other animals have been sucked into the tar to their death in this benign-looking pool. Some victims have stopped to drink the rainwater that often floats on top and slipped in accidentally, only to become helplessly mired. Some animals have charged into the pit to attack others who were trapped, only to become trapped themselves.

Not far from shore you see a woman fighting desperately to keep from sinking farther into the tar. She is panicked and struggling; her struggles only drive her deeper. She begs you to rescue her. But she is too far away for you to reach her with your hand. Only a few small tree limbs are within reach, all of them too fragile to help. You wonder if the tar is as sticky as it seems—could you rush in and grope your way back to safety with her? But she seems capable of grabbing you and miring you down with her. You might accomplish your rescue if you just leaned far enough out to her, or just put your feet out into the edge of the pit, where the tar seems more solid. If you blunder, though, you will both disappear without a trace. Should you give her the rational advice that she should float on her back on the surface until you can return with help for her? That does not seem like the heroic thing to do. If you do find help, however, you can be assured that you at least won't become so mired that you cannot be pulled out. What will you do?

An addiction is in many ways like that tar pit. It is a hundred feet deep, but without help one can drown close to the surface. A therapist can often struggle heroically across the pit to someone who is mired, but without social, technical, and treatment support, the client's weight of problems and despair quickly become dangerous to you both. You have only so much professional time during each week, and drug clients often need many hours each day of supportive help to combat their craving, their boredom, their withdrawal, their drug-using friends, and their pain. What will you do? Can you rescue them? Or should you throw them a float so that they can extricate themselves?

It is our experience that if you struggle very far out of your normal sphere of influence to save your clients, you will save some, and some will pull you and your practice apart, perhaps permanently. It is more realistic, over both the short and long run, to throw your clients the tools to save themselves. They will learn much more and will retain their learning much longer if you use educational and consultative approaches, rather than heroic interventions. Interventions that work against the client's will should be used only when the life of the client or the client's dependent is immediately at risk. Even in those circumstances, such interventions should be carried out only by an intervention team composed of trained professionals and family members who have received appropriate training.

If you are not a therapist in a chemical dependency center, we suggest that you decide how to get the best daily treatment help for your clients while you assess what you can do to further the process. You must also make and follow up on referrals to treatment, support clients' decisions, and educate clients about what to expect in treatment. Even though you work independently of the treatment center, you may still be able to visit the client in treatment, and work with in-house staff if necessary to provide clients with special expertise on specific emotional problems that may be complicating their chemical dependence treatment. You must work with clients' families so that they can support the decision-making process and be available to clients when they want to leave the center without completing treatment. Almost certainly, you will need to help the client continue after formal chemical dependence treatment to work on relapse dynamics and to provide a rational and objective appraisal of the client's unfolding family and occupational situation. Counselors who work with clients without accurately assessing their drug involvement may suddenly find themselves 30 feet out into a tar pit with a client. Without referral and expert supervision, counselor and client may actually sink more quickly together than the client would have alone.

Recall the first rule of counseling: Do no harm. When you work with clients who have problems for which you are poorly prepared, you can do harm in several specific ways. Most important of these is that, by working on peripheral counseling issues, you may enable the client to delay or avoid chemical dependence treatment completely. In some cases, such delay or avoidance may be an ulterior motive for psychotherapy. The client may learn how to further subordinate and rationalize his or her real problems to the detriment of all concerned.

Although therapists are not required by statute to predict the risk that a particular client behavior will occur, therapists are required by law, within the sphere of their training, to assess the client and the client's concerns accurately. Through that assessment, therapists must provide an accurate picture (conceptualization) of the general range of the client's impulsive, risky, and threatening behavior, including the risks to themselves and to others posed by the client's chemical dependency. For example, a client whom you are seeing for depression, but whom you have not assessed for alcoholism, leaves your office and immediately runs over a pedestrian. He fails a sobriety test at the scene of the accident, even though he seemed sober in your office; in fact, his blood alcohol level may be low enough for him to function adequately, despite his failing a sobriety test and being unable to drive legally or safely. Although you may successfully defend yourself against a suit by the pedestrian's family based on lack of adequate assessment, referral, and ongoing standard of care, you well may not.

Having emphasized some of the risks of working with chemically dependent clients who are not concurrently receiving structured treatment, however, let us now outline situations where counselors can reasonably feel more confident. In general, counselors who have access to supervision can work with chemically dependent clients who are not in a structured program under the following alternative circumstances. First, the client has been through a structured treatment program and wants to work with you on identifiable psychological or relapse concerns. Second, the client has had lengthy periods of recent sobriety and has a relatively stable and supportive job and social situation. Third, the client has clear goals of working on stress, family problems, or other personal issues that may play a role in relapse dynamics, and the client is working on a high quality program like AA or Rational Recovery. Fourth, the client has been assessed to be in the early stages of alcohol abuse, not dependence.

◆ Two Case Histories ◆

Although it is important for the counselor to have formal training in relapse prevention before accepting chemically dependent or abusive clients, the issues we have described are relatively clear and circumscribed. Let us look at the following two cases.

Ruth, a 19-year-old woman from a blue-collar family, presents herself at a community mental health center on the advice of her fiancé and her HMO physician. Assessment has included a variety of personality, psychopathology, and drug involvement measures, and a detailed clinical interview. Assessment indicates that she is in the early abusive phase of alcohol and other drug use. Ruth has maintained lengthy periods of sobriety in the immediate past, but she enjoys drinking and often frequents the bars. She is aware that her drinking and occasional use of other drugs are beginning to cause serious problems because her fiancé has broken up with her on several occasions over her risky and aggressive behavior when she drinks.

Ruth and her fiancé are now planning marriage again, and she has contracted with you to refrain from drinking or using any other drug during the six weeks of your continuing assessment, education, and consultation relationship. She is willing to be screened to verify her sobriety. She has mild withdrawal symptoms, and her cravings for the drug are not strong most of the day, even though she is often irritable and anxious or moderately depressed by the end of the day. She has the support of her fiancé and her family, and she indicates that she wants to explore why alcohol is so attractive. She has experimented with other drugs at parties and has used cocaine on one occasion. However, cocaine, and her friends who are involved with it, frighten her. She is clear about her goal to abstain from alcohol, but feels she needs to understand her situation better before she can make a final decision about how to proceed. She has had blackouts while drinking, and those have provided added motivation since her father, who also has a history of blackouts, was injured as the result of a car accident during a blackout. Finally, she is willing to attend a non-AA abstinence group that meets twice each week to see what the group has to offer.

In this scenario, the client may be appropriate for assessment outside a treatment center and, possibly, treatment outside a center, because she is motivated, is moving through contemplation of change into preparation, and has a history of affecting positive change when she is clear about the objectives. She has intact coping mechanisms and social support in the form of friends, fiancé, and family. She has come to assessment and treatment willingly, even though she may turn out to be resistant in some areas. She is not, so far, using drugs as a primary component in emotional and sexual regulation. She can express herself and her commitment openly, and you have been given open access by the client to people in her life (such as her fiancé) who are willing to confirm independently that she is not drinking or using other drugs. Finally, you have made a contract with the client and her partner that she will take a referral to a more structured treatment setting if she does not maintain her abstinence.

Clearly, counselors with chemical dependence training and proper supervision can work independently with clients like Ruth who are highly motivated to abstain, who have shown they can abstain, and who have peer and family support. It is also possible to work nonconcurrently with clients who have had effective prior treatment and who want to work on problems of living and relapse, as well as those who have just begun their chemical abuse careers and who want and need information, support, education, and counseling for both abuse and psychosocial problems. In Ruth's case, she is able to pull herself away from the edge of the tar pit with professional help; she needs further education in order not to wander too close again. Like Ruth, many clients have one foot on solid ground and one foot in shallow tar. They are thirsty, and the rainwater on top of the tar is particularly satisfying to them. But they sincerely want a road map to a less risky lifestyle, some support on the journey, and education about how to live near the attractive spot without forgetting the dangers of "accidentally" falling back in. Relapsers and early abusers are especially rewarding to work with in unstructured settings because their self-change processes are intact, and they can make excellent progress without heroic interventions. Such clients are able to take responsibility for their behavior and, with proper support and challenge, can usually learn to help themselves cope more effectively.

Those who we decide do need a structured program are more difficult but are equally rewarding to work with in therapy as individuals and families, concurrently with structured treatment for their long-term abstinence concerns. Let us look at the following case of a client with whom we would not feel comfortable working unless she were in a concurrent structured program including both group and family therapy:

Jan is a 21-year-old white female and the eldest of three siblings. Very popular in high school because of her good looks and exuberant personality, she was elected to the homecoming court and numerous class offices. Her grades were also excellent and she intended to follow her father into the medical profession—a plan she dropped in college. She has been described as perfectionistic and has struggled for the past five years with bulimia in an effort to "control her weight." Jan began drinking at parties in junior high school; her drinking continued every weekend during high school, escalated in college, and has not abated since graduation. She has had numerous fights with her friends and her roommate—a friend since high school—and sometimes drinks alone. She is presently working in an insurance office as a sales representative. Peers often have to care for her when they are socializing because she may drink to drunkenness. She has had several DUIs and her coworkers have begun to worry that she will be forced to resign if she loses her driver's license. Jan has had numerous blackouts, during which she has had unwanted sexual experiences, and one serious accident, during which she suffered a head injury.

Jan's mother and father are college-educated professionals with a ready supply of cash and criticism of their children. Both are perfectionistic and demanding. Jan's mother appears to have little understanding of, or empathy for, her children, and continually threatens to cut off the youngest two from their monthly allowances that keep them in college.

Jan's younger brother and sister both abuse alcohol, marijuana, and other drugs, including cocaine. Although her parents claim to drink socially and in moderation, her paternal grandfather died of alcoholism at an early age. Recently, Jan's friends and coworkers will not take her anywhere that alcohol is served because of her impulsive actions when she drinks. She also becomes dependent and sad or angry when she drinks, and, if she is out with one of her several boyfriends, is always in the process of fighting, breaking up, and tearfully reuniting.

Jan says that she needs to learn to control her drinking and that she should be able to do so, given that "control" is one of her family's central issues. She is known, however, to make promises that remain unkept, to miss work appointments, to be unaware of other people's feelings, and to be involved with her present employer in a seductive and exploitative way.

It is important in Jan's case to consider carefully the various concerns for assessment and diagnosis and how they will be integrated into a conceptualization of the case before we consider referral to a structured treatment setting and concurrent psychotherapy alternatives. Considerations that you will need to specifically address in your theory of the case are Jan's (1) potential dual-diagnosis status: eating disorder, long-term effects from head trauma, dysfunctional personality traits; (2) current lack of insight and social exploitation; (3) extensive history of drug abuse and alcohol abuse and dependence; (4) lack of family support and guidance; and (5) poor cognitive and affective coping styles. Jan also has a variety of strengths that make her a candidate for concurrent psychotherapy. Consider the specific strengths and problems that Jan may bring to concurrent psychotherapy, and develop an outline of actions from which you might proceed with her as a client.

In conclusion, no matter how final the counselor's assessment and conceptualization of a client's problem may seem, they are hypotheses that must be tested over time in treatment. As Shaefer and Neuhaus (1985) pointed out, these hypotheses are generated from biological, sociological, psychodynamic, and behavioral perspectives on the client's drug and general life problems. Such hypotheses help the counselor make efficient use of time, keep the counselor from prematurely ceasing to collect data on the client, and provide a stimulus to explore neglected questions about the client (Lazare, 1979). Our hypotheses are always partial formulations that should be open to change because drug use is overdetermined—in other words, it has multiple and competing causes. However, a word to the wise may be in order here: however sure you may feel that you know why a client is using drugs, never underestimate the power of the drugs themselves in the causal chain, regardless of the immediacy and salience of presenting psychological characteristics.

STUDY AND DISCUSSION QUESTIONS

1. What are the basic foundational building blocks of chemical dependence assessment (chemical dependence testing, personality appraisal, client history, clinical interview)?

2. Describe the critical decisions counselors are likely to make with clients who reveal alcohol or other drug problems to them, and outline how they might approach their decision at each important juncture.

3. What are the prominent components of the mental status exam?

4. How do we separate immediate substance use, abuse, or dependence dysfunction from other areas of mental functioning?

5. What criteria would you use to decide whether to refer a client to psychotherapy or to structured chemical dependence or abuse treatment?

6. What individuals most clearly need to establish total abstinence as a goal?

7. What are the most important features of the chemical dependence clinical interview?

8. Review the indicators of specific drug use and abuse (see Worksheet 2.2).

9. Commit to memory the questions from the Brief MAST (see Worksheet 2.3), and practice asking these questions during a clinical interview role-play.

ADDICTION SEVERITY INDEX (ASI)

The ASI is a semistructured interview designed to address seven potential problem areas in substance abusing patients: medical status, employment and support, drug use, alcohol use, legal status, family/social status, and psychiatric status. In 1 hour, a skilled interviewer can gather information on recent (past 30 days) and lifetime problems in all of the problem areas. The ASI provides an overview of problems related to substance, rather than focusing on any single area.

Target Population

Adults

The ASI can be used effectively to explore problems within any adult group of individuals who report substance abuse as their major problem. it has been used with psychiatrically ill, homeless, pregnant, and prisoner populations, but its major use has been with adults seeking treatment for substance abuse problems.

Administrative Issues

Approximately 200 items, 7 subscales

Pencil and paper self-administered or interview

Time required: 50 minutes to 1 hour

Administered by technician

Training required for administration. A self-training packet is available as well as onsite training by experienced trainers.

Scoring

Time required: 5 minutes for severity rating

Scored by technician

Computerized scoring or interpretation available.

The ASI provides two scores: severity ratings are subjective ratings of the client's need for treatment, derived by the interviewer; composite scores are measures of problem severity during the prior 30 days and are calculated by a computerized scoring program.

Normed on the following treatment groups— alcohol, opiate, cocaine: public, private; inpatient, outpatient—and the following subject groups: males, females, psychiatrically ill substance users, pregnant substance users, gamblers, homeless, probationers, and employee assistance clients.

Source: From "Assessing Alcohol Problems: A Guide for Clinicians and Researchers," by J. P. Allen and M. Columbus (Eds.), for the *National Institute on Alcohol Abuse and Alcoholism Treatment Handbook Series 4,* NIH Publication No. 95-3745, pp. 168–175, 1995, and from Lewis, Dana, & Blevins, published by Brooks/Cole Publishing, 1993.

Psychometrics	Reliability studies done:
	    Test-retest
	    Split half
	    Internal consistency
	
	Measures of validity derived:
	    Content
	    Criterion (predictive, concurrent, "postdictive")
	    Construct

Clinical Utility of Instrument	The ASI has been used extensively for treatment planning and outcome evaluation. Outcome evaluation packages for individual programs or for treatment systems are available.
Research Applicability	Researchers have use the ASI for a wide variety of clinical outcome studies.
Copyright, Cost, and Source Issues	Public domain—supported by grants from the Veterans Administration and the National Institute on Drug Abuse. No cost; minimal charges for photocopying and mailing may apply. A free computerized scoring disk is provided with the training materials. Copies of the ASI and related materials may be obtained from DeltaMetrics/TRI ASI Information Line: 800–238–2433 A computerized version of the ASI is available from: Quickstart Computer Company at 214–342–9020. Cost for the Base ASI Module is $990.
Source Reference	McLellan, A. T.; Luborsky, L.; O'Brien, C. P.; Woody, G. E. An improved diagnostic instrument for substance abuse patients: The Addiction Severity Index. *J Nerv Ment Dis* 168:26–33, 1980. McLellan, A. T.; Kushner, H.; Metzger, D.; Peters, F.; et al. The fifth edition of the Addiction Severity Index. *J Subst Abuse Treat* 9:199–213, 1992.
Supporting References	McLellan, A. T.; Luborsky, L.; Cacciola, J.; and Griffith, J. New data from the Addiction Severity Index: Reliability and validity in three centers. *J Nerv Ment Dis* 173:412–423, 1985. McLellan, A. T.; Kushner, H.; Peters, F.; Smith I.; Corse, S. J.; and Alterman, A. I. The Addiction Severity Index ten years later. *J. Subst Abuse Treat* 9:199–213, 1992.

Hodgins, D. C.; and El, G. N. More data on the Addiction Severity Index: Reliability and validity with the mentally ill substance abuser. *J Nerv Ment Dis* 180(3):197–201, 1992.

Stoffelmayr, B. E.; Mavis, B. E.; and Kasim, R. M. The longitudinal stability of the Addiction Severity Index. *J Subst Abuse Treat* 11(4):373–378, 1994.

ADDICTION SEVERITY INDEX
SEVERITY RATINGS

The severity ratings are interviewer estimates of the patient's need for additional treatment in each area. The scales range from 0 (no treatment necessary) to 9 (treatment needed to intervene in life-threatening situation). Each rating is based upon the patient's history of problem symptoms, present condition and subjective assessment of his treatment needs in a given area. For a detailed description of severity ratings' derivation procedures and conventions, see manual. Note: These severity ratings are optional.

Fifth Edition

SUMMARY OF PATIENTS RATING SCALE

0 - Not at all
1 - Slightly
2 - Moderately
3 - Considerably
4 - Extremely

I.D. NUMBER ☐☐☐☐

LAST 4 DIGITS OF SSN ☐☐☐☐

DATE OF ADMISSION ☐☐☐☐☐☐

DATE OF INTERVIEW ☐☐☐☐☐☐

TIME BEGUN ☐☐ : ☐☐

TIME ENDED ☐☐ : ☐☐

CLASS:
   1 - Intake
   2 - Follow-up ☐

CONTACT CODE:
   1 - In Person
   2 - Phone ☐

GENDER:
   1 - Male
   2 - Female ☐

INTERVIEWER CODE NUMBER ☐☐

SPECIAL:
   1 - Patient terminated
   2 - Patient refused
   3 - Patient unable to respond ☐

GENERAL INFORMATION

NAME _____

CURRENT ADDRESS _____

_____

_____

GEOGRAPHIC CODE ☐☐

1. How long have you lived at this address? ☐☐ ☐☐
   YRS.   MOS.

2. Is this residence owned by you or your family? ☐
   0 - No   1 - Yes

3. DATE OF BIRTH ☐☐☐☐☐☐

4. RACE ☐
   1 - White (Not of Hispanic Origin)
   2 - Black (Not of Hispanic Origin)
   3 - American Indian
   4 - Alaskan Native
   5 - Asian or Pacific Islander
   6 - Hispanic - Mexican
   7 - Hispanic - Puerto Rican
   8 - Hispanic - Cuban
   9 - Other Hispanic

5. RELIGIOUS PREFERENCE ☐
   1 - Protestant   4 - Islamic
   2 - Catholic   5 - Other
   3 - Jewish   6 - None

6. Have you been in a controlled environment in the past 30 days? ☐
   1 - No
   2 - Jail
   3 - Alcohol or Drug Treatment
   4 - Medical Treatment
   5 - Psychiatric Treatment
   6 - Other _____

7. How many days? ☐☐

ADDITIONAL TEST RESULTS

Shipley C.Q. ☐☐☐

Shipley I.Q. ☐☐☐

Beck Total Score ☐☐

SCL-90 Total ☐☐☐

MAST ☐☐☐

_____ ☐☐☐

_____ ☐☐☐

_____ ☐☐☐

SEVERITY PROFILE

	PROBLEMS	MEDICAL	EMP/SUP	ALCOHOL	DRUG	LEGAL	FAM/SOC	PSYCH
9								
8								
7								
6								
5								
4								
3								
2								
1								
0								

MEDICAL STATUS

1. How many times in your life have you been hospitalized for medical problems? *(Include o.d.'s, d.t.'s, exclude detox.)*

2. How long ago was your last hospitalization for a physical problem   YRS.   MOS.

3. Do you have any chronic medical problems which continue to interfere with your life?
0 - No
1 - Yes _____
Specify

4. Are you taking any prescribed medication on a regular basis for a physical problem?
0 - No   1 - Yes

5. Do you receive a pension for a physical disability? *(Exclude psychiatric disability.)*
0 - No
1 - Yes _____
Specify

6. How many days have you experienced medical problems in the past 30?

FOR QUESTIONS 7 & 8 PLEASE ASK PATIENT TO USE THE PATIENT'S RATING SCALE

7. How troubled or bothered have you been by these medical problems in the past 30 days?

Comments

8. How important to you now is treatment for these medical problems?

INTERVIEWER SEVERITY RATING

9. How would you rate the patient's need for medical treatment?

CONFIDENCE RATINGS

Is the above information significantly distorted by:

10. Patient's misrepresentation?
0 - No   1 - Yes

11. Patient's inability to understand?
0 - No   1 - Yes

EMPLOYMENT/SUPPORT STATUS

1. Education completed *(GED = 12 years)*   YRS.   MOS.

2. Training or technical education completed   MOS.

3. Do you have a profession, trade or skill?
0 - No
1 - Yes _____
Specify

4. Do you have a valid driver's license?
0 - No   1 - Yes

5. Do you have an automobile available for use? *(Answer No if no valid driver's license.)*
0 - No   1 - Yes

6. How long was your longest full-time job?   YRS.   MOS.

7. Usual (or last) occupation.

_____
(Specify in detail)

8. Does someone contribute to your support in any way?
0 - No   1 - Yes

9. (ONLY IF ITEM 8 IS YES) Does this constitute the majority of your support?
0 - No   1 - Yes

10. Usual employment pattern, past 3 years.
1 - full time (40 hrs/wk)
2 - part time (reg. hrs)
3 - part time (irreg., daywork)
4 - student
5 - service
6 - retired/disability
7 - unemployed
8 - in controlled environment

11. How many days were you paid for working in the past 30? (include "under the table" work.)

How much money did you receive from the following sources in the past 30 days?

12. Employment (net income)

13. Unemployment compensation

14. DPA

15. Pension, benefits or social security

16. Mate, family or friends (Money for personal expenses).

17. Illegal

Comments

18. How many people depend on you for the majority of their food, shelter, etc.?

19. How many days have you experienced employment problems in the past 30?

FOR QUESTIONS 20 & 21 PLEASE ASK PATIENT TO USE THE PATIENT'S RATING SCALE

20. How troubled or bothered have you been by these employment problems in the past 30 days?

21. How important to you now is counseling for these employment problems?

INTERVIEWER SEVERITY RATING

22. How would you rate the patient's need for employment counseling?

CONFIDENCE RATINGS

Is the above information significantly distorted by:

23. Patient's misrepresentation?
0 - No   1 - Yes

24. Patient's inability to understand?
0 - No   1 - Yes

DRUG/ALCOHOL USE

	PAST 30	LIFETIME USE	
	Days	Yrs.	Rt of adm.
01 Alcohol - Any use at all			
02 Alcohol - To Intoxication			
03 Heroin			
04 Methadone			
05 Other opiates/ analgesics			
06 Barbiturates			
07 Other sed/ hyp/tranq.			
08 Cocaine			
09 Amphetamines			
10 Cannabis			
11 Hallucinogens			
12 Inhalants			

13 More than one substance per day (Incl. alcohol).

Note: See manual for representative examples for each drug class

* Route of Administration: 1 = Oral, 2 = Nasal 3 = Smoking, 4 = Non IV inj., 5 = IV inj.

14 Which substance is the major problem? *Please code as above or 00-No problem; 15-Alcohol & Drug (Dual addiction); 16-Polydrug; when not clear, ask patient.*

15. How long was your last period of voluntary abstinence from this major substance? *(00 - never abstinent)*   MOS.

16. How many months ago did this abstinence end? *(00 - still abstinent)*

* 17 How many times have you:

Had alcohol d.t.'s

Overdosed on drugs

* 18 How many times in your life have you been treated for:

Alcohol Abuse:

Drug Abuse:

* 19 How many of these were detox only?
Alcohol

Drug

20 How much would you say you spent during the past 30 days on:

Alcohol

Drugs

Comments

21 How many days have you been treated in an outpatient setting for alcohol or drugs in the past 30 days *(Include NA, AA)*.

22 How many days in the past 30 have you experienced:
Alcohol Problems

Drug Problems

FOR QUESTIONS 23 & 24 PLEASE ASK PATIENT TO USE THE PATIENT'S RATING SCALE

23 How troubled or bothered have you been in the past 30 days by these:
Alcohol Problems

Drug Problems

24 How important to you now is treatment for these:
Alcohol Problems

Drug Problems

INTERVIEWER SEVERITY RATING

25 How would you rate the patient's need for treatment for:
Alcohol Abuse

Drug Abuse

CONFIDENCE RATINGS
Is the above information significantly distorted by:

26 Patient's misrepresentation?
0 - No   1 - Yes

27 Patient's inability to understand?
0 - No   1 - Yes

LEGAL STATUS

1. Was this admission prompted or suggested by the criminal justice system (judge, probation/parole officer, etc.)

   0 - No   1 - Yes

2. Are you on probation or parole?

   0 - No   1 - Yes

How many times in your life have you been arrested and charged with the following:

* (03) - shoplifting/vandalism
* (04) - parole/probation violations
* (05) - drug charges
* (06) - forgery
* (07) - weapons offense
* (08) - burglary, larceny, B & E
* (09) - robbery
* (10) - assault
* (11) - arson
* (12) - rape
* (13) - homicide, manslaughter
* (14A) - prostitution
* (14B) - contempt of court
* (14C) - other

(15) How many of these charges resulted in convictions?

How many times in your life have you been charged with the following:

* (16) Disorderly conduct, vagrancy, public intoxication
* (17) Driving while intoxicated
* (18) Major driving violations (reckless driving, speeding, no license, etc.)
* (19) How many months were you incarcerated in your life?   MOS.

20. How long was your last incarceration?   MOS.

21. What was it for? (Use code 3-14, 16-18. If multiple charges, code most severe)

(22) Are you presently awaiting charges, tria, or sentence?
   0 - No   1 - Yes

(23) What for (If multiple charges, use most severe).

(24) How many days in the past 30 were you detained or incarcerated?

Comments

(25) How many days in the past 30 have you engaged in illegal activities for profit?

FOR QUESTIONS 26 & 27 PLEASE ASK PATIENT TO USE THE PATIENT'S RATING SCALE

(26) How serious do you feel your present legal problems are? (Exclude civil problems)

(27) How important to you now is counseling or referral for these legal problems?

INTERVIEWER SEVERITY RATING

(28) How would you rate the patient's need for legal services or counseling?

CONFIDENCE RATINGS

Is the above information significantly distorted by:

(29) Patient's misrepresentation?
   0 - No   1 - Yes

(30) Patient's inability to understand?
   0 - No   1 - Yes

FAMILY HISTORY

Have any of your relatives had what you would call a significant drinking, drug use or psych problem- one that did or should have led to treatment?

Mother's Side	Alc	Drug	Psych
Grandmother			
Grandfather			
Mother			
Aunt			
Uncle			

Father's Side	Alc	Drug	Psych
Grandmother			
Grandfather			
Father			
Aunt			
Uncle			

Siblings	Alc	Drug	Psych
Brother #1			
Brother #2			
Sister #1			
Sister #2			

Direction: Place "0" in relative category where the answer is clearly no for all relatives in the category; "1" where the answer is clearly yes for any relative within the category; "X" where the answer is uncertain or "I don't know" and "N" where there never was a relative from that category. Code most problematic relative in cases of multiple members per category.

FAMILY/SOCIAL RELATIONSHIPS

(1) Marital Status ☐

    1 - Married   4 - Separated
    2 - Remarried   5 - Divorced
    3 - Widowed   6 - Never Married

2 How long have you been in this marital status? YRS. MOS.
(If never married, since age 18).

(3.) Are you satisfied with this situation? ☐
    0 - No
    1 - Indifferent
    2 - Yes

• (4.) Usual living arrangements (past 3 yr.) ☐
    1 - With sexual partner and children
    2 - With sexual partner alone
    3 - With children alone
    4 - With parents
    5 - With family
    6 - With friends
    7 - Alone
    8 - Controlled environment
    9 - No stable arrangements

5. How long have you lived in these arrangements. YRS. MOS.
(If with parents or family, since age 18).

(6.) Are you satisfied with these living arrangements? ☐
    0 - No
    1 - Indifferent
    2 - Yes

Do you live with anyone who:
    0 = No   1 = Yes

6A. Has a current alcohol problem? ☐

6B. Uses non-prescribed drugs? ☐

(7) With whom do you spend most of your free time: ☐
    1 - Family   3 - Alone
    2 - Friends

(8.) Are you satisfied with spending your free time this way? ☐
    0 - No   1 - Indifferent   2 - Yes

(9.) How many close friends do you have? ☐

Direction for 9A-18: Place "0" in relative category where the answer is clearly <u>no for all</u> <u>relatives in the category</u>; "1" where the answer is clearly <u>yes for any relative within the</u> <u>category</u>; "X" where the answer is <u>uncertain or</u> <u>"I don't know"</u> and "N" where there <u>never was a</u> relative from that category.

9A. Would you say you have had close, long lasting, personal relationships with any of the following people in your life:

    Mother
    Father
    Brothers/Sisters
    Sexual Partner/Spouse
    Children
    Friends

Have you had significant periods in which you have experienced serious problems getting along with:

0 - No 1 - Yes

	PAST 30 DAYS	IN YOUR LIFE
(10) Mother		
(11) Father		
(12) Brothers/Sisters		
(13) Sexual partner/spouse		
(14) Children		
(15) Other significant family _____		
(16) Close friends		
(17) Neighbors		
(18) Co-Workers		

Did any of these people (10-18) abuse you: 0 = No; 1 = Yes

18A. Emotionally (make you feel bad through harsh words)?

18B. Physically (cause you physical harm)?

18C. Sexually (force sexual advances or sexual acts)?

(19.) How many days in the past 30 have you had serious conflicts:

A with your family?
B with other people? (excluding family)

FOR QUESTIONS 20-23 PLEASE ASK PATIENT TO USE THE PATIENT'S RATING SCALE

How troubled or bothered have you been in the past 30 days by these:

(20) Family problems
(21) Social problems

How important to you now is treatment or counseling for these:

(22) Family problems
(23) Social problems

INTERVIEWER SEVERITY RATING

(24) How would you rate the patient's need for family and/or social counseling? ☐

CONFIDENCE RATINGS

Is the above information significantly distorted by:

(25) Patient's misrepresentation? ☐
    0 - No   1 - Yes

(26) Patient's inability to understand? ☐
    0 - No   1 - Yes

Comments

PSYCHIATRIC STATUS

[ ][ ][ ][ ]

• (1) How many times have you been treated for any psychological or emotional problems?

In a hospital [ ]

As an Opt. or Priv. patient [ ][ ]

(2) Do you receive a pension for a psychiatric disablity? [ ]

0 - No   1 - Yes

Have you had a significant period, (that was not a direct result of drug/alcohol use), in which you have:

0 - No   1 - Yes

	PAST 30 DAYS	IN YOUR LIFE
(3) Experienced serious depression	[ ]	[ ]
(4) Experienced serious anxiety or tension	[ ]	[ ]
(5) Experienced hallucinations	[ ]	[ ]
(6) Experienced trouble understanding, concentrating or remembering	[ ]	[ ]
(7) Experienced trouble controlling violent behavior	[ ]	[ ]
(8) Experienced serious thoughts of suicide	[ ]	[ ]
(9) Attempted suicide	[ ]	[ ]
(10) Been prescribed medication for any psychological/emotional problem	[ ]	[ ]

(11) How many days in the past 30 have you experienced these psychological or emotional problems? [ ][ ]

FOR QUESTIONS 12 & 13 PLEASE ASK PATIENT TO USE THE PATIENT'S RATING SCALE

(12) How much have you been troubled or bothered by these psychological or emotional problems in the past 30 days? [ ]

(13) How important to you now is treatment for these psychological problems? [ ]

THE FOLLOWING ITEMS ARE TO BE COMPLETED BY THE INTERVIEWER

At the time of the interview, is patient:

0 - No   1 - Yes

(14) Obviously depressed/withdrawn [ ]

(15) Obviously hostile [ ]

(16) Obviously anxious/nervous [ ]

(17) Having trouble with reality testing thought disorders, paranoid thinking [ ]

(18) Having trouble comprehending, concentrating, remembering. [ ]

(19) Having suicidal thoughts [ ]

Comments

INTERVIEWER SEVERITY RATING

(20) How would you rate the patient's need for psychiatric/psychological treatment? [ ]

CONFIDENCE RATINGS

Is the above information significantly distorted by:

(21) Patient's misrepresentation?
0 - No   1 - Yes [ ]

(22) Patient's inability to understand?
0 - No   1 - Yes [ ]

INDICATORS OF SPECIFIC DRUG ABUSE

	Alcohol	Marijuana	Inhalants	Depressants	Stimulants	Narcotics	Hallucinogens
Odor	Acetone/alcohol	Burned rope	Bad breath/ inhaled matter		Bad breath		
Nose	Reddish		Runny nose Nosebleeds Sneezing	Depressed respirations	Rapid respir. Dry (amphet- amine) Runny (cocaine)	Slow, shallow respirations Runny/itchy nose	Rapid, shallow breathing (PCP)
Eyes	Bloodshot Glazed	Red Glassy Poor depth perception Slow glare recovery	Watery Large pupils (mydriasis)	Involuntary movement Smaller pupils (miosis)	Enlarged pupils (mydriasis) Poor focusing	Pinpoint pupils (miosis) Watery Reduced vision	Large pupils (mydriasis except PCP) Light sensitive Rapid movement Blank stare
Speech	Slurred	Loud, rapid, incomplete sentences	Slurred	Slurred	Garbled Talkative	Slowed	Slurred Incoherent
Coordination	Poor Slow reactions	Poor balance w/eyes closed Slow reactions	Uncoordinated gait Poor muscle control	Poor Slow reactions Stumbling	Poor Increased reflexes Tremor	Jerky Muscle spasms	Poor Numb extremities

Orientation	Short-term memory loss	Disoriented Confused	Disoriented Dizzy	Paradoxical excitement Disoriented Confused Forgetful	Often confused Manic Overoriented Stereotypic	Vague Good connections Good continuation	Poor perception of time/distance
Blood Pressure		Changes w/ body position	Above norm	Below norm	Above norm (148/105)	Below norm	Above norm (falls during overdose)
Pulse		Increased	Increased	Decreased	Increased	Decreased	Increased (falls during overdose)
Temperature		Below norm			Above norm		Above norm
Mental State		Apathetic Poor comprehension Poor math		Interest loss	Excitable Restless Paranoid	Apathetic Can be volatile Can be impulsive	Anxious Restless
Appetite	Poor	Eating binges Thirsty	Poor		Very poor	Poor but craves sweets	
Physical Signs		Dry mouth and throat	Appears tired and drowsy	Clammy skin Sometimes a rash Paradoxical excitement Yawning	Hyperactive Licking lips Weight loss Grinding teeth Scratching nose Sweaty	Moist skin Cool skin Frequent yawns Insensitive to pain Constipation Ulcerative colitis Withdrawal symptoms: pain, diarrhea, cough	Trancelike looks Drooling Flushed Trembling Sweaty

Note: MDMA (called Exstacy, X, Adam, Eve) is a combination of stimulants and hallucinogens. It causes the symptoms of both but also results in temperatures far above norm, fear, tight jaw muscles, and peculiar rhythms of the pulse.

CHEMICAL DEPENDENCE ASSESSMENT INVENTORIES

Michigan Alcoholism Screening Test (MAST)

The MAST is one of the most widely used measures for assessing alcohol abuse. The measure is a 25-item questionnaire designed to provide a rapid and effective screening for lifetime alcohol-related problems and alcoholism. The MAST, which can be used in either a paper-and-pencil or interview format, has been productively used in a variety of settings with varied populations. Several briefer versions of the MAST have been offered (see below).

Target Population	Adults
Administrative Issues	25 items, 0 subscales
	Pencil and paper self-administered or interview
	Time required: 10 min
	Administered by practitioner or self
	No training required for administration
	Also available are briefer versions of the MAST, including the 10-item Brief MAST (Pokorny et al., *Am J Psychiatry* 129:342–345, 1972), the 13-item Short MAST (SMAST) (Selzer et al., *J Stud Alcohol* 36:117–126, 1975), and a 9-item modified version called the Malmo modification (Mm-MAST) (Kristenson and Trell, *Br J Addict* 77:297–304, 1982). A geriatric version of the MAST, called the MAST-G, also has been developed (Mudd et al., *Alcoholism Clin Exp Res* 17:489, 1993).
Scoring	Time required: 5 minutes
	Scored by staff
	No computerized scoring or interpretation available
	No norms available
Psychometrics	Reliability studies done: Test-retest Internal consistency
	Measures of validity derived: Content Criterion (predictive, concurrent, "postdictive")

Source: Adapted with permission from *Journal of Studies on Alcohol, 36,* No. 1, January 1975, 117–126. Copyright © 1975 Journal of Studies on Alcohol, Inc., Rutgers Center of Alcohol Studies, Piscataway, NJ 08855.

Clinical Utility of Instrument	To screen for alcoholism with a variety of populations.
Research Applicability	Useful in assessing extent of lifetime alcohol-related consequences.

Copyright, Cost, and Source Issues	No copyright
	
	Cost: $5 for copy, no fee for use
	
	Source:
	   Melvin L. Selzer, M.D.
	   6967 Paseo Laredo
	   La Jolla, CA 92037

Source Reference	Selzer, M. L. The Michigan Alcoholism Screening Test: The quest for a new diagnostic instrument. *Am J Psychiatry* 127:1653–1658, 1971.
Supporting References	Zung, B. J., and Charalampous, K. D. Item analysis of the Michigan Alcoholism Screening Test. *J Stud Alcohol* 36:127–132, 1975. Skinner, H. A. A multivariate evaluation of the MAST. *J Stud Alcohol* 40:831–844, 1979. Zung, B. J. Factor structure of the Michigan Alcoholism Screening Test in a psychiatric outpatient population. *J Clin Psychol* 36:1024–1030, 1980. Skinner, H. A., and Sheu, W. J. Reliability of alcohol use indices: The Lifetime Drinking History and the MAST. *J Stud Alcohol* 43:1157–1170, 1982. Hedlund, J. L., and Vieweg, B. W. The Michigan Alcoholism Screening Test (MAST): A comprehensive review. *J Operational Psychiatry* 15:55–65, 1984.

The Brief MAST

Questions	Circle Correct Answers	
1. Do you feel you are a normal drinker?	Yes(0)	No(2)
2. Do friends or relatives think you are a normal drinker?	Yes(0)	No(2)
3. Have you ever attended a meeting of Alcoholics Anonymous (AA)?	Yes(5)	No(0)
4. Have you ever lost friends or girlfriends/boyfriends because of drinking?	Yes(2)	No(0)
5. Have you ever gotten into trouble at work because of drinking?	Yes(2)	No(0)
6. Have you ever neglected your obligations, your family, or your work for two or more days in a row because you were drinking?	Yes(2)	No(0)
7. Have you ever had delirium tremens (DTs), severe shaking, heard voices or seen things that weren't there after heavy drinking?	Yes(2)	No(0)
8. Have you ever gone to anyone for help about your drinking?	Yes(5)	No(0)
9. Have you ever been in a hospital because of drinking?	Yes(5)	No(0)
10. Have you ever been arrested for drunk driving or driving after drinking?	Yes(2)	No(0)

Alcohol Abstinence Self-Efficacy Scale (AASE)

The AASE assesses Bandura's construct of self-efficacy and evaluates an individual's efficacy (i.e., confidence) to abstain from drinking in 20 situations that represent typical drinking cues. These situations form four subscales, comprising five items each, examining cues related to negative affect, social/positive, physical and other concerns, and withdrawal and urges. In addition, these same items can be assessed to evaluate an individual's temptation to drink, providing a measure of cue strength to relate to the efficacy evaluation. Both efficacy and temptation are rated on 5-point Likert scales ranging from not at all to extremely. Individuals are asked to give a current estimate of temptation and efficacy. These scales can be used to evaluate individuals entering treatment, progress during treatment, relapse potential, and posttreatment functioning.

Target Population	Adults
	The AASE would be especially helpful to treatment personnel and in treatment programs where the goal of intervention is abstinence. It could also be used to evaluate AA program participation. These measures would be helpful for outcome evaluations and program evaluation. The AASE also could be used for adolescents if the goal for these individuals was alcohol abstinence.
Administrative Issues	20 efficacy and 20 temptation items, 4 subscales
	Pencil and paper self-administered
	Time required: 10 minutes
	No training required for administration
Scoring	Time required: 5–10 minutes
	Hand scored by staff
	No computerized scoring or interpretation available
	Normed on outpatient substance abusers
Psychometrics	Reliability studies done: Internal consistency
	Measures of validity derived: Construct
Clinical Utility of Instrument	The AASE yields clients' evaluations of their perceived temptation to drink and their efficacy to abstain in 20 common situations. Individuals who score high in temptation and low in efficacy across all situations are more dependent. Individuals who respond differentially to specific situations could be given more specific interventions. Clinicians could

also give the measure repeatedly to assess progress in treatment in terms of these self-evaluations. Finally, relapse prevention programs could use these estimates of temptation and efficacy to individualize and guide treatment.

Research Applicability

Self-efficacy can be used as either an outcome measure or a mediator of drinking outcomes. This scale is comparable to ones used for smoking cessation, diet, and substance abuse, so self-efficacy could be comparably evaluated across behaviors. The measure can also be used to track progress during treatment. Scores can be used in latent growth analyses as well as in more traditional multiwave analyses. Efficacy scores have been found to vary with stage of change and to be responsive to relapse threats, so they could be used in relapse studies.

Copyright, Cost, and Source Issues

No copyright and no cost

Available from:
    Dr. Carlo DiClemente
    Department of Psychology
    University of Houston
    4800 Calhoun
    Houston, TX 77204–5341

Source Reference

DiClemente, C. C.; Carbonari, J. P.; Montgomery, R. P. G.; and Hughes S. O. The Alcohol Abstinence Self-Efficacy Scale. *J Stud Alcohol* 55:141–148, 1994.

Supporting References

Ito, J. R.; Donovan, D. M.; and Hall, J. J. Relapse prevention in alcohol aftercare: Effects on drinking outcome, change process, and aftercare attendance. *Br J Addict* 83:171–181, 1988.

Project MATCH Research Group. Project MATCH: Rationale and methods for a multisite clinical trial matching alcoholism patients to treatment. *Alcoholism Clin Exp Res* 17:1130–1145, 1993.

DiClemente, C. C.; Fairhurst, S. F.; and Piotrowski, N. Efficacy in the addictive behaviors. In Maddux, J. E., ed. *Self-Efficacy, Adaptation and Adjustment: Theory, Research, and Application.* New York: Plenum Press, in press.

Alcohol Abstinence Self-Efficacy Scale (AASE)

Client ID ___/___/___/___/___/___/___
CRU   ___/___/
Date   ___/___/___/___/___/___
Session   ___ (0 = baseline; 1=3 MoFU);
                3 = 9 MoFU; 5 = 15 MoFU)
Location   ___ (1 = onsite; 2 = offsite)

___DE ___V

Listed below are a number of situations that lead some people to drink. We would *first* like to know:

1. How tempted you may be to drink in each situation.

Circle the number in each column that best describes the feelings of *temptation* in each situation *at the present time* according to the following scale:

1 = Not at all tempted
2 = Not very tempted
3 = Moderately tempted
4 = Very tempted
5 = Extremely tempted

Situation	*Tempted*				
	Not at all	*Not very*	*Moderately*	*Very*	*Extremely*
1. When I am in agony because of stopping or withdrawing from alcohol use	1	2	3	4	5
2. When I have a headache	1	2	3	4	5
3. When I am feeling depressed	1	2	3	4	5
4. When I am on vacation and want to relax	1	2	3	4	5
5. When I am concerned about someone	1	2	3	4	5
6. When I am very worried	1	2	3	4	5
7. When I have the urge to try just one drink to see what happens	1	2	3	4	5
8. When I am being offered a drink in a social situation	1	2	3	4	5
9. When I dream about taking a drink	1	2	3	4	5
10. When I want to test my willpower over drinking	1	2	3	4	5

1 = Not at all tempted
2 = Not very tempted
3 = Moderately tempted
4 = Very tempted
5 = Extremely tempted

Situation	*Tempted*				
	Not at all	*Not very*	*Moderately*	*Very*	*Extremely*
11. When I am feeling a physical need or craving for alcohol	1	2	3	4	5
12. When I am physically tired	1	2	3	4	5
13. When I am experiencing some physical pain or injury	1	2	3	4	5
14. When I feel like blowing up because of frustration	1	2	3	4	5
15. When I see others drinking at a bar or at a party	1	2	3	4	5
16. When I sense everything is going wrong for me	1	2	3	4	5
17. When people I used to drink with encourage me to drink	1	2	3	4	5
18. When I am feeling angry inside	1	2	3	4	5
19. When I experience an urge or impulse to take a drink that catches me unprepared	1	2	3	4	5
20. When I am excited or celebrating with others	1	2	3	4	5

Drinking-Related Locus of Control Scale (DRIE)

The DRIE is a 25-item self-report questionnaire presented in a forced choice format. It is adapted from the conceptual model and assessment method developed by Rotter to define an individual's beliefs about the extent to which the outcome of important life events are under personal control (internal locus of control) or under the influence of chance, fate, or powerful others (external locus of control). The DRIE assesses these beliefs specifically with respect to the individual's perceptions of control over alcohol, drinking behavior, and recovery. The scale is multidimensional, having empirically defined factors assessing perceived control over interpersonal, intrapersonal, and general factors associated with drinking. Alcohol-dependent individuals have been found to be more external in their drinking-related locus of control than nondependent drinkers. An external locus of control is associated with more physical, social, and psychological impairment from drinking. The perception of control appears to become more internal over the course of alcohol treatment; individuals with more external perceptions are also more likely to drop out of treatment prematurely. Following treatment, alcoholics having an internal drinking-related locus of control are less likely to relapse, drink less and have a shorter prolonged drinking episode if they do relapse, and have a better overall drinking-related outcome than alcoholics with an external DRIE score.

Target Population	Adults, especially adult alcohol abusers and alcohol-dependent individuals
Administrative Issues	25 items, 3 subscales
	Pencil and paper self-administered
	Time required: 10 minutes
	Administered by staff
	No training required for administration
Scoring	Time required: 5–10 minutes
	Scored by staff
	No computerized scoring or interpretation available
	No norms available
Psychometrics	Reliability studies done:
	Split half
	Internal consistency
	The DRIE total scale has been found to have a high degree of reliability, with alpha and split-half reliability coefficients of 0.77 and 0.70, respectively.
	Measures of validity derived:
	Criterion (predictive, concurrent, "postdictive")
	Construct
	The DRIE has been found to differentiate between alcohol-dependent and nondependent individuals;

to be related to drinking patterns and alcohol-related physical, social, and psychological impairment among alcohol-dependent individuals; and to be predictive of posttreatment drinking behavior. It is also related to measures of generalized locus of control, but at relatively low levels. Fact analysis indicates that there are three meaningful dimensions of drinking-related locus of control: Interpersonal, Intrapersonal, and General.

Clinical Utility of Instrument

The DRIE can be used to assess the individual's perception of personal control related to alcohol, drinking behavior, and recovery. More external scores, suggesting less personal control and a greater influence of chance, fate, or powerful others, have been shown to be related to more rapid return to drinking, more drinking during the initial lapse episode, a greater likelihood of an initial lapse escalating into a more serious relapse, and overall poorer drinking-related outcomes following treatment. A possible focus of interventions would be to modify the perception of control through cognitive-behavioral approaches, with an anticipated shift toward a more internal locus of control.

Research Applicability

The DRIE can be used as a predictor of treatment compliance and outcome, an indicator of severity of alcohol dependence, a moderator of the relationship between reasons for drinking and relapse, and as one component of a constellation composed of perceived locus of control, alcohol-related outcome expectancies, and self-efficacy expectancies. The scale has also been adapted to assess substance-specific control orientations of cocaine abusers and cigarette smokers.

Copyright, Cost, and Source Issues

No copyright

No cost

Source Reference

Keyson, M., and Janda, L. "Untitled Locus of Drinking Control Scale." St. Luke's Hospital, Phoenix, AZ, unpublished.

Supporting References

Oziel, L. J.; Obitz, F. W.; and Keyson, M. General and specific perceived locus of control in alcoholics. *Psychol Rep* 30:957–958, 1972.

Oziel, L. J., and Obitz, F. W. Control orientation in alcoholics related to extent of treatment. *J Stud Alcohol* 36:158–161, 1975.

Donovan, D. M., and O'Leary, M. R. The drinking-related locus of control scale: Reliability, factor structure, and validity. *J Stud Alcohol* 39:759–784, 1978.

Kivlahan, D. R.; Donovan, D. M.; and Walker, R. D. Predictors of relapse: Interaction of drinking-related locus of control and reasons for drinking. *Addict Behav* 8:273–276, 1983.

Abbott, M. W. Locus of control and treatment outcome in alcoholics. *J Stud Alcohol* 45:46–52, 1984.

Jones, J. W. Predicting patients' withdrawal against medical advice from an alcoholism treatment center. *Psychol Rep* 57:991–994, 1985.

Mariano, A. J.; Donovan, D. M.; Walker, P. S.; Mariano, M. J.; and Walker, R. D. Drinking related locus of control and the drinking status of urban Native Americans. *J Stud Alcohol* 50:331–338, 1989.

Bunch, J. M., and Schneider, H. G. Smoking-specific locus of control. *Psychol Rep* 69:1075–1081, 1991.

Oswald, L. M.; Walker, G. C.; Reilly, E. L.; Krajewski, K. J.; et al. Measurement of locus of control in cocaine abusers. *Iss Ment Health Nurs* 13:81–94, 1992.

Prasadarao, P. S., and Mishra, H. Drinking related locus of control and treatment attrition among alcoholics. Special Series I: Alcohol and drug use. *J Pers Clin Stud* 8:43–47, 1992.

Strom, J. N., and Barone, D. F. Self-deception, self-esteem, and control over drinking at different stages of alcohol involvement. *J Drug Issues* 23:705–714, 1993.

Koski-Jannes, A. Drinking-related locus of control as a predictor of drinking after treatment. *Addict Behav* 19:491–495, 1994.

Drinking Related Internal-External Locus of Control Scale

Instructions for the DRIE Scale

These are questions to find out the way in which certain important events in our society affect different people. Each item consists of a pair of alternatives lettered a or b. Please select the one statement of each pair (*and only one*) which you more strongly *believe* to be the case as far as you are concerned. Be sure to select the one you actually *believe* to be more true rather than the one you would like to be true. This is a measure of personal belief: obviously there are no right or wrong answers.

Please answer these items carefully but do not spend too much time on any one item. Be sure to find an answer for every choice. Find the number of the item and circle either letter a or b, which ever one you choose to be the one more true.

In some instances you may discover that you believe both statements or neither one. In such cases, be sure to select the *one* you more strongly believe to be the case as far as you're concerned. Also try to respond to each item independently when making your choice; do not be influenced by your previous choices. Please begin.

Drinking Related I-E Scale

1. a. One of the major reasons why people drink is because they cannot handle their problems.
   b. People drink because circumstances force them to.

2. a. The idea that men or women are driven to drink by their spouses is nonsense.
   b. Most people do not realize that drinking problems are influenced by accidental happenings.

3. a. I feel so helpless in some situations that I need a drink.
   b. Abstinence is just a matter of deciding that I no longer want to drink.

4. a. I have the strength to withstand pressures at work.
   b. Trouble at work or home drives me to drink.

5. a. Without the right breaks one cannot stay sober.
   b. Alcoholics who are not successful in curbing their drinking often have not taken advantage of help that is available.

6. a. There is no such thing as an irresistible temptation to drink.
   b. Many times there are circumstances that force you to drink.

7. a. I get so upset over small arguments that they cause me to drink.
   b. I can usually handle arguments without taking a drink.

8. a. Successfully licking alcoholism is a matter of hard work; luck has little to do with it.
   b. Staying sober depends mainly on things going right for you.

9. a. When I see a bottle, I cannot resist taking a drink.
   b. It is no more difficult for me to resist drinking when I am near a bottle that when I am not.

10. a. The average person has an influence on whether he drinks or not.
    b. Oftentimes, other people drive one to drink.

11. a. When I am at a party where others are drinking, I can avoid taking a drink.
    b. It is impossible for me to resist drinking if I am at a party where others are drinking.

12. a. Those who are successful in quitting drinking are the ones who are just plain lucky.
    b. Quitting drinking depends upon lots of effort and hard work (luck has little or nothing to do with it.)

13. a. I feel powerless to prevent myself from drinking when I am anxious or unhappy.
    b. If I really wanted to, I could stop drinking.

14. a. It is easy for me to have a good time when I am sober.
    b. I cannot feel good unless I am drinking.

15. a. As far as drinking is concerned, most of us are victims of forces we can neither understand nor control.
    b. By taking an active part in our treatment programs, we can control our drinking.

16. a. I have control over my drinking behavior.
    b. I feel completely helpless when it comes to resisting a drink.

17. a. If people want to badly enough, they can change their drinking behavior.
    b. It is impossible for some people to ever stop drinking.

18. a. With enough effort we can lick our drinking.
    b. It is difficult for alcoholics to have much control over their drinking.

19. a. If someone offers me a drink, I cannot refuse him.
    b. I have the strength to refuse a drink.

20. a. Sometimes I cannot understand how people can control their drinking.
    b. There is a direct connection between how hard people try and how successful they are in stopping their drinking.

21. a. I can overcome my urge to drink.
    b. Once I start to drink I can't stop.

22. a. Drink isn't necessary in order to solve my problems.
    b. I just cannot handle my problems unless I take a drink first.

23. a. Most of the time I can't understand why I continue drinking.
    b. In the long run, I am responsible for my drinking problems.

24. a. If I make up my mind, I can stop drinking.
    b. I have no will power when it comes to drinking.

25. a. Drinking is my favorite form of entertainment.
    b. It wouldn't bother me if I could never have another drink.

Scoring of the DRIE   **I – E Answer Sheet**

External options are <u>underlined.</u>

1.	a	<u>b</u>		14.	a	<u>b</u>
2.	a	<u>b</u>		15.	<u>a</u>	b
3.	<u>a</u>	b		16.	a	<u>b</u>
4.	a	<u>b</u>		17.	a	<u>b</u>
5.	<u>a</u>	b		18.	a	<u>b</u>
6.	a	<u>b</u>		19.	<u>a</u>	b
7.	<u>a</u>	b		20.	<u>a</u>	b
8.	a	<u>b</u>		21.	a	<u>b</u>
9.	<u>a</u>	b		22.	a	<u>b</u>
10.	a	<u>b</u>		23.	<u>a</u>	b
11.	a	<u>b</u>		24.	a	<u>b</u>
12.	<u>a</u>	b		25.	<u>a</u>	b
13.	<u>a</u>	b				

The DRIE is scored in the <u>External</u> direction by summing the number of external response options endorsed.

Total Score
   Sum of external items endorsed across the entire scale.

Factor 1—Intrapersonal Factor
   Sum of external endorsements on items #9, 11, 13, 14, 16, 17, +25

Factor 2—Interpersonal Factor
   Sum of external endorsements on items #3, 4, 6, 7, 10, 22, +23

Factor 3—General Control Factor
   Sum of external endorsements on items # 5, 8, +20

3

CASE CONCEPTUALIZATION, TREATMENT PLANNING, AND TREATMENT

Understanding the factors involved in referring a client to structured treatment requires an accurate case conceptualization. Conceptualization requires that we know the important psychological, sociological, physiological, and technical (chemical dependence) aspects of the case in great detail. Accurate case conceptualization also requires that we understand how these various factors interact to produce the client's cognitive and affective schemas, the client's available processes for change (including coping resources and strategies; see also Tables 1.1 and 1.2), and the client's movement within (and cycling back and forth among) particular stages of change.

The content, depth, and breadth of our theory of the case informs our treatment planning in several ways. First, in-depth conceptualization allows us to understand what kinds of experiences and experiments may be most useful to facilitate client change. Second, case conceptualization allows us to determine what feedback from the client will allow us to conclude that interventions have been successful. Unless we can make reasonable treatment hypotheses and assess the congruence between the hypothesis and the actual outcome, our understanding of exactly which therapeutic activities led to treatment success is impaired.

Chemical dependence case conceptualization differs from conceptualization of other sorts of counseling cases because we must develop an accurate model of the relationship between the drug (and activities and people surrounding the drug) and psychological features of the client's life, such as cognitive and emotional coping and change. Among clients who are moving through ever accelerating processes of drug abuse into drug dependence, drugs have begun to play a variety of formative and (dys)functional roles. These include, for example, an introjective role (the drug becomes friend, lover, parent, child), a projective role ("like me, everyone really uses drugs or wants to"), a behavioral role (license to give up impulse control), a cognitive role ("I think more clearly now!"), an emotional role ("only the drug can free me from despair"), and a regulatory role ("without the drug, I will fall apart"). If we do not take account of the drug's meaning in the client's life, we will fail to conceptualize the problem accurately, and therefore we will fail to plan effectively for treatment. If we underestimate the power of the primary drug of choice in the client's life we will remain ignorant of the dynamics that may develop during treatment.

LOCATING THE CLIENT IN THE
CHEMICAL DEPENDENCE PROCESS

In its narrowest focus, accurate conceptualization implies that we understand what is causing a problem—we understand its etiology. Our work is rarely that simple, however. The conceptualization of dependence for a particular client, for example, implies that we understand not only the biological roots and the general physiological course of the process, but also that we understand the client's unique history with the problem, family situation, peer support network, insight into the problem, and personality features that may impact treatment and relapse prevention. We must also understand the conditions under which psychotic exacerbations take place, the history of therapeutic drugs used in treatment (such as Antabuse and Narcan), and, finally, the client's change processes and immediate stage of change. Many other important features might, of course, be usefully identified. Although it is important to understand addictions in general, our conceptualization depends on whether we have an intimate knowledge of this client's dependence in particular; that is, we must understand the person and his or her place in a functional (or, more aptly, dysfunctional) set of interacting systems.

Learning the family's contribution to a client's chemical dependence necessitates answering the following questions, among others: Does the client's chemical dependence have biogenetic roots in the family? How has the family traditionally responded to the challenge? Have other family members been chemically dependent? The questions on the MAST can be generalized to include the family (see Worksheet 2.3 at the end of Chapter 2) to help you determine other family members' chemical dependence. You should also complete a structured kinship diagram or genogram, describing each person in the family from the client's great-grandparents on down (McGoldrick & Gerson, 1985). How were drugs dealt with in prior generations? How does the family usually enable drug abuse and dependence behavior? Other systems to consider are the dyad of the client and his or her spouse or partner, and the client's social, work, academic, and cultural contexts.

Important questions that can locate the individual client in the chemical dependence process include the following: Can you identify the client's position in the dependence cycle? In other words, have you assessed the duration and pervasiveness of the client's use, associated risky behavior patterns, and the client's preoccupation with the drugs, for example? What is the client's current stage of change? What do these stage indicators mean to treatment? What does the client's developing dependence mean to the client? How has the client managed to keep his or her self-esteem intact in the face of what looks like a degenerative disease process? What was the client's life like sober? How did the client maintain sobriety? Has the typical split into a good self (not necessarily sober but not acting out publicly) and bad self (the abusive, acting-out self) taken place? This peculiar splitting process allows the client to salvage some ego intact: Is that process working? What buried relapse triggers has the client put in place so that relapse becomes inevitable unless the triggers are defused? Typical triggers ("I can drink again when . . .") include a divorce's becoming final, or the death of the client's parent, who then will no longer be able to judge the client's behavior. How much about these triggers is known (and typically enabled) by family members who may be asked by clients to play parts in the client's relapse psychodrama? What existential awareness does the drug defend against? How does the client's personality predict the client's particular drug or drugs of choice? Is there a self-medication element? How does the drug allow the client to answer unmet primitive drives, often sexual or narcissistic?

Each of these questions requires a shorter cognitive-behavioral answer and an in-depth, intrapersonal answer. A thorough conceptualization requires that you understand both answers and that you work to understand the relationships between them. If you do not work to answer these questions you will lose interpersonal power in your relationship with the client and will be more subject to manipulation. Counter-transference problems often arise through faulty conceptualization of the client's relationship to the counselor.

Drug Alteration of Instinctual and Social Drives

As Gold (1994) indicated, chemical dependence leads to changes in personality because drug use alters basic instinctual processes and drives. Use of chemicals reinforces and redirects those drives so that the drugged state is continued and use escalates. Addictive drugs operate differentially on exactly those areas of the brain—particularly the hypothalamus, hippocampus, and the limbic system (Julien, 1995; Miller et al., 1987)—in which the drives originate and through which they are regulated and reinforced. Drives are primarily unconscious and are difficult to regulate through conscious ego mechanisms, even though behavioral and cognitive-behavioral techniques can and do affect them. However, to the degree drug use becomes tied to primitive drives—sexuality, for example—it is less under conscious control and more closely connected emotionally to personal survival. The longer drugs are used, the more closely drug use becomes attached to the most primitive biological needs, so that stopping use becomes more threatening to basic ego structures.

Many of the effects that drugs have on neurotransmitter systems may be very long-lasting; some effects may be permanent. Therefore, when drugs start to clear from the system, the brain produces a cascade of potentially self-defeating internal and interactive stimuli, including gratifying drug dreams, enticing memories of drug use, cues, triggers, thoughts, and feelings that powerfully reinitiate and reinforce continued drug use. These feelings and thoughts help evoke a relapse dynamic because opposing cognitive and emotional processes are less available and sometimes unavailable.

Drug alteration of drives is thought to create a long-term psychiatric syndrome predisposing the person to relapse (Gold, 1994). Thus, if clients weren't mentally ill before they became addicted, they often seem so after becoming addicted, especially if a dissociative dual self—composed of the sober, prosocial self on the one hand and the abusing, antisocial, crisis-oriented self on the other—has emerged. The antisocial self is enlisted to help preserve drug use, which has become directly tied to the individual's identity. Unfortunately, self-preservation becomes deeply tied to continuation of drug use. Clients often equate treatment of their drug use with a personal attack, raising deeply held, usually unconscious, defense reactions.

As we have indicated, the dual nature of chemical dependence (good me versus bad me) is an ego defense, which may keep at least some of a client's self-esteem and self-efficacy intact. Unfortunately, this creative process culminates in regression and degradation of prosocial drives. Social needs appear to be pitted against narcissistic needs, interdependence against dependency needs, responsibility against antisocial thinking, and rational patterns against irrational (borderline) ones. In short, regressed and self-serving needs may ultimately win out over needs for interpersonal support. This altered self-system may attain the level of a pervasive personality disorder in its own right—one that affects, orders, and sustains mood, cognition, behavior, and consciousness, and around which other areas of personality and life functioning must navigate if the individual is to remain existentially intact. The influence of chemical dependence on personality can be compared to the influence of living on a mountain. Living in such a place, which is difficult to access, influences every life action and must be constantly taken into consideration. But rather than elevating life, as a residence in the mountains might, chemical dependence chronically and pervasively lowers every other aspect of a person's life to the lowest biological, libidinal denominator. To misunderstand the basic psychodynamic aspects of an addiction is to misunderstand how to use the cognitive and behavioral techniques that are our tools in chemical dependence treatment.

Clients are also swamped by the sociological component of addictions. Social needs have often been reordered to service the addiction. The chemical dependence requires the development of a social system of enablers and codependents. Even though primitive needs drive the social relations of chemically dependent clients, their narcissism gives them heightened interpersonal power (of which therapists are often aware, but which they are not trained to deal with in treatment). Although chemically dependent clients' wants may ultimately prove adolescent in nature, clients are usually able to exercise effective social control over relatively normal peers, parents, partners, and therapists.

STRUCTURED TREATMENT AND CONCURRENT PSYCHOTHERAPY: A CASE HISTORY

Let us look at the assessment, conceptualization, and treatment planning concerns that arise in the following case.

Joel was a 28-year-old, single, Jewish man from the City. His presenting problems at the student health center included headaches, anxiety, problems with his departmental peers, and alcohol relapse. During the preceding weekend he had drunk himself unconscious, and he appeared Monday morning at the university counseling center remorseful and depressed. He had been sober for one year preceding the binge. He was presently a graduate student in creative writing at a major university.

Joel had a twin brother who was a physician and an older sister who was a musician. Joel's mother taught music at a prestigious university. His father had also been a musician, a music professor, and an untreated alcoholic who died of alcoholic cardiomyopathy (alcohol-induced heart problems) when Joel, then 15, was in reform school for drug abuse. His mother and brother blamed Joel for precipitating his father's fatal heart attack. Joel had an exploitative relationship with his enabling sister, who had paid Joel's treatment and drug bills at various times.

Joel was identified early in life as the family's major problem. Even as a very young child, Joel resisted his parents and received many severe beatings. Rather than defend himself against the family dysfunction by overly conforming as his brother and sister did, Joel continually acted out. Drinking as a preteen, he quickly moved on to narcotic drugs as a teenager. He was truant from school, performed badly, got along poorly with his peers, and got into many scrapes with the law.

Joel's most significant memories were as follows. First, he remembered his drunken father's attacking the 12-year-old Joel with a knife over his grades. Second, he recalled that his mother could have kept him from being sent to reform school at the age of 15 by telling the truth about his whereabouts during a burglary he claims he did not commit, but she would not testify in his behalf. Third, he recalled the family's turning him in to the police after he escaped from the reform school and returned home for an important family holiday.

Joel received extensive drug education and completed a GED while in reform school. Because he had a very high IQ and was creative, he managed to work his way through an undergraduate curriculum while on financial aid. During those undergraduate years he had several relapses into narcotic and alcohol use. He saw his acceptance into a creative writing graduate program both as vindication and salvation, but now his social relationships and creative work in the department had begun to deteriorate.

Joel vacillated interpersonally in his attachment pattern between compulsive self-reliance (dismissing others) and anxious dependence. He believed that he was rejected by his mother at an early age because he was a difficult, colicky baby, whereas his twin was less demanding. He blamed his mother for his problems but had not been able to improve or sever his relationship with her. Joel had had few satisfying relationships with women because he so completely dominated the interaction. If conflict developed, he pushed women (and anyone else) away. Historically, Joel had become more frequently sexually impotent as his relationships with women progressed. He had embraced and then rejected involvement with Alcoholics Anonymous and Narcotics Anonymous at various times, and he cycled between the contemplation and action stages without structured preparation for changes crucial to his recovery.

Developmental Concerns and Personality Dynamics

From an object relations standpoint, Joel's early object (parental) introjects clearly were insufficiently warm and consistent. As a toddler, he was not allowed to develop a close dependence on his mother, his primary caregiver; as a result, he did not develop the emotional interdependence necessary to explore his social and physical environment independently without excessive fear. This lack of exploration was reflected in his lack of individuation and stalled identity development. Thus, as angry as he became at them, Joel had great difficulty psychologically separating from his family. Rather, he acted as though other family members were unruly extensions of himself. Like his ambivalent, hypercritical, and dismissive mother, Joel saw himself as a good person when he was being good, and bad when he was bad; there was little middle ground and little to counteract this black-and-white, all-or-nothing thinking. When Joel was sober, the good self was sober and the bad self was an addict to be despised. When Joel was drinking or using narcotics, the good Joel was high, free, and expressive, while the bad Joel was straight and a cop-out to a society that he despised for punishing him as a teenager.

During the first session, Joel defined his bottom line: He would not enter an inpatient treatment center. He would refrain from drinking or using as long as possible and agreed to tell me when he relapsed. He also indicated that he would check every recommendation made in therapy with the student health center physician who referred him for substance abuse evaluation and treatment, which suggested a well-developed paranoia about treatment—not exactly a promising start!

Critical Therapy Decisions

Would you work with this client? Even though Joel had many competing problems, he was bright and functioned at a relatively high level. He had a history of relapses each year that seemed to be triggered by both social and internal factors. He clearly stated that he would not accept a referral to inpatient treatment, even if the referral was reasonable. Perhaps you would decide, despite your limited experience with dual-diagnosis clients, that you would work with him for a limited number of sessions to assess his situation more fully so that a meaningful treatment plan could be designed.

How might your earlier experiences with alcohol and other drugs influence how you would relate to Joel? What are the critical elements in your decision? How would you remain objective if Joel began to resist the imposition of the structure necessary to treatment? Would you refer Joel to a structured outpatient program or work with him on your own?

Although we were willing to complete an extended intake on Joel and work with him on his stated emotional and relapse concerns, we indicated we would not undertake long-term treatment without his investing energy in concurrent structured work—the least intrusive structured alternative. Because Joel could not afford private treatment, he was referred to an evening group therapy program offered through a community treatment facility. Because of his negative experiences with group treatment at the reformatory, Joel strongly resisted the idea of group therapy. After we worked through his fears and explained in detail the importance of group exposure, Joel agreed to attend at least two meetings. He also agreed to focus during the first week on the following: first, his anxiety during his group meetings; second, the here and now, not past problems; third, crisis intervention; and, finally, the contribution of his problems with people to his immediate relapse. We scheduled one-hour meetings with Joel each day for the next three days.

Crisis Management   During the remainder of our scheduled first session, Joel developed a reasonable plan for the rest of his day and we role-played some of the stressful issues concerning his upcoming therapy group meeting. We also made a clear plan for the remainder of Joel's week. As insurance, Joel asked his physician at the health center to prescribe Antabuse. Antabuse sets off a dramatically aversive reaction if one drinks by restricting the metabolism of acetaldehyde so that toxic symptoms, including nausea and headache, begin immediately. Joel had a history of relapse drinking, followed by taking Antabuse. Then he would discontinue his Antabuse after several months and begin drinking in earnest again.

In contrast to his behavior during previous relapses, Joel attended the structured evening program and continued in psychotherapy. We contracted for six weeks of therapy, meeting twice each week. We encouraged Joel to visit Alcoholics Anonymous with one of his therapy group members. After many fits and starts, he began to enjoy and find growing emotional and educational support for his developing sobriety.

Dual-Diagnosis Concerns   Although Joel's psychiatric problems—immaturity, anxious attachment pattern, hypervigilance, manipulativeness, and lack of social skills—began to emerge early in our first meeting, he was also bright and interesting, and he had displayed surprising resilience over the years. Although we felt comfortable working with him, it was clear that some members of his treatment group would respond negatively to his passive-aggressive style. Joel's incompetence and underlying angry ambivalence in social interaction usually led to his being rejected; this rejection led to depression, and depression led to relapse. Therefore, we focused our energies on limiting the behavioral cues that set off Joel's rejection-depression cycle and branching into a detailed analysis of social stressors that could be organized into a hierarchical stress management program.

Cultural and Sexual Issues   Even though his interaction style was the most immediate cause of his social rejection, Joel was convinced that people did not like him because he was Jewish. This useful fiction produced secondary gains for Joel, because his creative writing centered on these themes. We first broached this issue by concentrating on how this background might influence our counseling relationship. As our work together progressed, Joel was encouraged to check out how his peers viewed his cultural background. After much foot-dragging, he was surprised to learn that none he asked in his graduate program knew anything about his background at all; they had avoided him because of his explosive temper.

Joel's sexual difficulties also complicated his therapy. He had been sexually abused by an adult male while in the reformatory. Added to the psychological and physical abuse he had suffered from his parents, this experience had eroded his masculine self-image. Joel distrusted men and women, and his hypervigilance exacerbated his fear of losing control in social interactions. We decided to work with these concerns as they arose in our interaction, particularly as they were reflected in his concerns for power and control. Joel was willing to make clear behavioral contracts because they gave him a sense of equality in our relationship. He was always ready to remind us of specific provisions in the contracts he had made if he felt any of these provisions were not being fulfilled by either party.

Conceptualizing This Client's Intrapersonal Dynamics

Developmentally, Joel had not successfully navigated several of the early Eriksonian stages. He compensated for his lack of developmental continuity by becoming overly developed in thinking, vigilance, and verbal activities, which he identified with adulthood. Because his early nurturance, narcissistic, and exploratory needs were not met, he had great difficulty trusting himself or others. His ability to function autonomously was stunted, and in relationship with others he vacillated between dependence on and rejection of others' attempts to care for him. Shame about his person, especially his sexuality, and doubt about his actions (and the actions of others) were fundamental to his social incompetence and his inability to exert self-control. As is typical of personality disorders instigated in very early childhood or infancy, his self-image was highly distorted by unstable emotional schemas that were not successfully compensated by more mature coping mechanisms. He appeared cognitively over-controlled while at the same time emotionally out of control. He particularly lacked control over depressed emotional states that triggered his alcohol (and heroin) relapses.

Joel compensated for lack of ego boundaries and growing unconscious libidinal pressures in a variety of important ways. First, on the negative side, without object constancy, Joel became angry and vengeful when he perceived that others were trying to control him, even though they may only have been trying to enter his life in a positive way. This tendency limited his positive social interaction and, therefore, his social learning. Second, more positively, he wrote poetry and music, which gave form and expression to his chaotic inner world. However, images and primitive thoughts often intruded beyond his repression boundaries, suggesting to him frightening actions and especially physical harm to himself concurrent with drug use.

Joel's narcissistic and self-destructive traits clearly had to be worked on concurrently with his drug problems. Most important, treatment needed to encourage trust, ego and identity development, and better cognitive control over the conditions that reinforce his cyclical relapse dynamic.

Treatment Planning

During the first several meetings with a client who has just entered intensive outpatient treatment, individual therapy should provide intervention, support, and crisis management; individual therapy should also involve behavioral contracts concerning drug use and suicide, and should take account of rebound anxiety and depression. Supportive and consistent confrontation of distorted thinking processes, especially those that may negatively influence intensive group work, are very important for clients like Joel. As threatening as it is, group work is very important because it allows clients to recapitulate their dysfunctional family dynamics in relative safety. Although individual therapy is important for a client like Joel, positive group experiences are invaluable in helping such clients learn how to overcome their immediate relational difficulties. Individual therapy must support group work in such cases.

Levels of confrontation are often very high in group therapy during family role reenactment. Interactional, interpersonal pressures arise at a time when clients are only tentatively accepting more responsibility for their actions. Thus, it is preferable to begin by helping the client with immediate problem-solving and self-efficacy issues, rather than concentrating on deeper identity or existential issues. First, this concrete approach leads to better crisis management; second, unless the etiology of a psychiatric problem is particularly obvious, we often cannot tell whether presenting psychological problems are part of an underlying psychiatric syndrome or the product of chemical dependence or protracted withdrawal. Immediate withdrawal, polydrug use, and protracted relapse dynamics often complicate the diagnostic picture.

Treatment should focus quickly on developing a stress-reduction plan, because relapse risk is directly associated with rising stress. Controlling stress necessitates plotting the paths of the emotional, cognitive, and behavioral incidents that have led to the present relapse. Then we must use our understanding of these incidents' hierarchical importance to help the client design a more specific and effective self-control contract or plan. Most of us work to relieve stress by controlling the environment that presents us with stressors (stimulus control). If we are overloaded at work, for example, we try to restructure our workload or change our job. It is rare that we can effectively control the behavior of coworkers to relieve stress, but we can exert important control over the environment in which their behavior takes place and how we respond to their stressful actions. People do what they do, but we can adapt ourselves and our situation.

Chemically dependent clients quite reasonably try to control others' behavior directly in order to relieve their own stress in interacting with these others. Such attempts, however, more often raise clients' stress levels, because direct interpersonal control is rarely possible over the long run. As internal stressors build, clients exert their utmost efforts to control others. Each controlling action exacerbates the problem rather than solving it, however, pulling the client into a circular pattern of self-defeating control and over-control. For example, as we learned in our first few sessions, Joel attempted to form social relationships with members of his department. Often he would be rebuffed because of his dominating, aggressive style. Rather than backing off, Joel would try even harder to dominate an interaction that was escaping his grasp. The more he tried to set things right, by controlling events, the worse things got. As his control failed, Joel's anger increased and he began to act out by telling people off—exactly what he did in his family of origin. By telling them off, he reduced his most immediate anxious and angry feelings, but he set himself up to be even more soundly rejected. He also found himself called on the carpet by the department chairman, whom Joel also failed to dominate, but whom he did not fail to alienate.

Buried Relapse Triggers   Like many chemically dependent people, Joel had buried triggers that activated cognitive-emotional schemas, which in turn caused him to re-initiate drug use. When a certain point on his anxiety escalation curve was reached, he covertly visualized (planned) drug-using holidays that would, finally, remain under his control. This visualization acted to alleviate his immediate anxiety (he always felt a rush of self-confidence when he imagined controlled drinking or controlled use of heroin, with the visualization acting like a placebo). These plans served, in his own mind, to punish everyone around him for having unwittingly set up the emotional conditions for his lapse. Our work with Joel unearthed an important covert plan to pull a fatal trigger upon learning that his academic career was "hopeless." He believed his career would be hopeless if he lost his graduate fellowship or failed an important course. He also tied failure to rejection by the department chairman, whom he respected as a writer and looked up to as a father figure. If this ultimate and potentially fatal relapse trigger was at the top of the stress curve, what organization had Joel set up in his own mind concerning all the minor and moderate stressors in his life?

Cognitive-Behavioral Contracts   Joel's movement along the relapse trajectory was accelerated not only by external crises but by his own inadequate personality; his irrational, black-and-white thinking; and his lack of long-term relapse prevention planning. Our treatment pressed Joel to develop a specific contract for each important stressor and trigger. The contracts included detailed countermeasures to be invoked at each progressively more stressful behavioral and emotional step in his relapse dynamic. Although self-control contracting may seem overly mechanistic or simplistic, remember that clarity, simplicity, and concreteness are great virtues, especially during the first few weeks of treatment. Unfortunately, we have only limited power to help clients discover an uninjured emotional space where their self-efficacy remains intact.

In the first several weeks of their treatment, clients must have specific tasks to do, goals to accomplish, and stress-reduction activities to perform if they are to learn to intervene early in their relapse dynamic. These techniques should be taught and practiced during the therapy session in the early stages of treatment, not left up to the client to perform at home without supervision. The greatest threat to Joel's continuing progress in structured group treatment, for example, was his inability to deal with confrontation from others, especially without support from the rest of the group. Therefore, we worked hard on reducing Joel's stress concerning confrontation by role-playing what might appear to him in group as threatening talk. We looked in particular at how Joel decided what people meant when they confronted him, and we looked for antidotes for his unusually sensitive reactions. At the same time we analyzed how Joel could reduce his stress in the writing department. A central concern was to address his felt need to control his interpersonal interactions. In a short time, Joel came to see the connection between his problems in group and his problems in his department. Over succeeding sessions, as Joel better adapted to his treatment group, we put more and more time into identifying each critical step in his many stress escalation curves. We worked to find alternatives to lower his stress and, therefore, the compulsive acting-out and escalation to higher anxiety and acting-out.

As we have indicated, a control contract is an agreement between therapist and client that the client will perform an alternative behavior, designed to reduce stress, by following an agreed-upon hierarchical self-management schema. There is nothing magical about a stress-reduction, abstinence, or suicide contract. The power of behavioral contracts lies in the fact that most clients can quickly reduce crisis-producing behaviors if new and expected behaviors are divided into manageable, digestible action steps that can be practiced consistently both in treatment and in clients' everyday lives. Contracting also decreases clients' risk by helping them become more aware of the routinely self-defeating cognitions that tend to precede their self-defeating behavior. To be effective, stress-control contracts (or any cognitive-behavioral contract) should contain a structured, instrumental plan that includes action steps that clients help develop and in which they have a personal investment. The plan cannot be imposed from the outside, without the client's participation. It is crucial that clients process in depth not only what the contract says and what the action steps are, but what these steps mean. Unless the meaning is clearly understood, clients cannot commit themselves to the process. Although counselors certainly cannot control the level of client motivation, they can work to increase the client's understanding and commitment—the primary constituents of motivation. These objectives are crucial in the first several days and weeks of concurrent group and individual psychotherapy, whether the psychotherapist is employed by the treatment center or is working with the client through another agency or privately.

CRITICAL DECISION POINT: INPATIENT OR OUTPATIENT REFERRAL?

Referral is one critical decision stemming from the treatment planning process. Once a decision has been made to refer a client to structured treatment, the question is whether to refer the client to inpatient or outpatient treatment. This decision depends on answers to a variety of questions we have examined in regard to Joel's case, which are developed in the course of a thorough assessment and conceptualization process.

Outpatient Treatment Referral

Criteria for client referral to structured outpatient treatment programs include the following:

1. The client has failed to find quality sobriety in less structured therapy (least intrusive alternative [LIA]; Lewis, Dana, & Blevins, 1994), including either individual, group, or family therapy, and regardless of whether chemical dependence therapy was a central focus of overall treatment.
2. The client has had long periods of sobriety during the past several years. The client's history has been characterized more by sobriety than by relapse.
3. The client is psychiatrically stable; that is, the client has demonstrated self-control and self-management in a variety of relatively stressful settings. Impulse control problems and antisocial activities do not appear to be central psychiatric concerns.
4. The client has demonstrated in work with you and in other treatment settings that he or she can function effectively in an intensive outpatient group setting.
5. The client does not have a medical or dual-diagnosis medication problem that would require 24-hour medical attention over the course of treatment.
6. The client has typically been able to resolve his or her detoxification and withdrawal problems in the immediate past without experiencing medical complications.

Inpatient Treatment Referral

We suggest the following general guidelines for inpatient referral. Dual-diagnosis clients who are chronically mentally ill, HIV-positive, or homeless also require special consideration because they so often need referral to a partial hospital setting.

1. The client has failed to discontinue drug use after a reasonable period of structured outpatient treatment to which he or she was clearly committed.
2. The client has failed to discontinue use during the education and evaluation phase of your work together, and your evaluation is (a) that the client is at particularly high risk for peer and family pressure, (b) the client has not succeeded in conforming to the principles of a well-constructed control and stress reduction contract, or (c) the client has special needs for structure because he or she has had very limited time periods of sobriety during the preceding months and (usually) years.

3. The client has severe physical problems (seizure risk or high risk for delirium tremens, for example) or concurrent psychiatric problems (schizophrenia or bipolar disorder, for example) that may make the availability of around-the-clock nursing and pharmacological care by an addictionologist necessary. If the client's medical or psychiatric problems have been severe, the client may need treatment in a medical hospital setting, not simply an alcohol and drug inpatient setting with access to a physician.

4. The client's psychiatric and drug problems are reciprocally reinforcing each other to the extent that you cannot make progress in individual therapy until the client is taken out of his or her daily routine, including employment, which may be exacerbating his or her combined problems.

5. The client has been found to be incapable of working in an intensive group therapy condition without exacerbating his or her psychosis.

6. The client has a concurrent antisocial, narcissistic, or other sociopathic personality disorder. Clients who are mandated into treatment by the courts should be referred only to treatment centers with a history of providing proper care for these high-risk clients.

TREATMENT PLANNING ISSUES FOR OUTPATIENT AND INPATIENT SETTINGS

Treatment planning consists of finding both immediate and long-range strategies to meet both client and therapist goals in light of the therapist's assessment and conceptualization developed with the client's direct involvement. For treatment to be successful, these goals must be negotiated, understood fully, and shared between therapist and client in a meeting of the minds. Goals must also be reasonable and practicable. If the client's goal is to establish better control over alcohol, and the therapist's goal is to move the client into a total abstinence contract, the client is not likely to follow the treatment plan, even if there is surface agreement.

Setting Goals

As a counselor, you have an obligation to help your clients reach their stated and implied goals. That does not mean, however, that your goals for treatment must always be secondary. You should fully discuss possible negative implications of the client's goals; you may be able to restructure these goals through counseling interaction. Counselor goals should be stated up front and kept in plain view. Given your assessment and conceptualization of the case, if the client's long-term goals are clearly unattainable or potentially damaging and you find that you cannot in good conscience commit yourself to them, you should strongly consider referring the client.

Remember, however, that if clients could easily identify reasonable and attainable goals, they probably would not be in therapy with you. You have an obligation to help clients identify goals that are attainable, responsible, and healthy, not just help them accomplish goals they have previously identified. If the client wants to work toward controlling his or her drinking or other drug use, and you firmly believe that the client needs to abstain, then, if education does not refocus the client's goal and you cannot accept moderation as a goal, please do not try to convert the client through using your own knowledge and sobriety as a kind of religious text. Instead, refer the client to someone who will try to work with the client toward risk reduction. The client will either succeed or fail at that objective. Many such failures lead clients back into treatment that is focused on abstinence.

Individuals who most clearly need to establish or maintain abstinence as a goal are (again) those who have any of the following general traits:

1. They are using any drug whatever that is illegal.
2. They are suffering physical, emotional, or behavioral problems that are tied in any way to legal or illegal drug use.
3. They have been identified earlier as dependent on or addicted to any drug.
4. They have a family history of illegal drug use or legal prescription medication dependence.
5. They have any physical, emotional, or behavioral problem that is concurrent with drug use.
6. They have never begun drug use in the first place.
7. They are not adult.
8. They are, plan to become, or are at risk to become pregnant.

Total abstinence goals must be met through steps that are identifiable, owned by the client, doable, and mutually agreed upon by client and therapist. These goals must be capable of division into realistic cognitive, emotional, and behavioral action steps whose accomplishment both counselor and client can readily evaluate. Remember, although behavioral steps are the most easily identified, cognitive and emotional steps must also be planned. Also, negative behaviors, biases, and feelings (resistances) that presently block the attainment of designed steps must be identified and addressed. An effective way to begin that process is to work with rather than against the resistance. Identify the resistance with the client's help and explore its meaning to the client. Finally, therapist and client must be explicit about the disadvantages of actually attaining abstinence goals; the secondary gain that drug users derive from treatment failure must be routinely discussed. For example, sobriety may and often does lead to the reorganization of relationships. Sabotaging treatment may be seen as a way of saving one's marriage. We may hope that treatment will encourage primary relationships to prosper, not disintegrate. You must help your client plan, however, for the effects of changing roles, power bases, alliances, and triangulations in the immediate (and later the extended) family constellation.

Working with a Treatment Center

Your continued concurrent work with the client will vary greatly depending on whether you refer the client to an inpatient or outpatient structured program. Most inpatient settings do not make their facilities available for independent practitioners to provide cooperative psychotherapy unless the counselor has a prearranged cooperative relationship. Therefore, you will often be working with clients after their inpatient residence, usually on relapse prevention, psychological problems, or problems of living. In many cases, of course, you will be providing concurrent care for clients whom you have referred to outpatient care or partial hospitalization. It is important for therapists to develop close relationships with chemical dependence treatment centers and to work out cooperative arrangements that will allow therapists not only to see centers' clients concurrently, but also to continue to develop therapists' own chemical dependence treatment skills.

Concurrent Therapy with Outpatient Clients

Concurrent psychotherapy differs in a variety of important domains that we will discuss in more detail. These areas include the following:

1. *Client confidentiality:* Relatively open communication is needed with a client's cocounselors, employers, family, and important peers.
2. *Drug testing:* Counselors need permission and cooperation to share information on drug screening.
3. *Written summaries of the client's week in therapy:* Include individual, group, and family work; attendance at AA, NA, or Rational Recovery meetings; and occupational compliance.
4. *Behavioral contracting:* The client needs to evaluate relapse, depression, craving, mania, and suicide risks on five-point Likert-type scales from very high to very low each session.
5. *Counselor evaluation of the client's distorted or outright criminal thinking:* The counselor needs to confront clients' twisted thoughts concerning their uniqueness, specialness, entitlement, or grandiosity—or, in contrast, their guilt, shame, or need to abase or punish themselves.
6. *Saturation with treatment or self-help groups:* The counselor needs to assess in an ongoing way whether treatment activities are continuing to be useful to the client.

Communication   Providing optimum concurrent therapy requires practitioners to communicate effectively and often. That means that clients must complete both general and specific consent forms for the necessary reciprocal flow of information between center staff and therapist. Concurrent therapy places an added burden on each therapist to clearly define what his or her scope of practice activity will include. Therapists must also identify potential areas of overlap and anticipate conflicts that might arise. Counselors can easily be triangulated by clients who wish to escape the pressure they feel in each setting. This triangulation usually sounds like this: "Well, yes, we're working on that in group. I think I'd rather keep it in the group." Of course, the client may not be working on the problem in either setting. The client's impulse to divide and conquer therapy, rather than actively participate in it, may lead to a loss of crucial information if therapists do not routinely share information. For example, a client may "forget" to inform the concurrent psychotherapist that the client failed a drug screen at the treatment center.

To avoid such therapeutic tall tales and mirages, it is important to keep close track of each client's weekly progress in outpatient group. At the same time let your cocounselor know how your work is progressing. With appropriate releases in place, we usually keep in touch with clients' significant others, parents, or employers to continually monitor and assess how sobriety is affecting client's work and family life. Unless extreme circumstances arise (a spouse is selling drugs, for example), we maintain contact with the client's family members and involve them as directly as possible.

Although addictions develop both openly and in secret, relapse usually prospers best in secrecy. Clients are often reluctant to give up what they consider their privacy (read: secretive ways) because secrecy is fundamental to keeping their family's esteem, while hiding their continued drug use. Therefore, any mechanism that the counselor can use that is consonant with the ethical guidelines of the American Psychological Association and American Counseling Association should be used to destroy the walls of secrecy surrounding drug clients' lives. While we believe that real privacy needs are important, false privacy, like false pride, usually comes before a relapse.

Drug Testing   Therapists must be willing and able to send clients for drug testing. Many therapists have an unfortunate need to believe their clients are clean and sober as a way of believing that therapy is important to clients. Therapists all too often feel emotionally crushed when they learn, usually after the client stops coming to treatment, that the client was drinking or drugging during the course of their work together. We are trained to think the best of clients, to trust clients so that they can learn to trust themselves. There is no real contradiction, however, in trusting clients but not their drugs of choice. Trust but verify: It often seems that drugs think for the clients before the clients have a fair chance to think for themselves.

Further, although relapse is serious and will be discussed in great detail in Chapter 4, neither lapses nor relapses need to be seen as catastrophic. If they were, almost every client would be a catastrophe because many (if not most) will both lapse and relapse before they learn to stay clean and sober. If the relapse is a bad one, just say: OK, where do we go from here? From our perspective, drug screening shows that we care about the efficacy of therapy as well as about clients. If a screen turns out positive, and we have an honest relationship with our client, it becomes grist for the mill: We can work our way through the problem together, and treatment will usually be strengthened.

Sharing Treatment Summaries   Encouraging clients to prepare weekly written summaries of their progress in group and in other social relationships helps them achieve a sense of progress and success. Even very slow progress may seem remarkable to clients whose lives were rapidly going downhill prior to treatment. Summaries of client work also give the counselor necessary information about changes or challenges that are needed in the treatment plan. Although interaction problems in group therapy should be immediately handled in group, of course, it is reasonable to help the client learn how to respond with less defensiveness. Do not, however, interfere with group process. Don't rescue, triangulate, soothe, or otherwise try to save clients pain and embarrassment in their group work. Give clients firm support and confrontation, but do not diffuse or meddle with their relationships with their groups (although you should intercept attempts to scapegoat the group work). If you do meddle with the group relationships, you will enable clients to deflect group pressure more easily, whereas group pressure is the client's best friend. It is surprising how easily even experienced counselors unwittingly enable their clients to deflect responsibility for their treatment. For this reason, many treatment centers discourage concurrent treatment with therapists not directly affiliated with program.

Do not take it too hard when you first discover that you have helped a client circumvent treatment. Find ways to work more closely with structured programs so that you can help your clients better bridge the gaps in their recovery. Finally, remember that as hard as we may try, clients are always more in control of the therapy process than we are. Therapists must be prepared for the point at which clients attempt to exploit this knowledge as leverage against treatment rather than against their dependence.

Ongoing Assessment   The client's relapse potential, depression, anxiety, craving, and suicidal preoccupation should be assessed at least each week, and, depending on the client's situation, possibly each day. Depending on clients' risk, either ask clients where they think they are on a scale of 1 to 10 in each area or have clients document their status on a written self-report Likert-type scale. This information, along with a summary of the clients' progress with individual, group, and family work, should be entered in the therapist's treatment notes. Also, discuss and document relapse triggers that may have been unearthed during the week. Facing these uncomfortable concerns up front on a weekly basis may save great pain and suffering later on.

Counselors must make every effort to supportively confront clients' distorted and outright criminal thinking. Although the content of criminal thinking varies from culture to culture, the generation of these thinking traps is similar all over the world. Criminal thinking originates in patterns that are socially reinforced, often by family, in which individuals receive internal (or family) rewards for working against the norms of their social group. Instead of reforming their reference group in their own image, sociopathic people accept the image as it is and try to undermine the group values to meet their own narcissistic desires. Drug counselors often refer to this deviant cognitive processing as "stinkin' thinkin'." Any collusion with the client's often seductive bashing of society will sabotage and damage the therapy relationship. All distorted thinking must be confronted directly and completely.

TREATMENT: WEEKS 1–6

For practical purposes the first six weeks of concurrent treatment differ from subsequent weeks because therapy during those weeks focuses on providing encouragement, assessment, crisis management, referral to concurrent structured treatment, and continuity of treatment, and emphasizes immediate events, feelings, and self-defeating relapse thoughts and behaviors. Early sessions will often be scheduled more frequently than weekly. Although we will not attempt to provide a complete summary of the most basic counseling skills necessary to undertake substance abuse counseling, we will discuss techniques that are particularly important during the first 16 weeks of therapy. We encourage the counselor in training to read carefully or to reread *Interviewing Strategies for Helpers* by Cormier and Cormier (1991) and *Foundations of Therapeutic Interviewing* by Sommers-Flanagan and Sommers-Flanagan (1993). Cormier and Cormier discussed a wide range of techniques that lend themselves especially well to substance abuse counseling. Of particular importance are the behavioral protocols for goal setting, emotive imagery and other forms of covert modeling, cognitive modeling and thought stopping, cognitive restructuring, reframing, stress inoculation, meditation and progressive muscle relaxation, systematic desensitization, and self-management. Cormier and Cormier also set out useful general strategies for working with clients' resistance. Sommers-Flanagan and Sommers-

Flanagan (1993) provided an excellent overview of the intake and interview process; of particular importance, their book contains detailed information on the mental status examination and suicide assessment, intervention, and contracting.

Although written material on counseling in general, and alcohol and other drug counseling in particular, is important, if you listen and observe carefully, your clients will teach you more about therapy than anyone else can. Unfortunately, the learning process is often painful because it involves counselors' failures to teach and counsel as well as clients' failures to learn. These failures often result in relapse. You must be prepared to learn from both success and failure.

Innovation is the basis of both personal and social change. The client must think new thoughts, develop new behaviors and a new lifestyle, and create a wider emotional range. The counseling relationship becomes the client's basic model for new social behavior. Without the necessary emotional support, the client is unlikely to develop innovative attitudes and behaviors. Innovation must eventually stand the real-world test of utility, but the testing process should not include immersion that is too rapid or unsupported. Client and counselor should seek to develop and apply these innovative responses to life in a planned, cooperative fashion. It is especially important for the counselor to help the client learn to forecast how these innovative responses may be received—that is, in a way that may actually increase the client's immediate risk of relapse.

Some Dos and Don'ts of Treatment

There are dos and don'ts in alcohol and other drug treatment that may seem obvious to the reader; but even obvious mandates are not always easy to put into practice with chemically dependent clients. Some of these mandates—such as forming a relationship—are the same as in other forms of counseling. Some are not; some take on added or disguised significance. Let us look at some of these strategic activities.

Relationship Issues   Forming a relationship, a working alliance, is as important in drug therapy as in any other kind of therapy. Clients' addiction backgrounds, however, can make forming a truly egalitarian relationship more difficult. First, substance abusers are used to forming overly close, enmeshed relationships. They do so, of course, in order to exploit others so they can get and use drugs more freely. Second, substance abusers are used to being exploited (burned) by others when they do indeed form relationships. So, a relationship "dance"—a structured interaction with a covert purpose—easily develops around power, control, and personal boundaries. How do you keep your boundaries clear without pushing the client away from you? You can do so by maintaining your space, by showing respect for the client, by empathizing but not sympathizing, by disclosing who you are but not disclosing too much about your personal life, and by using your skills of active listening, immediacy, genuineness, positive regard, and supportive confrontation.

It is particularly important to know beforehand what is relevant for you to disclose about yourself and what is not. If the client asks you directly whether you are recovering or whether you drink or use other "recreational" drugs, you need to have a straight answer ready. From our perspective, an excellent answer is this one: "Let's explore why that is important to you. Do you feel that if I am not in recovery, I won't understand what you're going through?" Confronting the question in this manner usually allows clients to discuss their fears of not being understood without shifting the focus of therapy away from the client.

If your answer to a particular question feels phony to you, it probably will to the client. You may need to practice your responses to these kinds of personal questions with another counselor until you feel comfortable with them. If you feel that indicating your prior use status is necessary, be concise and direct. Understand, however, that the client can use any personal information about your current or past drug use to push against your boundaries. Clients' attempts to gain power over boundaries usually involve manipulating your personal feelings about, and investments in, the therapy relationship. Remember the West African adage: A handshake does not extend above the elbow.

Learning Issues   Individuals who are in early recovery often do not learn quickly or well because of the effects of drugs on the brain's memory systems. Drugs affect clients' abilities to listen, see, coordinate data, transfer information from short-term to long-term systems, and consolidate and retrieve data. Therefore, you must learn to be concrete, direct, focused, specific, and repetitive—and more repetitive—and even more repetitive. Save your deep insights into the client's psyche until much later and then introduce them into the client's program only in small batches. Address the obvious: depression, anxiety, anger, grief, and fear. The "kiss" principle holds: "Keep it simple, silly."

Monitor suicidal intent daily during the first week and then each following session. Work on the spontaneous anger that often underlies depression, but do not "pull" for it; that is, encourage the client to express strong feelings and then move on. Do not dwell on negative, self-defeating feelings; in AA lingo, do not let clients sit too long on the pity-pot. Examine instead who is in control of those feelings—the client, right?—and how the client intends to broaden his or her range of feelings without continually plumbing the depth of particularly negative (and often undirected) feelings. Enough powerful feelings will arise during the first few weeks of therapy to provide useful examples without helping the client write them in stone. There will be sufficient time down the road, between weeks 6 and 16, to focus more centrally on negative feelings. In our experience it is not productive to have clients beat pillows, whip beds, or hit one another in group with foam bats. Let clients learn to sit in their chairs and experience whatever feelings arise without pushing them toward greater catharsis. Because clients are apt to feel physically and psychically terrible as protracted withdrawal symptoms arise following the first blush of honeymoon sobriety, it is wiser to focus on achieving more rational self-management rather than to explore powerful negative emotions.

Practitioners of rational-emotive therapy (RET; Ellis & Velten, 1992) have been reasonably accused of directing clients to limit strong emotions (Okun, 1990). Rightly or wrongly, RET is, of course, designed to help clients limit strong negative feelings they wish not to experience. In early alcohol and other drug treatment especially, RET is very useful because it allows the therapist to make use of what might otherwise be viewed as a limitation on treatment. Drug abusers rarely learn much from catharsis. They often use the neurochemistry that is part and parcel of strong feelings (such as high levels of norepinephrine production) as a substitute for their drug of choice.

Learning to use silence effectively with clients in early recovery is not a straight-forward task. Many drug clients' families and partners have used silence as a form of punishment. Therefore, explore what silence traditionally means to the client and what it may mean if it occurs during treatment. We have found, for example, that clients in early recovery may be silent for long periods of time simply because little is happening either cognitively or emotionally. Remember that severely depressed clients who vegetate during therapy are not doing therapy; they are merely exhibiting symptoms.

Dealing with Depression   Depression is common among chemically dependent clients for a variety of reasons, including situational factors, extreme reactivity to negative concerns during withdrawal, and rebound cycles common in both depressant and stimulant drug use. Rebound depression usually lifts in relatively predictable incremental steps with time and therapy. Clients whose depression becomes incrementally more profound over the first four weeks, or who are progressively less and less able to profit from treatment due to their depression, should be evaluated by a psychiatrist for possible psychiatric drug therapy or referral to inpatient psychiatric treatment. Clients with converging signs of severe vegetative or endogenous depression, like all clients with double depression (dysthymia with a major depressive episode), are at heightened risk for suicide (Buelow & Hebert, 1995). Psychiatric and drug problems must be worked on together when that is feasible. As we have indicated, the order in which the two types of problems are confronted depends on the type and severity of psychiatric problems that are manifested, the particular drugs involved and the client's history of using those drugs, and their interaction effects.

Documentation Requirements   Treatment must be made concrete for the client and therapist in the form of written goals. To stand the test of time and legal challenge, goals must be meaningful, professional, understandable, shared, and updated. It is a truism that goals will change and, one hopes, develop as treatment progresses; the life history of that development must be reflected in the treatment notes for clinical, professional, and legal reasons.

As in all treatment modalities, chemical dependence treatment summaries should reflect behavioral milestones that indicate clients' progress or failure to progress. Impediments to progress should be clearly delineated, and plans for how you intend to confront those roadblocks should be indicated. If the family is a dominating problem, for example, case notes should reflect how you intend to work with family members or, in their absence, how the client may reduce their negative influences.

Thinking and Coping   Magical thinking is often chemically dependent clients' worst enemy. With added stress, such a pattern of solipsism escalates into crooked and sometimes criminal thinking. Clients' greatest allies are hard work, a willingness to endure emotional and physical pain, a desire to develop prosocial goals, a wish to communicate feelings, and constant examination of their own thinking patterns and cognitive schemas. Often it is less the development of new ways of thinking and coping than the rediscovery of older, more positive ways that leads most directly to clients' recovery.

Coping mechanisms are part of our natural defenses against stress and injury, both physical and psychic. Every possible avenue to increase natural resilience and hardiness must be explored, even when what is required is the long-term work of helping a client to develop a more adequate interpersonal attachment style. Many clients never fully accomplished late adolescent psychological separation. Clients' lack of separation often becomes obvious through their growing dependence on other clients or on their counselors, compulsive self-reliance, and fear of being emotionally swallowed up. The therapist should view clients' dependence or emotional flight as part of a developmental phase and not deflect or strongly insulate against that response. If clients' dependencies on their counselors are not handled as a normal part of treatment, the clients may simply shift that dependence to another client in treatment. Dependence on other clients can quickly lead to emotional or sexual exploitation, sexual or pseudosexual acting-out, and heightened risk of relapse.

Other Issues   Other treatment don'ts—within the limits of reason—include the following: Don't argue, scare, rebuke, or judge. Don't tell clients you respect them; show them by remaining objective and by caring about their views and feelings. Don't lecture; teach. Lecturing is telling what; teaching is showing how. As the old proverb goes: "I hear, I forget. I see, I remember. I participate, I know. I know, I gain wisdom." Don't replay drug-expert scripts you have heard back to clients; clients usually know more about their specific drug of choice than we do. Don't avoid issues, even when these issues include you. If an issue includes you, integrate the issue into the discussion, but work against using the session to do self-therapy. If you find yourself doing your own therapy in group, take a burnout holiday and recharge your batteries; you've had enough for a week or so, maybe more. Finally, don't get more pushy and confrontational because you feel that the client may be giving up. Sometimes giving up is a prelude to a deeper surrender to social influence; sometimes it reflects depression. You should look at the client's continuing emotional progress within an overall assessment-conceptualization framework, and not be overly reactive to daily ups and downs.

Suicide and Crisis Intervention

In general scope and outline, suicide intervention in cases of chemical dependence parallels such intervention in other kinds of cases—with several important differences. These differences account for the greater lethality among drug abuse clients. First, and most obviously, clients are likely to have recently used drugs and to have impaired impulse control and judgment. Drugs that mimic inhibitory neurotransmitters (alcohol and other sedatives, for example) impede higher-level cortical functions that might otherwise help establish an aversive reaction to risky thoughts and actions. Such drugs also increase clients' level of emotional response to events; like the child in the nursery rhyme, when clients feel good, they feel very good, and when they feel bad, they feel horrid (Steele & Josephs, 1990). The combination of bad feelings and poor impulse control is particularly lethal, and the chemically dependent commit suicide at a rate approximately four times the national average. Drugs that mimic excitatory neurotransmitters (cocaine, for example) often cause a dramatic rise in irritability without a correspondingly positive influence on mood. Thus, a client can be physically excited and irritable on the one hand, and suicidal on the other. This state is especially characteristic of clients with a long history of relapse. Also, stimulant-dependent clients are often suicidally depressed when the drugs have cleared their system because the cushioning excitatory neurotransmitters normally available have been suppressed by drug use.

Second, chemically dependent clients are often more labile (dramatic) in their mood swings, which may give an extremely uneven or unreal cast to their ideation and interaction. These clients may also seem comical to an uneducated public with a history of equating out-of-control behavior with humor. All threats, even those seemingly made in jest, must be taken very seriously because clients under the influence often use humor to deflect the self-hatred and loathing that is right under the surface. Rapid, angry mood swings are very common and difficult for crisis intervention teams to deal with successfully.

Third, chemically dependent clients' thinking processes (the reasoning faculty to which most direct appeals are made in crisis work) are more likely to be clouded either by the drug itself or by withdrawal from the drug. Therefore, explanations that seem clear and reasonable to you may seem garbled and difficult to comprehend for the client. Further, if clients are in a blackout or have anterograde memory problems due to their immediate drug use, they may not remember what you said only several seconds ago. A not so subtle tip-off may be that the client keeps asking you the same question over and over again. Clients in this predicament are not merely being resistant.

Fourth, drugs may be exacerbating (or uncovering) a concurrent (sometimes undiagnosed) mental illness. Cocaine, for example, may bring on a florescence of schizophrenia or other delusional disorder and may be associated with the first appearance of the illness. Also, the effects of psychiatric medications (tricyclic antidepressants, for example) may be complicated by an abused drug (with cocaine, for example, these medications may produce extreme mania); the combination may bring on atypical psychotic features of varying duration. Psychedelics, lysergic acid (LSD) and the psychedelic-anesthetic phencyclidine (angel dust) in particular, have been known to bring on psychoses of very long duration and have been called psychotomimetics for that reason.

Guidelines for Crisis Work   The following general guidelines should be followed in working with high-risk chemically dependent clients (and others as well) who are under stress, are in crisis, or may be suicidal.

1. If clients reach you by telephone, ask for their name, telephone number, address, and current location, and any other indicators of their present situation (who is present with them and whether they have harmed themselves or plan to). If clients will not reveal their name or location, you must decide whether or not to continue to work with them. This issue becomes very important for the therapist's state of mind if a client is intoxicated and threatening harm to self or others. Continue to work with the client over the phone if that is reasonable, but do not become involved in long-term psychotherapy. Assess the physical situation, assess the client's access to

help from immediate friends and family, and help the client make a clear and acceptable plan about how to make it through the crisis utilizing the client's own initiative and ingenuity. Work with the client to plan out in detail the next hour, the next 4 hours, the next 24 hours, or however long it will take before clients can see you or another counselor (their usual one). If the client has harmed himself or herself, or is threatening immediate harm to self or others, continue to talk with the client while you write a note to a coworker to have a trained emergency mental health worker or the police available to check on the client while you continue to talk with him or her.

2. Choose a safe place for a face-to-face interview as soon as possible—preferably at your office during regular working hours. Remember that meetings should not take place at your office at night or on weekends unless other trained professionals who can provide intervention and possible client transport to protective care are not only available, but actually present.

3. If you have arrived at the scene of a crisis—a client threatening suicide, for example—you need to remain calm and take charge. Find out whether other people present have been affected by the crisis and make plans for their care by others available to you. Unlike other counseling situations where you must let the client lead, you should be straightforward and directive. Tell the client clearly who you are and your purpose for being there. Sit down with the client, make good eye contact, speak at moderate volume and pace.

4. Gather information on what the client sees as the most immediate problem or on details of the current situation. If the person is panicking, ask the person to concentrate on what he or she want to happen next, not on how he or she feels. Don't facilitate more catharsis, which may lead to less emotional control. Encourage the client to focus on the present and help the client to break away from obsessive rumination on past events. Be present in the here and now. Don't get caught up with the past or the future. Stay centered on immediate issues of what and how, not why.

5. Don't give false assurances that everything will be fine. You don't know whether things will be fine or not, and the client usually knows it. It is likely, however, that what is not fine can be made better if not perfect, and suicidal clients should be reminded of that likelihood. Stick to what you do know. If you don't know something, say you don't know but that together you and the client can in all likelihood find a reasonable answer, or you can help the client access the resources necessary to find an answer.

6. Work with the client to identify past successful coping strategies that may be effective in the current situation. Then help the client follow through with those strategies. An example might be to help the client time his or her breathing so as to avoid hyperventilating.

7. The goal in crisis situations is short-term problem solving. Do not psychoanalyze the client or the situation, or attempt to continue your typical psychotherapy if the person in crisis is your client. Use your basic microskills to facilitate problem solving. Let the client know you care about him or her. Do not listen passively; don't simply reflect back to the client what he or she is saying, as is typical in Rogerian counseling. Listen carefully, but concentrate on using your active-directive skills,

while keeping confrontation to a minimum. You are there to help the client solve the immediate crisis problem, not to get stuck in existential dilemmas.

8. Don't take sides or assign blame. Acknowledge the client's perceptions without agreeing or disagreeing with the client.

9. Don't argue if the client criticizes you or something you said. Acknowledge that what the client is saying may be true. Then take another tack toward the same objective (such as deescalation of affect and immediate behavioral change). Don't be deterred by anger, sadness, or vague threats. Pay close attention, however, to direct threats.

10. Discuss the various options for action concerning each decision that needs to be made. Elicit the client's opinion. However, when you have come to a decision—such as that hospitalization is required—explain your rationale to the client, then follow through with the decision despite protests. You are in the best position to make the decision. Only new and significant information, not protests, should influence the carrying out of that decision. Do not talk about the option of hospitalization with a frantic client unless you have the means to execute the decision immediately.

11. Set goals with the client that are clear and achievable. Solutions must take into consideration what means are immediately available to implement those solutions. Break the present problem into manageable pieces. Get others who are present, or significant others who can be called into action, to support and help accomplish immediate tasks and short-term goals.

12. Never be afraid to consult with others, but remember that if you are dealing with your own client, you may know more about the developing situation than anyone else, even though you are not a crisis expert.

13. Finally, remember the following admonitions: (a) Time is generally on your side. Suicidal behavior is usually impulsive, and suicidal ideation will abate over time, at least in the short run; so keep the client busy with developing new problem-solving plans. (b) Work as part of a team when possible. (c) The profile of individuals with suicidal ideation is no different from the profile of attempters, including completers. Therefore, you cannot reasonably be asked to predict (as opposed to assessing) who will commit suicide and who will not, who will be violent and who will not. You can assess risk only within the limits of your training, and you are responsible only for reasonable judgments based on your assessment. (d) The police and emergency mental health workers are your friends and the friends of those in crisis. (e) You are probably not trained to restrain anyone, so don't try. If you hurt the client during a failed restraint, you may be sued and lose; if you are hurt, you will probably have to pay the medical expenses. (f) Do not transport clients unless you are trained, are paid to do so, and have at least one backup person in the vehicle to help you. (g) Do not get between a suicidal client and a window—the client can take you through the window with him or her. Neither should you let a violent or suicidal client get between you and the only means of escape—usually an outside door. Keep an outside door near at hand open, and if possible have a police officer posted outside. (h) Do not try to disarm a client—leave and call the police from a secure location. Call the police or other available personnel to you if you are threatened in any way, or if the client is threatening himself or herself with immediate harm.

Finally, crisis work is interesting and rewarding for some, chaotic and threatening for others. If you find that you are not suited for it after a few trials with your difficult clients, let others take the lead.

Week 1 of Treatment

The crisis is averted. The client has decided to work with you toward assessment; conceptualization of the problem; treatment planning and referral, including possible concurrent therapy; and initial treatment. During the first week we usually see the client once each day or every other day. This intensive approach provides better continuity, impresses the importance of daily work on the client, and provides immediate feedback on the client's behavior. If the client is clearly unable to maintain sobriety during that first week and is not making significant progress during structured (group) outpatient sessions, we need to find a solution that works and possibly discuss inpatient referral. During the first week we focus on crisis management, client expectations for treatment and sobriety, immediate withdrawal symptoms, relapse stressors, and coping resources and emotional support. It is particularly important to stress cognitive awareness and rational processes because emotions are likely to be very labile as withdrawal symptoms firmly assert themselves. During early assessment and treatment phases, clients need to trust their cognitions more and rely less on emotions and intuition, which are often confused and brittle. In most cases, clients' emotions are instructing them to use the drug and relieve the symptoms, even in the face of competing desires for sobriety. It is important, however, to validate whatever feelings the client is having—grief at giving up drugs, for example—while working at the same time to reinforce prosocial, pro-self emotions. Drugs may be a bad friend; nevertheless, sobriety often feels to the client as though a friend is dying. Remorse must be validated without exacerbating self-criticism.

During the first week, the client is likely to be confused, disoriented, depressed, or anxious, depending on rebound effects from the drug of choice and the length of continuous drug use. Some, believing their troubles are over, are unrealistically joyous. Who can blame them? It is well to warn them, however, that their euphoria (the honeymoon) may not last. So many immediate issues will soon begin to arise for the client that looking deeply into the future or into the past is not usually constructive. As difficult as the here and now is for the client, and sometimes for the counselor, it is the only place where change can occur.

Nonsupportive confrontations—those that seem argumentative, reproachful, punishing, derogatory, demeaning, parental, judgmental, or rude—must be avoided. Confrontations that are supportive, realistic, face-to-face, authentic, egalitarian, and well timed can be useful if supported by additional education, explanation, and exploration of what the client gleaned from the interpersonal interaction.

Week 2 of Treatment

The second week is often when the honeymoon begins; the client's energy has returned and problems feel less immediate. We focus on both "positives" and negatives of clients' drug use, their expectations for sobriety, pressures that may develop between concurrent therapies, and stress reduction strategies. Honeymoon feelings usually result from rebound effects subsequent to taking a depressant drug. In this condition, global neurotransmission rises, producing a generalized antidepressant effect. This phase is usually short-lived, however, because the client's endogenous excitatory neurotransmitters rapidly become exhausted. Also, the reality of the client's social situation and intransigent personality issues begin to assert or reassert themselves. Reality for recovering people (which may include job loss, marriage problems, and loss of respect in the community, to name only a few examples) is quite reasonably very depressing, and it is best to be realistic about it. The energy of the honeymoon period should be used to orient the client to the difficulties ahead. Encouragement must be constant, particularly if a slip or lapse has taken place.

Benefits of Drug Use for the Client   Drug use has both positive and negative features. Everyone who uses drugs is engaged in a constant cost-benefit analysis. As the chemical dependence asserts itself, reducing the pain and emotional disorganization of withdrawal becomes the most salient benefit. Even though clients may be suffering greatly from their drug use, drugs continue to have positive importance of which the counselor may be unaware. Drugs are usually stabilizing to the physical and emotional system, their procurement arranges a time schedule around which everything else revolves, and they are a best friend. Drugs often supersede other erotic relationships and, therefore, may act as a substitute for clients' other potential love relationships.

Because drugs hold such power over the client, it does little good to minimize their importance and dwell exclusively on their negatives. The chemically dependent are as varied as the general population, and although some certainly are pushed toward drug use by their dysfunctional backgrounds, many are pulled into dependence because drugs satisfy many human needs for specialness, love, erotic expression, emotional support, and self-understanding. Although such insight is predominantly illusory, many clients appear to understand themselves much better on drugs than off them. In these cases drugs have become fused with the self. This fusion must be wedged apart without the client's feeling consistently attacked as the drug attachments and interpenetrations are slowly disengaged. This disengagement process is no small task. It is best accomplished by alternately working on life areas where drugs have been most destructive and supporting those that are relatively unaffected. Deeper personality reconstruction should take place only after the client has achieved a deeper and longer-lasting sobriety.

Like expectations in other life domains, each client's expectations for sobriety differ in important ways. Not only clients' but counselors' expectations for the daily process of structured and individual therapy must be made explicit. Both client and therapist may give weight to unexamined, covert rules, which need to be brought to the surface and realistically examined as to their meaning and potential positive and negative outcomes.

The Pressures of Therapy   As we have indicated, pressures often develop from the interplay of structured outpatient group therapy and concurrent individual therapy. Not only may clients feel overloaded by therapy, but feelings of commitment to the group can interfere with individual exploration. In our experience, however, few clients can actually receive too much therapy in an outpatient setting. Complaints about feeling overloaded may express clients' natural resistance to the somewhat imperfect and fragmented treatment foci and processes. In these cases, it is important to help clients work through (process in detail) their feelings about the lack of congruence and, sometimes, the divided loyalties that may develop. It may also be important to make clients aware of how time-consuming inpatient treatment really is; inpatient treatment ordinarily requires morning and afternoon group therapy sessions that may last several hours, an individual session with a therapist, family or couples therapy, an education session after supper, and perhaps an AA or NA meeting during the evening. Although clients may fight against time constraints, free time should of course be minimized, especially during the first few weeks of treatment. Every second of the day must be planned and contracted. Deviations from the contract must be carefully explored and the client's new contract closely monitored.

Stress Reduction   Stress reduction is particularly important during the first six weeks of concurrent therapy. Whereas most of us have multiple defense mechanisms against stressful external events and internal states, many drug abusers, and most drug-dependent clients, have relied on drug use as their primary defense for so long that other, more mature mechanisms are less active or completely missing. For this reason, when drugs are not available, chemically dependent clients often regress to defenses more primitive than might otherwise be expected. It is important, therefore, to work with the client not only to rediscover old defenses against stress and develop new ones, but also to find ways to actually reduce the number and intensity of incoming stressful events. This work takes place, unfortunately, while group therapy is raising the client's level of interpersonal stress.

When using standard stress reduction techniques—progressive muscle relaxation, creative visualization, meditation, and self-hypnosis, for example—remember that the defenses of many newly recovering people are not well enough consolidated to keep them from experiencing severe anxiety (and frequently anxiety attacks) as a result of the dissociative, out-of-control feelings that may accompany deep relaxation. Clients should be advised beforehand of this possibility and helped to work their way up to the stress point and through it during succeeding sessions. If clients are aware of low-level feelings of anxiety arising as they relax, it is not difficult to help them make small steps in the process. If clients wait until they are very anxious before signaling their discomfort, they may exacerbate their panic reaction.

Dealing with Anxiety and Depression   Many clients have self-medicated panic attacks with alcohol for many years. Alcohol is a very poor anxiolytic, however, because it leads to further lability of the arousal system and, ultimately, increases depression and rebound anxiety. Rebound anxiety, which is a common feature in the discontinuation of sedative hypnotic use, ultimately exacerbates panic attacks. Unfortunately, many anxious patients are prescribed sedative-hypnotic anxiolytic medications by nonpsychiatrist physicians when these patients actually need evaluation for psychotherapy instead. Sedative-hypnotic medications are addictive, and patients often end up in drug treatment for medication abuse while they struggle through their withdrawal difficulties. Many clients want to stop using these medications, but when they stop, the number and intensity of panic attacks increase, and their sleeplessness is exacerbated. Their newly virulent panic attacks and long periods of insomnia may immediately drive clients back to drug use for symptomatic relief. It is particularly important, therefore, to decrease the severity of these symptoms when possible by gradually weaning clients away from the drug. Self-help techniques and psychotherapy certainly decrease the severity of symptoms; however, clients in outpatient treatment must be informed that they may not sleep at all for several days or until their bodies readjust to a sleep schedule. It is wise to have a close, withdrawal-educated, nonjudgmental friend sit with clients during these first few evenings.

Depression usually follows discontinuation of stimulant drugs (such as amphetamines, cocaine, nicotine, and caffeine) because the body stops the manufacture of normal amounts of excitatory neurotransmitters when it senses the presence of an external supply of stimulants. Thus, when the stimulants are discontinued, neurotransmission levels are lowered, and depression usually occurs. Clients are less likely to interpret this rebound depression as catastrophic if they have been both forewarned and forearmed. To be forearmed requires that clients have worked to defuse the impact of the developing cognitive, behavioral, and emotional shutdown.

Although all depression elevates a client's risk status (for accident as well as self-injury), the twin reactions of anger and hopelessness are especially lethal. For clients whose primary activity during the first several weeks of sobriety is to punish themselves for lost time and relationships, crisis management and suicide prevention should be the first order of business. A lethal defense against renewed drug use for some clients, whose typical defense against change is to punish themselves, may be suicide. Many clients have ended their lives when their relapse seemed inevitable because of a lapse, even though the lapse often provides an opportunity to recognize clearly the pervasive power of the drugs and thus is the point at which real progress often begins.

As sensitive as the problem is, clients must come to understand that in and of itself, a lapse is not catastrophic. It is only when the client learns nothing from the lapse that it spells eventual relapse. Inevitably, of course, more narcissistic clients will believe that, since a slip is not catastrophic, they should test out their relationship with you as their therapist by lapsing a few more times. It is important to explore this form of self-defeating (sometimes criminal) thinking in depth. You must clearly and nonjudgmentally define your bottom line concerning referral to more structured therapy if the client continues a manipulative pattern of behavior.

Treatment: Weeks 6–16

Let's try an experiment. Sit down in a comfortable chair. Wait until the second hand of your watch is on the minute. Take a normal breath, and then hold your breath, remembering that the point of the exercise is not to pass out. Watch the clock without breathing. Watch the seconds slip away as you continue to read this. For about 20 seconds you have relatively little trouble holding your breath, even though you want to breathe. At 35 seconds you may feel a bit lightheaded and need to concentrate very hard to continue not breathing. At one minute you are beginning to seriously question whether this exercise is a good idea. You are probably sure now that it is not a good idea. Somewhere from deep inside the limbic system and brain stem a message begins to surface in your mind that you are a fool for not breathing, that the pain of not breathing is becoming excruciating, that you will pass out or die soon if you don't breathe. If you are feeling so faint you are about to black out, please take a breath. If not, continue to hold your breath for a few more seconds. Imagine as you hold your breath what it would be like to feel the way you do now for weeks and months and years into the indefinite future. Imagine what a struggle the rest of your life would be if you were to go through it with these feelings constantly gnawing at your body and mind. The few holdouts should breathe now. Fortunately, our bodies will not allow us to hold our breaths until we die. Unfortunately, our bodies will allow us to continue to use drugs until we die of complications.

Struggling to Not Breathe

If you can, imagine a craving to breathe many times more powerful than what you have so far experienced. During the first few days and weeks of withdrawal, the craving to use drugs, particularly alcohol and narcotics, is often as strong as a drowning person's desire to breathe. And like not breathing, not using drugs seems emotionally and intellectually counterrational for the chemically dependent. The person's biological and psychological systems feel as though they are coming apart, while at the same time the person's body is telling him or her how foolish it is not to use the drug of choice to solve what seems to be such a simple problem. The person begins to feel that surely he or she can control the drug without letting it control him or her. How long would you hold out unaided against such a barrage of conflicted, painful emotional, cognitive, and behavioral messages? Many of us, even with the best intentions and a rational understanding of what we are up against, would try to stop the experience by lapsing back into drug use. In effect, we would try to breathe even though we knew we were going to breathe water, not air—as drowning people certainly do.

Thawing Out

So it goes for the first few days or weeks of sobriety for many clients. Small wonder many relapse. However, after detoxification has taken place, the drug has cleared the system, and clients have been weaned away from the drug—after the first weeks of intense craving are over and the honeymoon from the intense pressure to use the drug (a period of unrealistic optimism) has begun to recede—clients begin to make real progress in a variety of life areas. Such clients often make us think of people who have thawed out after many years spent frozen. Their minds and bodies become more normally active rather than depressed or manic. They find it possible to concentrate more effectively. They try to catch up on what they have missed during the past several months or years. But they are also raw, hypersensitive, and hypervigilant.

Not so curiously, perhaps, having been stuck so long in cognitive and emotional stasis, clients who are in recovery often begin their emotional journey where they stopped development when they began using drugs as their primary emotional adaptation to life some years before. Those who began using drugs as teenagers discover that they have not gone through the ordinary developmental steps experienced by their peers. Many discover that they never psychologically separated from their parents, or that they have few ways of relating to their spouses that are not buffered by drugs. The emotional aspects of their marriages, like themselves, have often been in stasis. Clients have described this phenomenon as waking after many years of emotional sleep.

Burying Relapse Triggers

During the first few weeks of treatment, clients are more likely to use primitive, narcissistic defense mechanisms of denial, regression, or acting-out to defend against drug discontinuation and therapists' (or group members') interpersonal influence. Unless clients have complicating psychiatric problems or have been addicted to drugs for a very long time, however, they quickly begin to develop more mature defenses. These defenses will be used in the service of recovery on the one hand, but they also can be used on the other hand to manipulate codependents into enabling a relapse.

In the second phase of withdrawal (6–16 weeks), more subtle forms of internal self-encouragement to relapse arise. Memories of better, earlier times when drug use was a supportive social experience, for example, begin to come spontaneously into memory. Dreams, daydreams, and fantasies arise during which the client is using again with good new results, rather than bad old outcomes. Whereas earlier in their lives clients were naive and unsophisticated, now they may feel persuaded that they understand the drug better and know better how to control it. More primitively distorted thoughts about returning to use that occurred in the first few weeks are replaced by more complex, antisocial thinking patterns in which triggers are laid down to facilitate relapse.

The belief that drug-dependent people can return to lifelong moderate use is an irrational one. Perhaps one in a thousand might return—but are those good odds? Any plan to resume use in the future (whether introduced by the dependent person or researchers) is sabotage. These sabotage plans are usually drawn up, and activating triggers are buried in the mind and emotions, while the client is still using drugs. These more subtle pressures arise after the first intense struggles for sobriety have been won. They assert themselves during the more protracted withdrawal period. Triggers may take the form of ideas, smells, tastes, actions, and life milestones (anniversaries or deaths in the family, for example) that are tied in positive ways to relapse or in negative ways to sobriety. Triggers may also take the form of complex cognitive and emotional plans with many accompanying automatic self-suggestions, compulsions, and stratagems to continue use.

Supportive psychotherapy is insufficient to unearth buried plans, motives, triggers, and desires. Only continual, face-to-face, authentic, here-and-now, confrontational interaction with the client over months of sobriety serves this purpose effectively. This fact above all others, we believe, is why alcohol and drug specialists, especially those who are recovering themselves, tend so often to be overly confrontational. Knowing what they have buried themselves, they cannot accept that other recovering people have not buried a similar covert initiating structure or that clients will not resist, as intransigently as these counselors themselves did, the exposure of these mechanisms.

That is also why more active, confrontational cognitive and Gestalt therapies tend to predominate in chemical dependence settings. Triggers are held in place by powerful irrational-emotive forces that must be confronted by both rational and mature counteractive forces. Triggers will not yield to direct assault, however, and chemical dependence counselors must be taught how to provide pressure on these issues without causing them to become even more deeply buried. This uncovering process requires a gradual escalation of confrontation that is balanced by continual emotional and cognitive support. It requires scouting out the inner landscape where the triggers are buried and rationally defusing them. The client must be shown that these triggers are unnecessary for continued protection once self-efficacy has been shored up.

These issues must be addressed with nondependent but abusing clients as well. For such people, triggers are usually less deeply buried, but are not necessarily obvious or on the surface. Each person has his or her own unique way of initiating relapse dynamics. Because clients who are abusing drugs have not hit rock bottom in the dependence cycle, inoculation effects that provide resistance against fantasies of returning to drug use may be less operative. The belief that one can return to drug use in the indefinite future with better results cannot be overcome by a simple frontal assault. Such beliefs must be exposed, explored, and accepted as a normal part of treatment, and the myth must be gradually exploded.

Abusing clients who are far from bottoming out often have a related problem: Because detoxification may have seemed relatively easy, they come to believe that when they want or need to, they can always clean up. Of course, in reality, sobriety becomes harder to attain with each cycle, and binges usually escalate in severity. For this reason, many old hands believe that one must bottom out before reality sinks in. In contrast, we believe that treatment is more effective the earlier we intervene in the dependence cycle, but the intervention must be designed to take these effects into consideration.

THE FIRST LAPSE OR RELAPSE

Continually confronting daydreams and fantasies of drug use is a daunting experience for all clients. How client and therapist handle the first actual lapse will often define the course of subsequent aftercare. If the client has relapsed while involved in an outpatient treatment group, all reasonable means must be used to get the client back to the group despite the client's fear of the group's condemnation. Group therapists must show group members how to develop a nonpunitive stance and demonstrate support while not enabling continued relapse. Tough love asks us to love the sinner, but hate the sin. Supportive confrontation is necessary for both the client and the group, even if the client is going to be referred out of group to inpatient care. The rest of the group can face their own concerns about lapses and relapse by helping to uncover the forces at work in other members' relapse dynamics.

As a general rule, one isolated slip (versus a pattern of growing relapse dynamics) should not engender automatic referral to a more structured treatment setting. Although a lapse threatens the group, mastering the lapse can bring the group and the individual into closer touch with the true magnitude of relapse pressures that exist in the world. It is important for other members of the group to understand what set off the episode and what forces pulled and pushed their comember to return to the group. The group needs to answer a variety of questions: What did the member learn from the lapse or relapse that may be crucial for everyone involved to know? How will other group members deal in the here and now with their own fears of relapse? Will the member's lapse be repeated? How do the client and the group know whether the lapse will or will not recur? What new issues will have to be examined in group to buttress each member's sobriety? What pressures succeeded in bringing the client back to group or individual therapy? What might have kept the client from coming back? How does the client feel about returning to the group? How do other group members feel about the client's return?

Punitive gestures toward the relapser from the group (passive aggressiveness, for example) must be acknowledged and disarmed through exploration. Group members must be allowed to experience the punitive feelings but encouraged not to punish the client because of them. Learning to respond to slips this way is of crucial interpersonal importance and has value in many other areas of social life. In the same way, clients who have lapsed must be encouraged not to punish themselves. Even though moderate remorse may be helpful in surfacing buried feelings, remorse forms a weak basis for ongoing relapse intervention, because it so often degenerates into an orgy of self-blame. Self-blame reduces efficacy and self-esteem, and ultimately self-blame accelerates failure. The abstinence violation effect that often follows lapse and relapse must be overcome by finding support for the continuing development of self-efficacy. A more detailed presentation of relapse intervention will follow in Chapter 4.

STUDY AND DISCUSSION QUESTIONS

1. What is a case conceptualization, and what are its most important elements?

2. How does chemical dependence case conceptualization differ from other psychological case conceptualization?

3. How should conceptualization interact with assessment and treatment planning?

4. What are buried relapse triggers?

5. Define a relapse stress control contract and describe how it can be used.

6. What criteria would you use to refer a client to structured inpatient chemical dependence treatment versus structured outpatient treatment?

7. What common problems and concerns arise in concurrent psychotherapy with clients in structured treatment?

8. Outline common steps that should be taken during the first week of concurrent psychological treatment, while paying special attention to the steps and processes of crisis and suicide intervention and depression management.

9. How do problems during the first few weeks of concurrent and structured treatment differ from those of weeks 6 through 16?

4

Maintenance, Relapse, and Relapse Prevention

Rather than a static recovery of prior functioning, maintenance of sobriety must be an active and developmental process that extends throughout life. For the chemically dependent who are in recovery, maintenance cannot be seen as a finished product, because new challenges to sobriety and peak functioning are always present. Prochaska and DiClemente (1992) described the maintenance stage as one in which the client

> builds on each of the processes that has come before. Specific preparation for maintenance, however, involves an open assessment of the conditions under which a person is likely to be coerced into relapsing. Clients need to assess their alternatives for coping with such coercive conditions without resorting to self-defeating defenses and pathological patterns of response. (p. 168)

In their view, maintenance involves not recapturing what was lost, but rather becoming more the kind of person one wants to be. Unconsidered maintenance (sometimes referred to as white-knuckled sobriety) is more akin to precontemplation than to personal development; buried within it are triggers for relapse. Maintenance requires the existential qualities of directed, rational action; commitment; responsibility; an internal locus of control; and courage. During maintenance, a variety of insight-focused therapies can be used to help enhance the client's self-knowledge, acceptance, emotional range and depth, and social and familial responsibility. Even in the face of long-term developmental maintenance, however, some clients do lapse, and some who lapse also relapse into continued chemical dependency.

Relapse as a Problem of Sobriety, Not Treatment

Relapse is often narrowly conceived to be a return to drug use subsequent to treatment—implicitly, a result of failed treatment. From this perspective, if treatment is successful, relapse should not occur. Taking a much broader view, however, Gorski (1990, p. 127) described relapse as "the process of becoming dysfunctional *in sobriety due to sobriety-based symptoms* that lead to either renewed alcohol or other drug use, physical or emotional collapse, or suicide" (emphasis added). Relapse can occur, of course, at any stage of change.

Gorski's view is especially important because it stresses that relapse is a process, one that includes outcomes other than drug use (such as suicidal depression). Gorski's view also emphasizes that even though some relapses may ultimately be traced to specific failures in treatment application, relapse often results from problems that develop from present sobriety, not past treatment. Clearly, treatment cannot forestall all possible future threats to sobriety, any more than education can always forestall the transition from drug abuse into drug dependence. Also, most people relapse not after formal treatment, but after informal self-help. Since a majority use only self-help methods to intervene in their chemical dependence, understanding the reasons for their failures and successes is as important to our knowledge of the relapse dynamic as accounts of those who relapsed after structured treatment (Prochaska & DiClemente, 1982, 1986; Prochaska, DiClemente, & Norcross, 1992).

In many cases clients do not need better treatment; they need better aftercare, which includes lifelong learning about relapse risks and skills to combat them. We share Gorski's view that the dynamics of relapse should be a distinct focus of both research and aftercare intervention. Treatments that are effective for a limited time do not necessarily fail simply because lapses or relapses occur. Instead, lapses or relapses should focus our attention on the risk interactions that follow treatment so that we can design not only better relapse prevention but better intervention strategies.

THE RELAPSE DYNAMIC

Renewed drinking and drugging are the most obvious expressions of a relapse dynamic, but actual drug use episodes may be only the tip of the relapse iceberg. By the term *dynamic,* we imply that relapse is part of an active process that, once set in motion, is not self-limiting. The process usually continues until an internal or external intervention is successful. Lapses, individual drugging episodes, do not invariably lead to complete relapse. For relapse to occur, a lapse must be accompanied by further initiating physiological and psychological factors. Emphasizing the dynamic character of drug reinvolvement also calls attention to the fact that lapses, and the relapses that often quickly follow, are elements in an ongoing process of reengagement with self-defeating modes of irrational thinking, narcissistic (self-centered and omnipotent) needs, and risky actions. Interestingly, a majority of individuals who quit drug use do so on their own, and often relapse many times before becoming fully abstinent (Schachter, 1982). Apparently, some drug abusers are not intimidated by early failures, and their lapses sometimes lead to better long-term adaptation. It is likely that these setbacks, through the process of trial and error, provided much material for learning. Overcoming relapse setbacks, then, may have helped these people develop clearer thinking, more prosocial values, and less risky behavior over the long run. Relapse setbacks also carry threats to self-esteem and self-efficacy, however. Many relapsers become more likely to fail in the future with each failure at maintaining sobriety. Clearly, we need to know much more about relapse dynamics, how self-help processes affect relapse, the most important negative effects of violating abstinence, and how to help clients develop better resilience in the aftermath of relapse.

Self-help, treatment, and relapse intervention may take many possible forms. Individuals begin their early drug engagement innocuously enough. Over time and association with the drug, they move progressively through stages of risky use into drug abuse. Many, however, struggle against their drug abuse and through self-help maintain lengthy periods of complete drug avoidance. Often, however, self-help fails, and drug dependence becomes established. Even in drug dependence, though, many individuals are able to intervene on their own behalf and stay sober for varying periods of time before they lapse and relapse. Some are able to find a high level of sobriety on their own and do not continue to relapse. We know the least about this group, since they are difficult to identify and intercept for research purposes. Those in structured treatment are easiest to draft into research because of their proximity, and they are also usually more willing to discuss their problems.

It is clear that many chemically dependent people relapse chronically. Relapsers often try self-help again, go back into treatment, or rededicate themselves to support groups like AA or NA. Many of those who receive structured treatment (even well-planned treatment) lapse back into drug use after several months; many of those who lapse end up relapsing. The reasons for lapse, relapse, and the reestablishment of chronic drug use are many and complex.

Reasons for Optimism—and Pessimism

Whether we view relapse as failed therapy or failed posttherapy relapse prevention, lapse and relapse rates among the drug dependent are very high. Fewer than 10% of alcoholics receive formal structured treatment; probably, no more than that percentage of people dependent on other drugs receive treatment either. Those who do receive treatment, especially inpatient treatment, are more often clients with severe dependence and a variety of concurrent social and drug-induced problems. The more down and out clients are, the more likely they are to become recidivists (Brownell, Marlatt, Lichtenstein, & Wilson 1986; Schachter, 1982). About 33% (plus or minus 10%) of all treated alcoholics remain completely abstinent after initial treatment. Another one-third chronically lapse and relapse but maintain a relatively high level of sobriety, are able to work and maintain intimate relationships, and often achieve total abstinence during middle age (U.S. Dept. of Health and Human Services, 1993). A final one-third of treated patients, however, relapse to pretreatment alcohol intake levels. Members of this group often die from alcohol-related complications. This "thirds rule" appears to characterize the relapse dynamic for other addictive drugs as well (Marlatt & Gordon, 1985; Vaillant, 1983). Finally, about one-third of patients being seen in structured treatment have had one or more prior structured treatments, and many have had other forms of psychological treatment, self-help, or unstructured drug intervention as well (U.S. Dept. of Health and Human Services, 1993).

Whether one views the cup as half empty or half full depends on one's expectations about the difficulties of addiction treatment. Miller (1992) provided the following reasons for optimism and pessimism. On the down side, in a 40-year longitudinal study, Vaillant (1983) found that a large sample of men treated for alcoholism had about the same remission rates as those who received no treatment at all. It is unclear, however, whether those who received structured treatment were at higher risk in the first place—a typical confound in comparative studies. Other longitudinal studies have found intensive treatment to produce no better results than short-term unstructured treatment and in some cases no better results than one-shot provision of advice (Miller & Hester, 1986).

Despite these reasons for gloom, experience with high-quality treatment programs evaluated using well-conceived comparative designs provides many reasons for optimism (Marlatt & Gordon, 1985; Miller, 1992; Miller & Hester, 1986). First, clients with jobs and intact family support (usually clients with higher socioeconomic status) are more resilient over the long run, with more than half showing a good overall treatment prognosis (Miller, 1992). This group is also amenable to a variety of relapse prevention strategies. Such clients' ability to use treatment effectively apparently stems from their cognitive coping skills (education, for example) and coping resources (such as family support) and also from the fact that they are usually able to afford better, more inclusive, and more lengthy treatment and aftercare. Unfortunately, groups of lower SES clients apparently have recovery rates that range between 0 and 20% (Gorski, 1990). Not only are such clients less likely to get good treatment, they are worse off by the time they get it, have fewer coping resources when they receive it, capitalize on relapse prevention aftercare less well, and are subjected to a riskier social milieu after treatment. It is clear that pretreatment screening, dual-diagnosis management, specially designed individual and group treatments, and more intensive relapse prevention are needed for this highly vulnerable group.

Second, research studies often demonstrate unreasonably poor results when clients with a very poor prognosis are lumped together with those who have ordinary resilience both pre- and posttreatment (Miller, 1992). In this case the effectiveness of what might otherwise have been seen as useful treatments is "washed out," and treatments that are actually useful for specific groups appear to be ineffective. Also, when therapists and clients are properly matched along dimensions of cognitive complexity and treatment expectations (support versus over-directiveness, for example), success rates rise to around 80% fro levels around 20% for unmatched client-therapist pairs (Miller, 1992; Hester & Miller, 1989).

Third, as a general rule, the better the research, the more easily positive findings can be separated from concurrent negative findings. In other words, the more comparable the treatment groups and treatment variables under consideration are, the more interpretable the treatment and relapse prevention effect sizes are likely to be.

Fourth, not surprisingly, the better the inpatient and outpatient treatment program, the better the treatment outcomes. Research shows that full-spectrum centers that employ a variety of highly skilled practitioners and provide well designed aftercare group programs produce results that are much better than average. Also, narrow-spectrum programs designed for a well-matched group of clients with a specific type of problem (dual-diagnosis clients, for example) produce better results than those that are less focused.

Fifth, well-designed brief interventions often have very good immediate effects that equal those of more extensive treatment. As Miller (1992, p. 767) pointed out, this result can be interpreted to question the usefulness of longer-term treatments, or it can be viewed more conservatively as suggesting that "even relatively inexpensive interventions may have a beneficial impact." A final point to remember is that more difficult clients require closer matching of client, therapist, and treatment. When matching is not the result of thorough assessment, it will be made through much more expensive trial and error.

Relapse Risk Factors

Risk for posttreatment relapse is elevated by sociological, environmental, psychological, and biological factors. Any actual specific drinking episode, however, must involve psychological factors such as positive motivations to drink and positive drug use expectancies. Expectancies, both pro and con, and their operative drives are not well understood by either clients or psychologists (Buelow & Harbin, 1996; Prochaska & DiClemente, 1982; DiClemente & Prochaska, 1982).

The relapse dynamic is a set of separable feelings, beliefs, expectancies, and actions in which circularity and multiplicity of causation are typical. Thus, relapse is causally over-determined; that is, many system outcomes are caused by multiple system inputs and operations that contribute both individually and cumulatively. From a systems perspective, personal and environmental inputs (increasing irrational beliefs or family dysfunction, for example) affect operations (internal cognitive schemas), which affect outputs (such as the client's willingness to travel to the bar to play some pool and see old friends). All of these are affected or informed in turn by system feedback actions (such as education, appropriate danger signaling, cognitive restructuring). A preparative behavioral lapse (going to the pool hall) quickly leads to a full-scale relapse, because lapses are usually preceded by poorly controlled, compulsive, and irrational expectancies concerning environmental cues and the pros and cons of drug use. The problems clients experience with decisional balance feed into irresponsible actions, which act to defeat treatment-developed feedback warning systems. These dysfunctional processes of relapse may find an outlet not only in using drugs, but also, as Gorski (1990) pointed out, in family violence, physical or mental illness, or self-harm. Thus, prevention of drinking or drugging is not the single purpose of relapse therapy. From our perspective, if prevention is to be effective, it must include movement toward deeper moral understanding, affective awareness, and cognitive development—the very heart of traditional psychotherapy practice.

Theories About the Etiology of Relapse

Relapse prevention makes sense as a construct only when we view clients with a history of chemical dependence as needing to abstain completely and permanently from drinking or drugging. As counselors, however, we often encounter clients who want to continue drinking and who need counsel, advice, and education about risk reduction. A low-risk user—one who has not been dependent on a drug, for example—who wants to reduce the amount or frequency of intake can certainly be helped by some of the same methods used to help chemically dependent individuals become more resilient to risk. We encourage therapists to decide whether they will work with low-risk clients on "safe" drinking or drugging, and which if any of these techniques they want to use with their particular group. We will, however, remind the reader of

Gorski's (1990) comment, quoted in Chapter 1: there "is no convincing evidence that controlled drinking is a practical treatment goal for persons who have been physically dependent on alcohol"—nor, we might add, on any other drug.

As we indicated, our viewpoint on the etiology of relapse is conditioned by our theory of how people become dependent on alcohol and other drugs in the first place. There are at least two competitive models. One emphasizes the cumulative negative effects of drugging behavior, whereas the other emphasizes the threshold aspect of chemical dependence. In the cumulative model, it is presumed that many pleasurable but problematic behaviors must be controlled to avoid personal and social risks. Such pleasurable behaviors include eating, drinking alcohol, smoking, sexual activity, gambling, and recreational drug use. All of these behaviors are seen as reaching a point of habituation (learning) or compulsiveness, at which time adherents of this view say that the individuals have become addicted to the behaviors. As the word *addicted* is used by the over-learning or strictly behavioral group, however, it has no special connotation besides indicating that over-learning and risky use are taking place. Thus, no matter where clients are found along the use gradient, they can presumably always go back to pretreatment levels by learning to moderate the behavior to socially approved levels (Peele, 1992; Watson, 1991). These theorists believe that the behavior has been greatly over-learned (because the behavior is pleasurably reinforcing) and simply needs to be unlearned, relearned, behaviorally reduced, or refocused.

Threshold theorists, on the other hand, in whose camp we are not always completely comfortable but usually find ourselves, believe that at some point on the use gradient, one has become so physically dependent on a drug that control of, or moderated use of, the drug is so unlikely as to be effectively impossible. Those who are dependent on the drug are considered addicted to the drug; those addicted to alcohol are usually called alcoholics. Dimensional tests—the MAST for example—are designed to produce threshold scores for alcoholism.

Threshold theorists, then, usually say that individuals who abuse drugs and alcohol are problem drinkers or abusers, and those who depend on alcohol or other drugs are addicted to their drugs of choice, or, as DSM-IV summarizes, chemically dependent. Threshold theorists usually say that people who are self-defeatingly involved with food, gambling, or sexual acting-out are compulsives or obsessive-compulsive personality types, not addicts. Although there is some overlap between problem drinking and alcoholism (because some problem drinkers do become addicted and, therefore, alcoholic), most problem or heavy drinkers do not become dependent on or addicted to alcohol, instead moderating their drinking as they age and become more aware of the drawbacks of drug use and abuse (Vaillant, 1983). Even though there are behavioral similarities and neurophysiological pathways in common between addictions and compulsive behaviors, we believe that lumping these problems together does little to further our understanding of the individual processes or their manifestation within individuals. Finally, although we believe that over-learning and compulsion are important in both abuse and dependence behaviors, drug-addicted individuals have risk factors that disqualify them from attempts at controlled or regulated use (controlled relapse). Unfortunately, the natural history of alcoholism and other drug use indicates that problem drinkers usually moderate their drinking and other drugging as they age, whereas those who become dependent on alcohol or other drugs usually become fatally attracted to their drug of choice, deepen their dependence on it, and often expand their dependence to include to other drugs as well.

Risk and Relapse Models

Risks for relapse can be analyzed as those that exist prior to treatment, those that arise during treatment, and those that develop during posttreatment aftercare. Each of these three periods is affected by the interaction of intrapersonal, interpersonal, pharmacological, and other environmental challenges. The intrapersonal, internal dimension includes individual psychological and biological factors. Interpersonal risks may arise from any form of social interaction, but especially from those with intimate partners, parents, and peers. Because both positive and negative changes in interpersonal behavior cause stress, good times as well as bad may challenge sobriety, although good changes pose less of a threat. Dependent substance abusers generally recall a time when their substance use was more controlled and enjoyable. Hence they may believe that they can return to controlled use; they are thus vulnerable to relapse during times of positive stress, such as a wedding, a graduation, or the birth of a child.

Process or system risks include the interaction effects of each contributing factor, their unique syncretisms and potentiation, and their cumulative effects. From our perspective, relapse is greater than the sum of its parts. Moreover, understanding individual relapse components does not necessarily imply understanding the precipitating dynamics. For each hardy person for whom the effect of failed abstinence is positive self-knowledge, there is another for whom relapse failures act to destroy self-efficacy and the hope of eventual sobriety.

Though an understanding of risk factors is crucial to understanding relapse, risk of relapse is not the same thing as relapse. Many who are at high risk for relapse do not, whereas many at low risk do. Infinitely many intervening historical, cognitive, and affective variables lead to relapse in general; we must be satisfied with partial knowledge and a large degree of indeterminacy. When working with specific clients, however, we must work toward as complete an individual risk profile as is possible through the processes of assessment, conceptualization, and formative evaluation.

Marlatt and Gordon (1985) provided a useful model for many important aspects of the relapse dynamic, which is set out in Figure 4.1.

In concert with Bandura's view of self-efficacy, Marlatt and Gordon's (1985) model emphasizes lowered self-efficacy as the engine that drives relapse. As coping responses (the outcome of cognitive coping strategies and resources) are eroded by continued cognitive lapses (daydreams about using, for example) in the face of intra- or interpersonal challenges, self-efficacy suffers. This diminished sense of self-efficacy and self-esteem fuels lapses in both thought and deed. The actual lapse further lowers self-efficacy through the abstinence violation effect, which Marlatt and Gordon defined as the lessened sense of efficacy resulting from having violated one's self-given mandate to remain abstinent. Clients, then, suffer deeply from their view that their bad side triumphed over their personal conscience. Further, many clients fail to form positive expectancies for the future because of their current lapses. Unfortunately, relapsers have been found to tend to make more internal, characterological self-

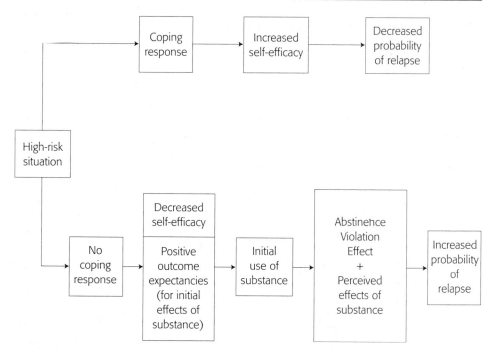

FIGURE 4.1   **The Relapse Dynamic** (From *Relapse Prevention* by G. A. Marlatt and J. R. Gordon, p. 38. Copyright © 1985 The Guilford Press. Reprinted with permission.)

attributions for their lapses or slips (Brownell et al., 1986), and these attributions erode self-efficacy. In contrast, clients who tend to lapse, but not to relapse fully, apparently blame outside circumstances for their lapses and, therefore, try to change the environmental conditions (cues) in which they tend to lapse—an excellent relapse prevention strategy. This externalization of responsibility may become detrimental once clients have fully relapsed, however, because they are less likely to have insight into their own personality dynamics and are less likely to feel accountable for their dependence.

Brownell and colleagues' (1986) attributional model also emphasizes the importance of cognitive coping processes, physiological and environmental factors (withdrawal and cue control, for example), and affect. Lapses may reinvigorate pretreatment feelings of guilt, shame, and self-loathing, which in turn reinforce negative cognitions about oneself. Positive views of self and coping skills go hand in hand. Thus, in order to internalize new coping skills, clients must be helped to develop a more positive self-image. Having positive emotional experiences, practicing self-control, reducing remorse, and raising commitment are important components of this process. Commitment is not merely a set of cognitions coupled with a propensity to act; these cognitions must be rational and reinforced by powerful emotional schemas that are congruent with self-protection and survival.

Intrapersonal risk characteristics include internal factors that increase an individual's likelihood of returning to drug use. Of particular importance are, first, relatively stable characterological problems, including self-defeating, borderline, antisocial, and egocentric personality styles, and, second, difficulties in regulating mood and affect. Studies indicate that nearly 70% of relapses occur during negative emotional states, including stress, depression, and anxiety (Brownell et al., 1986; Shiffman, 1982, 1984). Although negative emotional states propel lapses into relapses, however, the larger issue of inadequacy in mood regulation often sets the stage. In other words, feeling bad may occasion a momentary lapse, but the inability to counteract long-term negative states propels lapses into full-blown relapses.

High-risk relapsers usually demonstrate poor mood regulation and inadequate cognitive coping skills. Not only do they have fewer cognitive strategies for resisting internal and social pressures (habitual cues) to use drugs, but they also have a shallow understanding of how to use the skills they do have. For this reason, risk is highly correlated with cognitive complexity. Unfortunately, even though low cognitive complexity increases risk, high cognitive complexity does not give clients much protection against relapse if their commitment and motivation are low.

Commitment to practices important to sobriety is supported by positive emotions that are interwoven with positive cognitive-behavioral schemas. Therapists can reinforce commitment by helping clients build cognitive and emotional linkages and develop new coping skills and resources. Coping resources act like a bank account that can be draw upon when stress rises. Resources vary from client to client but may include, for example, sexual support, recreational activity, reading, learning, exercise, and participation in socially absorbing activities.

Interpersonal risk factors potentially include all social ties, but most dangerous to continued sobriety are drug-abusing or otherwise dysfunctional partners, family members, and peers. Although some few individuals suffer specific pressure to use, relapse occurs in the majority of cases because drug use is simply "business as usual" within the individual's primary reference groups (Oetting & Beauvais, 1987). This fact is illustrated by the finding that a significant number of lapses occur during supportive, enjoyable times; a person may begin to smoke or drink again during a party in his or her own honor, for example. Social pressure is clearly one causal factor in more than half of all relapses whether the pressure is active or passive. About one-third of these relapses are directly associated with positive interaction, whereas one-third are associated with interpersonal conflict (Brownell et al., 1986; Marlatt & Gordon, 1985; Shiffman, 1982, 1984).

Finally, it is clear that drug substitution (for example, drinking if one is a cocaine addict) increases one's risk of eventually relapsing to the original drug of choice. Alcohol use in particular raises one's risk of returning to tobacco. This risk is heightened in a variety of situations, including, first, habit reactivation, when drinking and smoking have been directly tied together historically—an example of over-learning (Peele, 1992); second, situations in which a person used to having the effects of one drug potentiate the good feelings from the other attempts to multiply pleasurable effects (using cigarettes and alcohol or speed and morphine together, for example); and, third, situations in which a drug (alcohol, for example) directly causes a loss of impulse control, which in turn leads to other drug use. Further, continued use of lower-risk smokable substances clearly increases the rate of relapse back to higher-risk smokable substances.

Clients with dual diagnoses are even more vulnerable to social pressures than other drug-dependent clients and suffer greater risks in all stressful social interactions. Overt interpersonal conflict creates the greatest stress, because it carries heightened negative affect. Long-term negative affect among dual-diagnosis clients often causes relapses in self-care and emotional and cognitive vulnerability (schizophrenic exacerbation, for example), which in turn diminish impulse control and accelerate drug use. Drug relapse, even though ultimately self-defeating, is often an effective short-term defense against entrenched negative moods and emotions. As Gorski (1990) pointed out in our original definition of relapse, reactivation of suicidal habits and mental illness are relapses in the same way that renewed drug use is. Finally, lapses are also cumulative; relapse in one important life area (a manic or depressive exacerbation, for example) potentiates relapse in others. In cases where relapses instigate a major collapse of the coping system, suicidal gestures and suicide are common.

Pharmacological risks of addiction vary by drug and by the individual's physical and psychological coping resources. Although self-medication is certainly not the primary reason people use drugs (Schinka, Curtiss, & Mulloy, 1994), a significant number of anxious and depressed clients do appear drawn to self-medicate and are then hooked into a cycle of emotion management through drugs. The more powerful euphoriant drugs like cocaine are such powerful reinforcers of continued use that clients return to them again and again, even after multiple treatments and seemingly well-tailored relapse control programs. Unfortunately, in the case of cocaine, clients' assessments of the cons of use rarely outweigh the pros; therefore, the decisional balance is usually not heavily weighted in a negative direction (Prochaska et al., 1994).

CRITICAL FACTORS IN RELAPSE PREVENTION

Clients experience relapse after both informal self-help and formal treatment. It is important to understand the progress clients make with self-help because successful strategies may be built upon it in structured settings. Even though self-help may not have been fully successful in preventing relapse, a clear understanding of client self-help strategies and cycles within stages of change may help with the specific client in question and also with understanding the self-help process in general. This understanding may help us design better formal treatments that maximize the effectiveness of self-focused techniques. In many respects, guided self-help can be viewed as the clinician's primary tool for facilitating change in both semistructured and unstructured treatment. Self-help principles also play an important role in formal substance abuse treatment. Inpatient clients who are unable to help themselves and continually rely on others frequently relapse, however professional their treatment structure or caring their counselors. A thorough assessment of the client's resistance to relapse must include an understanding of the structure and function of the client's self-help strategies. Such an understanding requires knowing the client's cognitive, affective, and behavioral coping skills and resources.

Assessing Clients' Coping Skills and Resources

Coping strategies include both resources and skills. Cognitive coping resources are the fund of knowledge and practices available for use by the client, whereas cognitive coping skills include the strategies clients use to put their resources into play. Even though therapists often emphasize coping skills (through such activities as rehearsing drug refusal, examining the ABCs of typical irrational beliefs, or dissecting the logic of recurrent irrational thinking into its constituent parts, for example), the client's fund of knowledge about alcohol and drug actions on the body and the mind is of supreme importance. Even though television ads are often visually interesting, sound bites rarely initiate personal change because they do not impart the quality or quantity of data upon which the decisional balance of drug use hinges. Clients need concrete, dependable information about drugs, their bodies, and their minds.

Understanding the cognitive and social coping skills that our clients typically use will also provide important information about whether self-help groups like Alcoholics Anonymous may be effective for them. AA and NA appeal to many clients who need social support, who are not put off by spiritually oriented doctrines, and who are relatively conventional in their outlook. Due to socioeconomic and drug-related deficits, clients may have difficulty understanding complex discussions of the etiology of addictions. Further, many may be actively searching for an emotional conversion to sobriety, rather than a deeper, psychodynamically based decisional balance. The best results, therefore, often stem from conventional, low-key, and highly structured training that is behaviorally oriented on the one hand while remaining emotionally attractive on the other.

Like cognitive coping, emotional coping includes both resources and skills domains. Emotional coping resources are limited by the width and depth of the client's emotional range; such resources include feelings, sensations, perspectives, emotions, memories, and meanings. Important questions that may help define resources include these: Are the client's feelings shallow and labile? Is the client aware of fine distinctions between often competing feelings? Upon what affective memory resources (emotive images of a happy childhood, for example) does the client typically draw during stressful times?

Emotional coping skills include clients' abilities to identify and access their feelings. Can clients readily explore feelings? Can they appropriately express their feelings to themselves and others? Emotions are not only vehicles through which we access our immediate world (a sensing network), but are important to the many processes of eliciting social support. Individuals who cannot readily express feelings become socially impoverished. Their social skill deficits lead to isolation, which in turn leads to depression, which accelerates the decline of social skills, which leads to further impoverishment, stress, and likelihood of relapse into drugs as a means of social support and affect management. Are clients able to use their emotions as sources of information, while understanding that emotions are not reliable directives for action?

Assessing our clients' emotional coping requires that we understand how they regulate both transient mood states and more stable emotional styles. Unfortunately, drug use is often the client's primary means for emotional coping and mood regulation. Clients will not necessarily step back into a pattern of healthy internal regulation when they stop using drugs, however. They typically use peers, codependent spouses, and dependent children to help them with emotional regulation. Clients who systematically use others as the linchpin of their coping strategies often become dependent on their therapists while they develop deeper resources. Such clients' external locus of control and powerful dependency needs should be worked through in both individual and group therapy, not avoided. These dependency needs are pressing and should be confronted concretely and supportively as a critical relapse concern.

Individuals' ability or inability to respond effectively to stressful internal and external events accounts for much of the variance in individuals' physical and mental health and in their propensity for relapse into drug use. Therefore, appraisal of coping skills and resources is a critical part of chemical dependence assessment. The clinical interview should include a thorough history of coping dynamics. In addition several useful paper-and-pencil stress and coping measures are also available to evaluate changes in a client's coping, including the Multidimensional Coping Inventory (MCI; Endler & Parker, 1990), Ways of Coping Questionnaire (WCQ; Folkman & Lazarus, 1985), and the Schedule of Readjustment Rating Scale (SRRS; Holmes & Rahe, 1967).

Goals, Motivation, and Emotion in Relapse

Although moods form an important affective base for emotions, emotions are intimately connected with specific goals because emotions are bound up with motivations. If one has a deeply held desire to be rich, for example, it is likely that the process of making or having money will be strongly associated with positive emotions—one will feel good when the money rolls in. Such feelings and their attendant goals become closely bound and reciprocally reinforcing. In contrast, if one has no special interest in wealth and achieving wealth is not a goal, feeling good is not directly tied to getting or having wealth, and feelings about money may be conflicted. Motivations consist of both cognitive and affective plans to achieve goals. Affective plans include daydreams in which one enjoys the positive emotion that stems from seeing oneself accomplish a valued goal. Cognitive plans, on the other hand, are behavioral maps for specific activities. Cognitions and emotions ordinarily reinforce each other so that goal attainment is maximized. Clients who do not have the motivational forces connected to a goal of sobriety are unlikely to succeed at sobriety over the long term. Fortunately, helping to motivate clients toward the goal of sobriety is not a mysterious process.

The therapist's role in helping clients develop motivation entails helping them to identify, plan, and act on the affective and cognitive components of goals. Methods easily adapted to this process include a variety of everyday, garden-variety counseling activities—including career development, social involvement or reinvolvment, and rational self-help, among other things. Useful creative motivational techniques include creative visualization, meditation, and Eriksonian hypnosis and suggestion.

RELAPSE ASSESSMENT AND REFERRAL

A difficult decision all chemical dependence counselors must make is whether (or when) to refer clients back into more highly structured treatment after working with them individually. This important decision should be made only following a thorough evaluation of the client's history of change and present motivation for change and an assessment of the client's understanding of treatment processes, relapse dynamics, dual-diagnosis concerns, and coping strategies. Individuals in full relapse should go through a detailed reassessment, one that looks closely at areas that may have been glossed over or omitted during the original intake. Relapse assessment should fully describe pretreatment, treatment, aftercare, and lapse-relapse phases and should set out a clear history of the client's typical cycles within the stages of change. Reassessment should provide sufficient depth and breadth to allow an accurate reconceptualization of the case, not a simple updating of the prior (often outsourced and inadequate) conceptualization.

Psychotherapists who intake clients for psychotherapy and learn of their chemical dependence later in therapy often have a broad but shallow knowledge of their clients' drug use history. That general knowledge may not provide an adequate understanding of the client's ongoing relapse dynamics. Furthermore, the prominence of personality factors may inhibit the psychotherapist's working understanding of the client's pretreatment motivation for long-term abstinence. Also, therapists who work exclusively with aftercare and relapse prevention groups frequently do not reassess (formatively evaluate) the client's pretreatment motivation for change and other underlying attitudes that may sabotage posttreatment group work. For that reason we encourage a detailed reassessment not only of prior treatment but pretreatment as well. Areas of reassessment should include the following:

1. *Pretreatment decisional balance:* Did the negatives (cons) of drug use ever truly outweigh the positives (pros)? Did therapy increase the pros? Was the actual decision to seek therapy internal to the client or generated through outside forces not owned by the client?
2. *Motivation:* What are (and were) the client's goals for sobriety? Are the client's stated goals the client's actual goals? What is the client's commitment to opposing goals? Can the goals be reached one day at a time, or are they fantasies? Has the client designed reasonable steps that can be followed each day, or are the steps so widely separated behaviorally as to be unmanageable?
3. *Attitudes:* Attitudes are self-constructs made up of belief, temperament, personality, and experience. Although more subject to change than temperament, attitudes are resistant to external challenge. We are not likely to change the attitudes that led us to a political party, for example, without good reason and strong social support. Clients are unlikely to reform basic attitudes about alcohol or other drugs without powerful cognitive and emotional interventions coupled with internal readiness for change.
4. *Cognitions:* What we learn about the world is highly conditioned by what we already know and believe. Knowledge about drugs grows only when information is presented in a rational, well-organized, and usually very concrete manner. Individuals who have a long history of self-serving and irrational thinking patterns in a variety of health-related areas certainly do not change their thinking patterns overnight; they may, however, stop discussing their views if they feel overwhelmed or unvalued. The more irrational clients' beliefs about drugs are, the more likely they are to be influenced by salient but misleading information and contradictory anecdotal evidence. Treatment must not only be concerned with straight thinking about drugs over the short run, clients must be taught to think more logically and critically in all important mental and physical health areas.
5. *Mood regulation:* Alcohol- and other drug-using clients often vacillate among external mood regulation systems, including not only drugs but, also, for example, charismatic people and religious cults. In the same way, clients turn to partners or therapists for mood regulation once they achieve early sobriety. Some clients

may actually appear to excel in treatment groups because they are able to dupe members (and the therapist) into helping the clients regulate themselves. They appear to have reached a high-quality sobriety and even appear to help other members with interpersonal concerns. They often have great difficulty in maintaining sobriety, however, unless they move immediately into a relapse prevention group after their treatment group terminates. Dependency problems should be worked through in long-term psychotherapy that focuses on underlying identity development.

6. *Plans:* Finally, it is crucial to ascertain whether the client actually planned to relapse after treatment. Were relapse triggers built into the treatment system? Was therapy used to provide the self-esteem necessary for the client to reenter the drug world with a new attitude but the same behaviors—a not uncommon pretreatment blueprint for failure? These self-defeating scripts should be a continuing focus of both individual and group treatment, but especially of relapse and aftercare therapy.

Evaluating Treatment in the Face of Relapse

Our close association with clients with whom we have a past therapeutic relationship may blind us to the unpleasant facts of their relapses. We must honestly ask, therefore, whether our individual and concurrent treatment was wrongly focused, whether the client, perhaps with our unwitting help, wriggled through weeks of group therapy without a clear commitment to change or without demanding help to learn the skills necessary to exercise useful control over (usually negative) interpersonal stress. We should ask the following questions, for example: Was family week a sham? Did the client bully or seduce the family behind the scenes to escape the full emotional impact of past behavior? Does the treatment center focus closely enough on resistance, or does it accept clients' reports without collecting objective measures that might or might not demonstrate positive change?

We must continually assess treatment effects by engaging in an honest, real-world dialogue with clients. We should also be willing to use drug testing on a continuing basis, as well as self-report instruments to measure client change. Although clients can avoid the truth, we are responsible for ongoing evaluation, including remaining open to feedback from significant others in the client's life. Again, in short, trust but verify.

AFTERCARE

Most broadly based chemical dependence treatment centers provide posttreatment aftercare. Aftercare is usually focused around regularly scheduled evening groups, after which clients are encouraged to attend self-help groups like AA, NA, and Rational Recovery. Relapse prevention groups, however, are only as sound as the center that sponsors them, the therapists who work in them, the supervisors who oversee them, and the commitment of the members within them.

Alcohol and drug relapse groups are, first and most important, groups. Therapists must be trained to work with groups, not thrown into aftercare to sink or swim.

Group dynamics can further either sobriety or relapse. Although recovering people with minimal formal training often do well with inpatient treatment groups that use a familiar 12-step structure, they often do less well with other sorts of aftercare groups in which myriad personality, identity, sexuality, and dual-diagnosis concerns arise. Although continuing sobriety should always be the primary focus of aftercare groups, deeper personality problems, unemployment, and stressful family interactions generated by deep structural problems are often significant concerns that must be addressed. As Gorski (1990) pointed out, most relapses are generated during the relapse prevention period itself, and personality, sexuality, and employment are typical problems during this highly vulnerable time. Counselors, therefore, should assess the history of clients' lapses and their relationship to relapse, the sobriety-based problems that may arise in clients' new lives, and the added stresses that may develop as clients begin to succeed. Unfortunately, nothing breeds failure among recovering clients like unexamined success. Finally, hearing the story of why a client relapsed is not an assessment. Understanding the reasons for relapse requires a reevaluation of the positive and negative processes operating within each step of developing sobriety. This understanding necessitates detailed research into the relationships among the client and his or her therapy, therapist, motivation, and life goals.

Effective aftercare strategies suppress relapse over the long run because they help clients develop alternative coping strategies and richer emotional lives. Successful aftercare strategies include, for example, (1) improved social and marital skills; (2) drug refusal, self-control, and self-management skills (including stress, conflict, and depression management); (3) employment training; (4) community reinforcement, including community reinvolvement or reentry groups (churches, for example) and clubs; and (5) using helping relationships, which should include proper matching between clients' and therapists' interpersonal styles and attitudes (Brownell et al., 1986; Marlatt & Gordon, 1985; Miller, 1992). Lifestyle changes should include proper doses of physical exercise, diet, meditation or contemplation, medication when necessary, and compulsion-free love and work.

Aftercare activities that do not appear to prevent relapse include (1) controlled (monitored) lapses in which clients are encouraged to lapse so they can work through the emotional outcome in a structured way; (2) extending treatment by adding periodic booster sessions of the same treatment; and, (3) adding more components to treatment without considering how they will be integrated into the overall treatment program (Brownell et al., 1986). Brownell and colleagues (1986) also indicated that lifelong recovery plans like Alcoholics Anonymous may have some negatives, including, for example, added expense and time. Others also feel that the AA view of oneself as continually recovering imparts a negative message that one is never cured of an addiction and sends a strong message that relapse is inevitable (Ellis & Velten, 1992). Although our experience indicates that clients' acceptance of themselves as recovering does not ordinarily entail their viewing themselves as weak or relapse as inevitable, therapists must probe whether specific clients are vulnerable to these self-defeating and irrational beliefs about their condition and help clients counteract the effects.

As we have indicated, Gorski (1990) and others (Miller, 1992; Brownell et al., 1986; Marlatt & Gordon, 1985) have emphasized that relapse is often the process of becoming dysfunctional in sobriety due to sobriety-based symptoms or causes. These symptoms may be affective, cognitive, and behavioral in nature. They include, in order of their relative importance, (1) personal (often depressing) job and marital stresses that may have been masked by more immediate drug use concerns and that are not the focus of posttreatment therapy; (2) long-term withdrawal dynamics for which no effective strategy has been developed; and (3) social and environmental cues, actions, and pressures for which no behavioral interventions (such as cue control or stimulus avoidance) have been designed (Shiffman, 1982, 1984; Brownell et al., 1986; Gorski, 1990). Although tackling these problems may not have been a priority during initial treatment, high-quality sobriety demands that these concerns be addressed quickly and effectively.

Let us look at the following case history of a client caught in an ongoing relapse cycle.

◆ THE RELAPSE CYCLE: A CASE HISTORY ◆

Frank is a 32-year-old, white male who was referred by a colleague for individual psychotherapy to your private practice. The colleague is presently leading a relationship group sponsored by a church in the City. Appropriate releases regarding confidentiality having been obtained, discussion with the group leader indicates that Frank, who has been working in group on the effects of his anxiety and depression on his romantic relationships, has expressed fears of relapse back into alcohol abuse and dependence. Rather than progress, Frank seems to be having greater difficulties, and much group time is now spent on his many problems. He has also attempted to form a romantic relationship with a female group member, and his attentions have not been welcomed. This issue has been addressed in group but not brought to a conclusion. He has been told that he will no longer be allowed to participate in group if he continues to focus on the female members.

Presently supported by a substantial trust fund, Frank comes from a wealthy family and patrician educational background, having attended private boarding schools from the age of 6. He has one brother and one sister, and the family usually assembles for one to two months during each summer at their beach house. Both siblings are successful professionals and apparently both are dependent on alcohol and other drugs. His father, a well-known entertainer, is also alcoholic and has been through a variety of treatment programs but continues to drink on a daily basis. His mother, highly esteemed for her charity work, takes a variety of prescription drugs, including Valium for sleep and Percodan for low back pain, and drinks heavily. Her children began drug use in their early teens by stealing tranquilizers and pain medications from their mother's large, constantly replenished supply. After a number of jobs in banking at which he failed because of his cocaine use, Frank has returned to the City to take private acting and screenwriting classes.

Although Frank has never been through an inpatient program, he has tried to complete structured 12-step outpatient chemical dependence treatment programs twice but left the programs without completing them. He continues to attend AA and NA, is presently active as a member, and has a sponsor who has seen him through many crises. Like his father, Frank is witty, entertaining, and handsome. He makes and loses friends easily, steering a course through life along the path of least resistance. His most immediate problem centers around his stage fright, anxiety attacks that are increasing in frequency as he tries to work in front of an audience. He admits that his "new" difficulty has pushed him into a therapy group that is not specific to his problems, and he has accepted a referral to concurrent individual psychotherapy for his relapse and sexuality concerns.

During the first session, Frank recounts a long (and in his view fruitless) history of working with a psychiatrist on emotional problems stemming from his drug use, bisexuality, depression, and family abandonment. Although he is a willing client, Frank's description of his prior therapy reveals that he has never worked a consistent recovery program (that is, he has never developed a daily strategy for self-development), has continually fought against what he considers outside control, and has glided through 12-step programs without facing the more demanding aspects of self-assessment. When his bravado and histrionic mask are dropped, Frank admits that he is truly frightened of relapsing back into alcohol and cocaine use and sexual acting-out. Although he has not fully relapsed back into drug use, he has lapsed into a variety of ongoing sadomasochistic, exploitative sexual fantasies around women and men from his past.

Clearly, Frank is a complex, high-risk case. Interestingly, however, despite his risks, he has achieved a great deal: He is presently sober and has been so for more than a year; he has applied himself to a new professional path that fits his personality and talents well; and he has attempted to find emotional support. Working against him are his history of crooked thinking, exploitative sexual relationships, family denial, inability to effectively utilize therapy alternatives, and lack of cognitive and affective coping strategies. Looking at his position in the stages of change, Frank has vacillated between maintenance and (re)action-relapse. Although he has managed to remain sober, he never developed necessary relapse intervention and prevention skills. His psychological problems continue to push him toward lapses in thought, and his relapses into sexual exploitation undermine his self-efficacy rather than raising his self-esteem. These sexual relapses, which involve either aggressive acting-out or victimization (and which are full-scale relapses in Gorski's view, even though drugs are not involved), continually trigger the abstinence violation effect and serve to decrease his self-esteem. Thus, even though Frank may be sober, he is not and does not consider himself "clean and sober" because he is not free of the shame and guilt from acting against his own best interests.

In brief, after a detailed clinical assessment, conceptualization, and treatment plan was completed and contracted for, Frank was referred to a structured outpatient relapse prevention group at a local chemical dependence treatment center and retained in concurrent individual treatment. He did not continue in his relationship group but was asked to attend a final meeting and to debrief the group on his reasons for seeking further treatment. Individual treatment focused, first, on crisis and suicide intervention planning; second, on weekly liaisons with his treatment center clinical director and therapist (including weekly drug screening); third, on depression, stress reduction, and anxiety management; fourth, on developing a long-term relapse deceleration plan; and, fifth, on identity development and sexuality counseling. Happily, Frank went on to conquer his stage fright. He developed a reasonable, doable relapse intervention and prevention plan, worked at psychologically separating from and forgiving his family, and became a successful actor and television writer.

Finally, we should reemphasize that not all clients, even those who are actively relapsing, come to us ready for action. Many continue to be mired in the contemplation stage and need more time and help concerning their personal decisional balance. Such clients may not have made a solid commitment to relapse prevention because they do not fully understand their problem, do not clearly understand long-term relapse dynamics, are unclear about the emotional and cognitive steps that have to be taken before they can achieve a high-quality sobriety, and are not clear that on many days the emotional cons of sobriety may appear to outweigh the pros. It is painful but important for therapists to understand that, although many clients lapse before they have considered their risks, others carefully weigh the benefits and risks of their drug use. The positive side to this reality is that well-informed clients understand their immediate risk and seek intervention. Unfortunately, the negative side is that many clients choose drugs over sobriety, perhaps believing in the fantasy that giving up to immediate gratification of the senses could never be a fair exchange for a demanding but developmental reality.

STUDY AND DISCUSSION QUESTIONS

1. What is the major thrust of Gorski's (1990) definition of relapse?
2. Why is it important to distinguish between lapses and relapses?
3. What is the "thirds rule," and why is it important not only for treatment but for treatment evaluation?
4. What does research tell us about chemical dependence treatment efficacy?
5. What are the most apparent relapse risk factors?
6. Define the term *relapse dynamics.*
7. Outline Marlatt and Gordon's (1985) relapse model, paying special attention to the abstinence violation effect.
8. What are the most critical intrapersonal and interpersonal factors and intervention strategies in relapse prevention?
9. How should we assess motivation to change?
10. What are the most salient factors in evaluating the effectiveness of aftercare treatment?

PART TWO

CHEMICAL DEPENDENCE
PRACTICE CONCERNS

5

Individual Treatment

All counseling theories do not lend themselves equally well to alcohol and drug treatment; neither do the specific strategies and activities that arise from these theories. To work well for chemical dependence treatment, a counseling theory must adequately address the many problems that arise in early intervention, crisis management, withdrawal, and initial treatment. The theory must also address the unique character of the relapse dynamic, critical decisions in referral to structured treatment, problems that arise in managing concurrent therapy, buried relapse triggers, and the difficulties in interaction with family members of chemically dependent clients, some of whom have been psychologically, physically, or sexually abused by the client. Each counseling theory has its own unique view of personality development, symptom etiology, and treatment planning, and its own approach to engaging clients and evaluating specific treatments. Clearly, although many theories are adequate for common psychological and developmental problems of ordinary living, those that are less proactive and directive are less suited for the early stages of chemical dependence treatment.

Directive Therapies in Chemical Dependence Treatment

Because so many crises arise during early withdrawal, and because of drugs' harmful effects on learning, memory, and motivation, the first several weeks of therapy are usually devoted to immediate problem solving, behavioral contracting, and supportive confrontation. For this reason, nondirective, client-centered approaches—although they may be very useful later in therapy—are not helpful in the early stages of therapy because they can lead an already confused client in self-defeating circles. Similarly, psychodynamic counselors, especially those who attribute addictions directly to unresolved unconscious conflicts and who delve immediately into these areas without paying direct attention to the immediate problems of maintaining sobriety, are likely to complicate problems rather than help clients resolve them. Later in treatment, however, a psychodynamic perspective can help us understand how clients have buried (or suppressed or repressed) triggers that may initiate relapse dynamics. Psychodynamic working through can also be helpful in disarming clients' growing resistances and self-protective defenses (Khantzian & Schneider, 1986; Bean-Bayog, 1986).

Clients in the early process of withdrawal are often confused, disorganized, unclear, disoriented, and in pain. Their memory is poor, their attention span and tempers are short, they are often either hyperactive or depressed, and their ability to structure and think through problems is limited. In addition to these deficits (which we may hope are temporary), such clients must handle a multitude of problems of daily living. Not surprisingly, straightforward problem-solving approaches are usually called for in early treatment. This beginning treatment stage, which focuses directly on intervention and crisis management, usually lasts for approximately a week following detoxification, depending of course on the duration and severity of the drug problem and the number of hours that the client is in direct, face-to-face treatment. If clients continue to have difficulty processing treatment information and managing interpersonal relations after a reasonable time, however, a neurological consultation is in order. "Soft," sometimes contradictory neurological signs are often present in clients who are not adapting well to treatment (Buelow & Hebert, 1995). Confusion and inconsistent problem solving can last many weeks for clients who have been drug dependent for many months or years. Unfortunately, deficits can last a lifetime because some drugs—particularly designer drugs (such as ecstasy), alcohol, and volatile inhalants—can cause permanent neurological damage if not death.

The Therapeutic Alliance

Time and energy spent concentrating with the client—on solving problems, relapse dynamics, and education about what alcohol and other drugs actually do in the body—not only serve those immediate ends; working with the client on these issues is also invaluable in developing a cooperative, trusting, and stable counseling relationship. Clients must feel the counselor's encouragement, support, and expertise early in treatment. Clients must sense that their problems will eventually be contained in magnitude, if not solved, and that the counselor understands not only their pain and suffering, but the basic biology, sociology, and psychology of their addiction.

Without a strong (and structured) therapeutic alliance, many clients drift quickly into a relapse dynamic. Working on the development of the therapeutic alliance is the responsibility of both parties. It is the counselor, however, who must initiate an attachment bond so that an alliance can develop. Attachment, which may be confused with emotional dependence (and therefore unwisely discouraged by some counselors) is facilitated by the counselor being present, nonjudgmental, authentic, considerate, and focused.

Rational-emotive therapy (RET) and Gestalt treatment strategies, tempered with a positive interpersonal process (through relationship building and the therapeutic alliance) are especially useful during the early and intermediate stages of therapy. Emphasis on the here and now, authenticity, responsibility, and self-support are all of prime importance to growth in the early stages of recovery. Particularly important to remember, though is, that strongly confrontational techniques, which may be called for later in therapy, should be tempered during the early treatment phases and used only while closely monitoring their effect on the client. Moreover, it is not necessary to practice RET in the distant, emotionally disengaged manner some RET practitioners propound. As clients succeed in sobriety and are able to handle greater stress, interpersonal confrontations can become more immediate, more experimental, and more vivid. Leaving clients adrift to accept responsibility for their drug dependence, while neither acknowledging and accepting the interpersonal dependence problems typical of those dependent on drugs nor helping clients develop adequate social support, represents a divergence from RET's humanistic roots.

Techniques designed to foster deeper personality change can be used during the mature counseling phases. By *mature* we mean, first, that the relationship has been built, tested, and found to be solid; second, that the client's commitment to sobriety is strong and has been verified by drug screening; third, that the client's relationships with others have taken on a mutually supportive character—that is, clients are able not only to utilize support from significant others, but to provide increasing support for themselves and others. This mature phase may be reached earlier for clients in inpatient treatment, where therapy is intense and continuous. However, the first few weeks after they are discharged, clients may feel the need to reengage (regress back to) early problem-solving techniques (especially those addressing relationship dependencies) before continuing with more unsettling, anxiety-provoking forms of therapy. Techniques oriented around deeper personality transformation are called for during late or mature psychotherapy and extended aftercare.

Psychological Separation and Individuation

In an important sense, clients must learn not only to maintain sobriety, but to separate from the drug psychologically. Separation from the drug is similar to the individuation from parents that generally is more or less achieved during late adolescence. Psychological separation is part of the overall individuation process (Bowlby, 1973; Hoffman, 1984). Individuation begins in infancy with the child's first moves toward independence and self-control, expands during childhood as greater autonomy is gained, and blossoms in late adolescence as children separate emotionally and physically from their parents in preparation for adult sexual partnerships with peers. Each stage is marked by the development of higher levels of responsibility for self and the ability to undergo emotional conflict with parents while remaining interdependent with them (Hoffman, 1984; Pistole, 1989, 1993).

Individuals who are dependent on drugs to enhance their emotional life have begun a cumulative process in which feelings engendered by the drug substitute for family reinforcements. Individuation stagnates (Brennan, Shaver, & Tobey, 1991). As clients become more dependent on drugs, their attachment to others is weakened. What appears to be a compulsive self-reliance develops; in fact, this is a compulsive reliance on the client's drug of choice. In their *Family Treatment of Drug Abuse and Addiction,* Stanton and Todd (1981) termed psychological separation concurrent with drug use *pseudoindividuation,* because the individuation process is distorted or delayed. Individuation from drugs must occur if healthy psychological separation is to follow.

Second, with late stage drug abuse or addiction, individuals go through psychological fusion with their drug, so that they cannot separate or often even imagine separating from it. The drug has become their primary emotional caregiver, and they attach to it in much the same way they attach to a human primary caregiver.

Therefore, movement away from the drug, as well as movement toward psychological separation, involves well-planned individuation exercises. Clients must be shown how to reach higher levels of developmental autonomy, while at the same time retaining a high degree of cooperation in therapy. These movements are not mutually exclusive and rely on a strong therapeutic alliance as well as confrontation with self and others. The self must be encouraged to present itself to others in treatment, no matter how infantile it may appear. Many clients appear to be emotionally in adolescence, even though they are middle-aged.

Individuation prospers when clients are taught assertiveness, conflict resolution, and communication skills. Provided that the client's personality is not severely disordered, the individuation process is always facilitated by group therapy concurrent with individual counseling. Groups are especially therapeutic in the psychological separation process to the extent that they can support members' attempts at authentic interaction and maintenance of group norms, while at the same time raising members' self-respect.

Continued psychological separation among recovering clients is more difficult if their personalities are inadequate or disturbed. Personality problems due to family role dysfunction and sexual or physical abuse are especially common among adult children of alcoholic or otherwise chemically dependent parents (whom we will refer to using the abbreviation ACOAs), who themselves are drug dependent. Such clients' emotional development has often been distorted by years of social and sex role confusion. ACOAs are particularly vulnerable to loss of autonomy, emotional dependence (codependence), and role stereotypy (Buelow, 1994b, 1995; Potter & Williams, 1991).

THERAPY WITH DUAL-DIAGNOSIS CLIENTS

Schuckit (1986), Solomon and Davis (1986), and Talbot (1986) estimated that around 40% of the chronically mentally ill (CMI) suffer from schizophrenia; 40% suffer from affective disorders, especially bipolar disorder; and 20% suffer from a variety of other problems. About 50% of this total group also suffer from alcoholism and other drug dependence, whereas approximately 75% of young CMI either abuse or are addicted to alcohol or other drugs (Schuckit, 1986; Solomon & Davis, 1986; Talbot, 1986). Although no clear genetic link between alcoholism or other addictions and major psychiatric diagnoses has been clearly established, clients who have a more treatable psychiatric problem (depression or anxiety, for example) tend to do well in substance abuse treatment, while those with poorer prognoses (schizophrenia and borderline personality, for example) tend to do very poorly. Further, clients with psychiatric problems of low severity do well in all kinds of alcohol and drug treatment programs, whether outpatient or inpatient; in contrast, individuals with highly severe psychiatric problems do poorly whatever the program type (Rounsaville, Dolinsky, Babor, & Meyer, 1987). Adolescent dual-diagnosis clients are most likely to be depressed and to be using alcohol and marijuana, both of which intensify depression, anxiety, and, among more severely disabled CMI, psychosis. Of a sample of teen substance abusers, 25% met DSM-III-R criteria for depression. Female gender, paternal psychiatric problems, and a history of physical or sexual abuse were good predictors of depression (Deykin, Buka, & Zeena, 1992).

Drug abuse is one of the criteria for DSM-IV (American Psychiatric Association, 1994) diagnosis of borderline personality disorder. In a study of 137 inpatients diagnosed as borderline, Dulit, Fyer, Haas, Sullivan, and Frances (1990) found that 67% abused drugs when alcohol and drug abuse were not included in their diagnosis. However, 23% of the 137 no longer met sufficient criteria for the personality disorder diagnosis and differed greatly from those who continued to meet the criteria. Interestingly, borderline clients tend to abuse depressants and hallucinogenics (sedative hypnotics 45%, alcohol 21%, cannabis and LSD 19%, as well as a mix of all of these drugs) even though these drugs are most likely to lead to worsening of borderline symptoms, not an amelioration as self-medication theory would predict. As with other patient samples, Dulit et al. (1990) indicated that borderline clients take drugs in order to increase their immediate gratification from feelings of impulsiveness and aggression, not to normalize their behavior.

Alcohol and other drug abusers are about five times more likely to attempt suicide than others (Craig & Olson, 1990). In these attempts, specific feelings of hopelessness and anger may be more important than overall depression. Compared to drug abusers who do not attempt suicide, attempters cope with stress poorly and are more likely to be antisocial, alienated, and withdrawn, as well as more distressed; attempters also have poorer judgment and use more primitive means of ego defense (Craig & Olson, 1990).

Although most of the CMI abuse alcohol and marijuana because they are most often available, many CMI will take whatever drug is available to them, including drugs known to cause relapses of their specific illness (such as cocaine among individuals with schizophrenia). Research has shown that 37% of a sample of 101 clients with a diagnosis of schizophrenia continued to use cocaine and amphetamines, which they knew from experience and chronic hospitalization increased their schizophrenia symptoms (Mueser, Yarnold, Levinson, Sengh, Bellack, Kee, Morrison, & Yadalam, 1990); 67% of borderline clients also met diagnostic criteria for abuse of alcohol or other sedative hypnotics, which are known to increase their acting-out and hospitalization (Dulit et al., 1990; Polcin, 1992b; Schneider & Siris, 1987). These findings bring the self-medication theory into serious question. As most chemical dependence treatment personnel have maintained for a long time, most CMI use drugs for the same reasons that non-CMI abusers use them—for their euphoric and disinhibiting effects.

About two-thirds of all CMI hospital admissions are precipitated by drugs or are exacerbations of illness concurrent with drug use. Drug-abusing teenagers with schizophrenia have their first hospitalization for their illness about four years earlier than teenagers who do not abuse drugs (Talbot, 1986). Drug-abusing teenagers are also more likely to be admitted more often, to stay longer in treatment, to abandon use of therapeutic drugs more frequently, and to have a poorer overall outcome with psychiatric drugs and with psychiatric treatment (Polcin, 1992a; Talbott, 1986). They also are more likely to leave treatment against medical advice, do not tend to refrain from drug use after substance abuse treatment, and do not continue with aftercare as readily. Unfortunately, the death rate for dual-diagnosis clients is significantly higher than for clients who have only one of these diagnoses.

Clearly, dual diagnosis places individuals at very high risk for relapse, hospitalization, joblessness, homelessness, poor physical health (including AIDs), and early death. Between 30% and 50% of CMI alcoholics are not diagnosed as chemically dependent during psychiatric treatment, even when the diagnosis of alcoholism is available in their medical records; medical records are often not assembled during treatment. Research has found that as many as 78% of dual-diagnosis CMI are polydrug users, and that they are more likely than other CMI to show hostility, disorganized communication patterns, suicide lethality, poor self-care, treatment noncompliance, and rehospitalization (Drake & Wallach, 1989).

Levels of alcohol or other drug use among the CMI that would not be considered abusive under DSM-IV should be considered abusive for this group, because even low-level and episodic use can heighten the risk of relapse, especially in people with schizophrenic, bipolar, and depressive disorders. As we find among the non-CMI, research indicates that alcohol use increases during periods of crisis and that CMI needing alcoholism counseling were two and one-half times more likely to need other drug counseling as well (Solomon & Davis, 1986). Because the dual-diagnosis clients are at clearly heightened psychiatric risk, a clear understanding of the specific nature of both their psychiatric diagnosis and their drugs of abuse is crucial to long-term treatment success. One size of treatment will not fit all. As Weiss, Mirin, and Frances (1992, p. 107) indicated:

> Patients with substance abuse and other psychiatric illness present with a wide variety of clinical problems and require a treatment approach that addresses their specific disorders.
>
> Examples of dual diagnosis patients include an alcoholic patient who remains depressed after being detoxified; a cocaine abuser with an eating disorder who secretly binges and purges while in the hospital for treatment of cocaine abuse and who thus does not focus on substance abuse treatment; an opioid addict who appears not to care about getting better; a patient with bipolar disorder who drinks heavily, begins taking lithium less regularly, and relapses into mania or depression; a patient who seeks treatment for depression but fails to improve because of substance abuse; and a patient with schizophrenia who knows that his use of cocaine could exacerbate the psychosis but takes that risk because of the allure of the drug-using lifestyle. Obviously, each of these clinical situations should be addressed differently.

Treatment Issues with Dual-Diagnosis Clients

Substance abuse, even casual use, can raise the risk profile dramatically even for those suffering from situationally driven emotional problems. Acutely depressed persons who drink may become suicidally depressed or paradoxically so disinhibited that they accidentally injure themselves. Acutely anxious people who take stimulants can become panicked or manic.

Substance-abusing clients who seek treatment for substance abuse as their primary focus should be continually evaluated for concurrent emotional problems in much the same way that counselors should continually evaluate whether their clients with emotional problems may also have concurrent (and underlying) substance abuse problems. Identification of a primary diagnosis does not absolve the counselor of the responsibility to look for and to treat another possible diagnosis effectively. Unfortunately, objective psychiatric tests like the MMPI diagnose early-treatment dual-diagnosis clients very poorly. Only 20% of participants in alcohol and other drug treatment continue to display psychiatric disorders several weeks into treatment, even though 80% may show severe pathology on the MMPI at intake (Balcerzak & Hoffman, 1985). Therefore, the therapist's assessment and diagnosis talents are at a premium. Diagnosis should be tentative (described as possible until ruled out) until the client's complete paper trail and family and social history are available.

Understanding a client's dual diagnosis client requires understanding each individual diagnosis alone and the interaction of these diagnoses. Emotional and substance abuse problems are synergistic; that is, they produce interaction effects that feed back into other problems, complicating these problems. Personality disorders and schizophrenia, for example, given their persistent and pervasive nature, make substance abuse treatment particularly difficult. When we neglect one part of the equation, we make the other more difficult to treat. Even though it may be hard to remember at times, clients with multiple problems are not simply the sum total of their various problems and illnesses. This matrix of problems and person is organized into a meaningful whole or gestalt—one that makes decisions, drives a car, and raises a family.

Drugs complicate the treatment of all other psychiatric problems. Drugs destabilize an already fragile neurochemistry. They lower impulse control, which is often not strong in the first place. They decrease or increase the potency of medications needed for stable functioning. Drugs are expensive, devouring any budget, no matter how large. Moreover, drug use also initiates a causal chain of dismissive behavior toward clients by health and mental health staff and is instrumental in alienating the client's family, the first line of defense against social isolation and relapse.

Paradoxically, drugs are often perceived by the emotionally disturbed as their best friend. Drugs provide relief from boredom, a cheap vacation, peer interaction, and, before psychiatric symptoms arise, a sense of power and control over their lives. All of the reasons and justifications that serve ordinary people who experiment with drugs serve the mentally ill as well. If their need for social stimulation, for novelty, and for control are not met through other forms of social interaction, clients will continue to attempt to meet these needs through drug involvement, regardless of the concurrent negative consequences of drug use.

Unfortunately, as Polcin (1992b) pointed out, dual-diagnosis clients are often rejected from alcohol and other drug treatment programs because of their mental status and rejected from psychiatric care because they continue to use drugs. People with dual diagnoses therefore are the most likely of all client populations to fall through the cracks and end up living on the streets. Their problems are exacerbated by therapists' difficulties in conceptualizing the complex effects of the interaction between mental disorders and substance abuse. Previously, many psychoanalytically oriented psychotherapists wrongly discounted the physically addicting properties of drugs, and too often attributed addictions to unconscious blocks or psychic injuries during infancy and childhood. Today, because of their narrow sample, chemical dependence treatment personnel are all too likely to take a diametrically opposite view—that drugs cause most mental illnesses (Levy, 1993). However, as we argued in Chapter 1, the truth is somewhere between these extremes. Drug addictions are caused by addictive drugs; but there are multiple behavioral, genetic, social, and personal gateways into the addictions and multiple pathways through them (Vaillant, 1983).

General Rules for Working with Dual-Diagnosis Clients

Although those with dual diagnosis share only some etiological characteristics in common, we can make the following summative observations:

1. We must carefully assess where the client stands on the spiral of both addictions and emotional problems. Emotionally troubled teenagers who are heavily influenced by peers (Oetting & Beauvais, 1987) and who have begun to abuse alcohol or other gateway drugs (predisposing drugs like cigarettes and marijuana) must be led carefully into treatment when possible, but mandated when necessary.
2. Dual-diagnosis problems must be treated jointly. Treatment must coordinate the activities and resources of all the parties concerned.
3. The positives of drug use should not be swept under the rug. All drug users and the mentally ill especially get powerful payoffs from drugs that must be discussed openly so that behavioral options can be designed, implemented, and reinforced.
4. Even though each drug of choice and psychiatric condition coalesce to create somewhat different treatment needs, client cognitive and affective needs are rarely unique.
5. The cognitive, emotional, and behavioral consequences of drug use must be dealt with together in therapy. One therapy will definitely not fit all clients. Drug counselors need to be aware of an even wider range of counseling, teaching, and consultative techniques than other sorts of therapists do.
6. Drug use can independently cause psychiatric injury. Many of the mental disorders caused by and through chemical dependence do not disappear because clients remain clean and sober. Moreover, clients who did not have emotional problems when they entered the dependence cycle have significant personal, partnership, marriage, and family issues to confront when they discontinue use. The modal view from experienced treatment professionals is that total abstinence is the only reasonable course of action for dual-diagnosis individuals (Beck, Wright, Newman, & Liese, 1993; Rounsaville, Dolinsky, Babor, & Meyer, 1987).

The sections that follow address specific types of dual-diagnosis clients.

Schizophrenia and Bipolar Disorders   Follow a less emotionally charged strategy, or one that does not call for high levels of emotional expression. When possible, work to lower the level of confrontation in the sessions by being supportive, concrete, and direct. Work especially hard to establish a warm and accepting working alliance (Siris, 1990). Make sure that the client is hospitalized if detoxification appears necessary. Remember that clients with suicidal ideation have the same essential characteristics as attempters; all ideation must be taken seriously (Craig & Olson, 1990).

Evans and Sullivan (1990) and Siris (1990) suggested the following general guidelines for working with clients with schizophrenia or bipolar disorder. Emphasize medication compliance, making a clear distinction between therapeutic medications and abusive drugs. Pay particular attention to anticholinergic medication abuse and abusive stimulants like amphetamine and cocaine. Stay simple and concrete. Use visual learning materials when possible. Repeat things often and practice (role-play) specific situations. Keep assignments short and doable. Work on structure. Avoid high levels of expressed emotion, which may tend to upset the apple cart. Emphasize the unmanageability of life with drugs and the manageability that proper medication makes possible. Focus on concrete things, places, and people who may actively participate in the healing process, rather than a higher power or mystical concepts. Deemphasize helplessness, and emphasize matters that are within the client's control. Attend to psychosocial concerns like housing, day care, and day treatment. Carefully talk out chemical use issues that may destabilize the client and medication regimes that may stabilize him or her. Emphasize group therapy with clients with similar psychosocial and medication compliance problems, and refer the client to group treatment when possible. Follow-up often on the client's progress with the client and, with proper consent, other treatment personnel.

Depression   In working with dual-diagnosis depression the following concepts should be emphasized (Beck, Rush, Shaw, & Emery, 1979; Buelow & Hebert, 1995; Evans & Sullivan, 1990). Remember that vegetative symptoms of depression occur in both endogenous (sometimes called primary) and exogenous (sometimes referred to as reactive or secondary) depressions and that the suicide rates in endogenous versus exogenous or reactive depression do not appear significantly different. Sadly, the suicide rate for dual-diagnosis people is approximately 30 times the rate for the general population (Levy & Mann, 1988) and, therefore, about 8 times the rate of those who are chemically dependent but do not have a dual diagnosis.

Do not try to fix the client's grief around giving up the abused substance; rather, help the client process that grief directly in therapy. Work to help clients build a social support system. Help clients make a bridge into an Alcoholics Anonymous, a Narcotics Anonymous, or a Rational Recovery home group that can provide a knowledgeable sponsor who has some experience with dual-diagnosis concerns and who will encourage psychiatric medication compliance. Do not discourage the use of antidepressants or other medications that your client may be taking for concurrent psychiatric illness, and be willing to assess whether an antimedication bias exists in any AA or NA group the client is attending. Be clear with the client, even if the client is biased against psychiatric drugs, that medications may be necessary to help relieve vegetative symptoms like early morning awakening, insomnia, poor appetite, anhedonia, and poor self-care.

Anxiety Disorders   For dual-diagnosis clients with anxiety disorders, the therapist should be aware of the following important issues. Carefully consider the addiction potential of the benzodiazepines (BZD; Otto et al., 1993) and discuss this issue with the prescribing physician if possible before BZDs are prescribed for a purpose besides weaning in alcohol withdrawal. Instead, consider referral to a known and competent addictionologist or psychiatric physician with specific training and experience in working with dual-diagnosis clients. A psychiatrist is more likely to properly prescribe (and follow up on) medications for anxiety attacks (such as propranolol, a beta-blocker) and for obsessive-compulsive disorder (heterocyclics like fluoxetine [Prozac] or sertraline [Zoloft], for example). Work with the client on relaxation, graded exposure, and anxiety management programs, especially programs with clearly structured protocols that both clients and therapists can fully understand (Barlow, 1988; Barlow & Cerney, 1988).

Youth   Where adolescents are concerned, it is important to focus on the drug of choice; but equally important are the processes of therapy and continuation in the abuse cycle, including disorders involving risk-taking, eating problems, or sexual act-ing-out (Chatlos, 1989). Work carefully on diminishing the immediate importance of relationships with drug-abusing peers, while reinforcing other important social con-tacts—especially the family, if the family is supportive (Oetting & Beauvais, 1987). Focus on the emotional support that teenagers derive from their drug of choice, and do not underestimate the power of that support. Find psychosocial interventions for psychiatric problems that may be complicating the chemical dependence treatment picture, and vice versa; small amounts of many drug classes can violently exacerbate teenagers' mood swings, dysphoria, suicide risk, and depersonalization—especially steroid use among young males.

Personality Disorders   As we find in couples and family counseling generally, for cli-ents with personality disorders one of the greatest threats to successful chemical de-pendence treatment is posed by intransigent characterological disorders among first-degree relatives with whom clients are in daily contact—especially clients' parents. Because personality disorders fundamentally affect clients' means of organizing all experiences, very disordered relatives must either be treated directly in both indi-vidual and family therapy or the influence of the individual in question must be in-sulated against while family therapy proceeds without that individual's participation.

Whatever their etiology, personality disorders cause distortions that color all the clients' thoughts, feelings, and behaviors, because the disorder is the basis for inter-pretation of incoming data and outgoing action. If all cognitions, emotions, and ac-tions are viewed as being filtered through the net of personality, a personality disor-der can be likened to a defect in the net's construction. Although the net catches some fish, many escape through holes or are not caught because of the net's inad-equate performance under water, such as twisting. A personality disorder may also be analogized to a volcanic mountain upon which the individual lives. The mountain is benign in some situations, but not in others. Even in the best of circumstances, the individual must adapt to the steep slopes and difficult terrain that separate the per-son from other people who live down on the more easily negotiable plain. More dra-matically, the volcano also may erupt without much warning, leaving the individual to pick up and start afresh after the eruption is over.

The DSM-IV (American Psychiatric Association, 1994) description of personality disorders emphasizes enduring patterns of cognition, emotion, and behavior that de-viate in important ways from social expectations. Such disorders tend to be inflexible, pervasive, and of long standing. They usually lead to distress and problems in both individual and social functioning. They are not the product of some other mental or physiological problem such as schizophrenia. Moreover, even though substance abuse and dependence are considered diagnostic traits for antisocial and borderline per-sonality disorders, the disorder is not due to the direct effects of substance abuse.

Because substance abuse commonly occurs alongside personality disorders and is typical to several disorders in which impulse control is a primary psychiatric feature, it is not always clear whether the personality disorder will abate when the substance abuse has been treated. Many individuals who have been diagnosed as having pos-sible personality disorders are reclassified after treatment. MMPI scores often change so dramatically between intake and release among the chemically dependent that pretreatment scores should be taken as very tentative.

Many of the diagnostic criteria of antisocial personality disorder are common to drug-dependent individuals, who did not display these characteristics before they began their drug abuse and dependence. DSM-IV 301.7 (A) lists the following features of antisocial personality disorder, which are also typical of many clients who are drug dependent: (1) failure to conform to social norms or laws; (2) conning; (3) impulsivity or failure to plan ahead; (4) irritability and aggressiveness; (5) reckless disregard for self or others; (6) consistent irresponsibility; (7) lack of remorse as indicated by rationalizing.

Clients who abuse and are dependent on drugs often manifest all seven characteristics. Therefore, many drug abusers will be diagnosed as having antisocial personality disorders when more accurately their antisocial traits and states are part and parcel of their drug abuse. Over time, many drug clients display the traits we have come to recognize as characterological. In fact, most drug-dependent clients have altered and dysfunctional personalities before undergoing drug treatment and long-term aftercare. Unfortunately, some clients are altered permanently by their drug use.

Under DSM-IV definitions of borderline personality disorder, we find the following diagnostic traits typical to both personality disorder and drug dependence syndromes: fear of abandonment, unstable relationships, identity disturbances, impulsivity, recurrent suicidal gestures, mood instability, chronic boredom and emptiness, inappropriate anger, and paranoia. Under the DSM-IV description of the histrionic personality we find the following traits: uncomfortable at not being the center of attention, sexually seductive or provocative, emotionally shallow, excessively impressionistic, theatrical, suggestible. Because of the overlap between these disorders and chemical dependence syndrome, and the difficulty removing the personality disorder labels once they are attached to the client's paper trail, we should be cautious in attaching psychiatric labels to chemical dependent clients until they have reached at least a moderately functional level of sobriety.

Let us look at the following dual-diagnosis case in the light of this discussion:

◆ DUAL DIAGNOSIS: A CASE HISTORY ◆

Baird is an 18-year-old, single, white male referred by the high school principal for truancy and lack of cooperation in classes. He is currently a high school senior who is unlikely to graduate on time. He presently lives at home and rides a motorcycle to school or drives a car that does not meet inspection standards and that is uninsured.

A large, raw-boned young man, Baird usually wears blue jeans, T-shirts, and motorcycle boots. He speaks slowly and seems to measure the effect his communications have on the listener. On first meeting he appears to be shy and introverted, yet upon further discussion, Baird is able to express himself well and in a distinctively confrontational fashion. On intake Baird described his general behavior as good, but as aggressive and sometimes mean when drinking. Baird states that he is not a gang member, but rather a loner, that he is easily provoked and does not have a high tolerance for teasing. He is quick to answer insults and has been involved in numerous fights. Baird, who is very muscular, has a record of assaults against both men and women when under the influence of alcohol. Those he has assaulted describe his behavior as relatively distant but not unfriendly when not drinking, yet unpredictable when intoxicated. Baird is aware of and seems somewhat pleased with this description. Assaultive behavior when not drinking has not been documented but is not ruled out. He has been arrested for numerous minor traffic violations, usually because lights on his car are not working properly. He has been arrested for disorderly conduct and assaulting a police officer, but these charges were dropped because he was a minor at the time.

Baird is the third of six children, none of whom has graduated from high school. He describes his family as poor but taking care of their own. Baird states that he does not know who his father is—a source of frustration and anger to him. His other siblings were fathered by two other men. He expresses anger at having been referred to by a teacher as a bastard. This incident, he states, has involved him in a number of fights with his classmates. Baird describes his mother as a hardworking woman. Yet he becomes quiet and soft-spoken when recounting that his mother has a live-in boyfriend of another race. He feels that this man is using his mother and does not care about either him or his siblings.

Baird states that his older brother, who also has a history of violent behavior, did not finish high school, but ran away from home and joined the Army. His oldest sister became pregnant as a junior in high school and left school to get married. She has since been divorced and has had a second child by another man. Baird states that he has been expected to take care of his three younger brothers and sisters, and sometimes his sister's children. He states that he resents this and that his mother leaves with her common-law husband, expecting Baird to take care of the children for days at a time, during which episodes he misses school. Baird indicates that alcohol is used often in his household. Friends of his stepfather come to the house to drink and gamble. During these times he is subjected to teasing and told he cannot hold his liquor. When he refuses to drink—not often—he is made fun of. As a preteen, Baird had alcohol poured on him and was forced to drink. When his mother leaves the house or is too drunk to attend to him, Baird often steals alcohol and drinks alone. He states that he has become drunk on a number of occasions and has been praised and encouraged to drink more by the older people gathered in his home.

Baird began to drink heavily with his peers as he entered junior high. He also began to drive his mother's car, even though he did not possess a driver's license. On one occasion, the police stopped him and charged him with underage consumption and driving without a license. Although he resisted arrest, he was not charged with this crime. Earlier in the year, Baird was found guilty of assaulting a police officer who stopped him for a traffic violation. He was put on probation but has made no effort to comply with the terms of his probation. Baird reports that people at a party called him a redneck and that he has long felt he is made fun of by others, especially women, whom he feels are prejudiced against him because of his impoverished family. He is often involved in arguments with girlfriends as a result of defending his family. As a teen, Baird became strongly interested in women both younger and older than himself. He states that he has a very strong sex drive and that a number of much younger girls are more than willing to be involved with him. Yet, when he becomes intoxicated, he describes himself as forcing himself on them and refusing to take no for an answer. He has been arrested for assault. As a result of his arrest, Baird spent five days in jail, but the young woman failed to press charges, and he was released.

Early in the interview, Baird was quiet and calm. Yet he becomes angry and upset when discussing his father, whom he claims not to know. He describes this man as having deserted his mother and as ruining her life. Baird describes others, especially teachers, as being prejudiced toward him and other "lower-class" students in his school. He expresses pleasure in being able to physically dominate other people, especially men. Baird also expresses feelings of being looked down on by the people of his small, rural community because of the behavior of his mother and her boyfriend. He feels that "no one has a chance in the rich man's world." He reports that early exposure to and availability of alcohol caused him to depend on the drug for relief and release. He states that he uses alcohol because it makes him feel more normal and because it is easy to obtain.

From the information available, is this short case description sufficient for a tentative diagnosis? What other information would you need in order to rule out a dual diagnosis of alcohol dependence and antisocial personality disorder? Is Baird's behavior while drinking consistent with your tentative evaluation of his personality dynamics? What direction would you take with a clinical interview if Baird were referred to you for an assessment? What direction might you take in concurrent treatment if you decided upon concurrent psychotherapy after referring Baird for structured chemical dependence treatment?

Assessment of dual diagnosis should be done without haste, should use multiple assessment strategies, and should hinge, finally, on the presence of psychiatric features prior to onset of chemical abuse and dependence and subsequent to adequate long-term aftercare. If chemical dependence was eliminated as a diagnostic trait, many clients who would otherwise be diagnosed as antisocial or borderline, for example, would not be classified simply because they would not meet a sufficient number of criteria (Dulit et al., 1990).

RATIONAL-EMOTIVE THERAPY IN CHEMICAL DEPENDENCE TREATMENT

RET, which combines philosophical rationalism, humanism, and learning theory, was developed by Albert Ellis during the early 1950s (Dryden & Ellis, 1988). It is an important force in the armamentarium of cognitive approaches. Many of its themes and practices are central to chemical dependence therapy across the nation and the world, because RET stresses rational control, self-responsibility, and action.

Central to RET is Epictetus' view that people are disturbed less by events that happen to them than by their perspective on those events. A lack of attention to the more positive aspects of strong emotions and an overemphasis on helping clients control negative affect has been one of RET's weaknesses (Corey, 1991). RET has been further elaborated in a number of books, articles, and research publications by a variety of RET practitioners as well as by Ellis himself (Ellis, 1962, 1971; Ellis, McInerney, Digiuseppe, & Yeager, 1988; Ellis & Grieger, 1986; Ellis & Whiteley, 1979; Ellis & Velten, 1992).

Like many therapies, the practice of RET took much of its early character from its developer, who appears to be very confrontational, argumentative, direct and directive, humorous, detached, rational, and curious. Although Ellis himself, perhaps due to his charismatic nature, does not seem to need to stress the development of a warm relationship, the development of a warm and cooperative working alliance with the client is certainly compatible with RET. Ellis may not consider transference a necessary or wise condition for good therapy, however, because he prefers to avoid the client's becoming dependent on the therapist. RET stresses self-reliance and self-help;

philosophical disputation of negative and self-defeating thoughts; living in the here and now; rational, nonmagical thinking; deemphasizing the history or etiology of personal problems; and hard work.

Important basic tenets of RET are, first, that we are neither good nor bad but we do have the power to rate ourselves as worthy or unworthy. Unhappy people seem to value themselves negatively as unworthy of love and happiness, whereas happy, better adjusted people, realizing there is no better judge than they themselves, tend to evaluate themselves as worthy of love and happiness.

Second, Ellis points out in a variety of his writings that people are born with the tendency to think, feel, and act in ways that are self-defeating or that have self-defeating consequences. Their innate tendency toward irrationality leads them to hold irrational beliefs. Irrational beliefs are based on inaccurate or incomplete knowledge, and rigid judgments of right and wrong ("the world *should, must,* or *ought to be* the way I want it"). These beliefs are self-defeating and lead to less competent problem solving, irresponsible behavior, negative emotions, and underachievement (Ellis & Harper, 1975). Rational beliefs are more relative (situationally determined) and are usually expressed as wants, wishes, likes, and dislikes, rather than as perfectionistic needs.

The primary goal of RET is to help people think more rationally (scientifically, clearly, flexibly), feel more appropriately (less violently and negatively), and act more functionally (more efficiently and less self-defeatingly). Subgoals of RET are self-interest, social interest, tolerance, acceptance of uncertainty, commitment, self-acceptance, risk-taking, long-range hedonism, non-utopianism, high tolerance for frustration, and self-responsibility for disturbance (Ellis, 1971; Ellis & Velten, 1992).

The ABCs of Rational-Emotive Therapy

To accomplish these goals, Ellis devised the ABC approach to understanding how our irrational beliefs undermine our rational actions toward meeting our wants and needs. Although we refer the reader to the books listed in the bibliography for a more complete explanation of RET by Ellis himself and to Corey's *Theory and Practice of Counseling and Psychotherapy* (1991, pp. 324–368) for an excellent synopsis, the essentials are basically as follows.

We are used to thinking that certain actions cause particular consequent feelings and actions. Ellis pointed out, however, that our feelings are strongly affected by intervening thought processes that often determine the intensity and direction (from positive to negative) of those feelings. Ellis recounted the following example: A man is walking down the street. Someone from a window nearby shouts down at him, "You are a stupid jerk!" Our walker immediately gets angry.

If we examine what precedes the immediate anger, we will find some self-statements of the form: "This person must know me, even though I can't quite make him out. He shouldn't be saying those things to me. He himself is a no-good bastard. He has no right to treat me this way." Proceeding on his way, however, our walker notices that he is passing by a mental hospital. He realizes that the person who has been yelling out the window is an inmate. His anger quickly vanishes—replaced by pity, perhaps, or only mild irritation. Prior to his anger dissipating, however, our walker said something to himself on the order of: "That was only a poor, demented man who couldn't possibly know me personally. So, therefore, I should pity him. What he said had nothing to do with me personally. I need not be angry."

Ellis's point, and the point upon which all cognitive therapies hinge, is that it was not the original *Action* (the shout) itself that caused the walker's *Consequent* (angry) feeling. It was the intervening *Belief,* in this case an irrational one, that the shouter knew the walker, was speaking directly to the walker, had no right to be calling the walker names, and was wrong and insulting. The walker's anger followed on his belief that he was being personally insulted, not from the mental patient's yelling out the window. Further, the walker's loss of anger followed from his new and more rational view, initiated by seeing the sign for the mental hospital, that the person's actions had nothing to do with him in particular. Thus, negative and dysfunctional affect was diminished by a more rational view of the situation. Accordingly, RET attempts to teach people to replace these intervening and dysfunctional thoughts and beliefs with more empirically justifiable, rational, and self-serving ones.

Ellis makes the point in all of his writings that *Activating* events, mediated by irrational *Beliefs,* often lead to negative *Consequences.* However, if we *Dispute* the irrational beliefs, this disputation process will lead to a more *Effective,* more rational belief, which will in turn lead to new *Feelings.* Thus, the ABCDEF cycle of action is proposed. Rational-emotive therapy, then, is the process of intervening with clients in the ABC cycle by helping them learn how to dispute their own irrational beliefs, self-defeating habits of thought, and unscientific thinking more effectively.

The primary diagnostic focus of RET is on discovering clients' beliefs, philosophies, and affective patterns that lead to their disturbances, assessing how these contribute to disturbances, and helping clients set realistic goals to diminish the negative affect accompanying these habitual and dysfunctional forms of thinking, behaving, and feeling. Central to helping clients is showing them the dysfunctional effects of their demands, their "awfulizing," their "I-can't-stand-its," their negative self-ratings, and their "musturbation"—the omnipresent belief that "things *must* be as I want them, or I just can't go on with life."

Like other existential approaches, but unlike more behavioral approaches, RET acknowledges that insight is necessary to profit most from therapy. Clients need enough insight to understand how their current thoughts and beliefs interlock with their emotional upsets, how to accept responsibility, how to accept themselves as fallible and often gullible human beings, how to work to change their beliefs, and how to recognize therapeutic gains (Ellis & Velten, 1992).

Strengths for Chemical Dependence Treatment

RET has many strengths that make it appropriate for alcohol and other drug treatment (Ellis & Velten, 1992; Ellis et al., 1988). First, RET is simple to teach to clients, and clients can then be shown how to work on further concerns through homework assignments and reading. Many simple exercises can be designed to help clients uncover their irrational beliefs concerning alcohol and other drug behavior. For example, many drug abusers irrationally believe that they can give up drinking but not change their overall lifestyle. Many believe that they can return to the bar and dance hall scene, for example, without initiating the drinking cycle again—not very likely, is it?

RET helps clients own the fact that life is not always going to be the way they want it. Clients frequently obsess on the lack of fairness that they were vulnerable to alcoholism while others were not. From an RET perspective, life is not fair. Some people get better luck than others: better bodies, better brains, and better families. If you can't seem to get more of what you want, however, success in life amounts to doing the best you can with what you have. It is irrational and self-defeating to believe that you deserve or are entitled to special (or even fair) treatment in life.

RET works in the here and now. For drug abusers especially, worrying about the past is a one-way ticket to wallowing in remorse over misdeeds committed while drunk or high on drugs. From an RET perspective, the past is gone. Learn from it, and live with it. Since you can't change the past, it makes better sense to take an objective, nonjudgmental view of your prior behavior. The future is also nonexistent. Without hard work in the here and now, our future will not be much different from what we presently experience. Better, then, to work with what we have, when we have it. Learning to better predict the consequences of our actions means working now, not constantly daydreaming about the future. Although it is not unreasonable for clients to show concern about the future, they must be shown how to accept it as it comes—not create self-fulfilling prophecies of failure, have unrealistic expectations, and make unreasonable demands upon the future.

RET techniques to help clients identify and dispute irrational beliefs are Socratic questioning (What does it actually mean?), empirical analysis (What are its facts?), functional analysis (What roles does it serve?), humor (What is its context? Does it really matter?), paradox (What are its ultimate limits?), imagery (What does it look like cognitively and emotionally?), and risk-taking (How far can I reasonably push it?). Each of these techniques is meant to bring clients into closer contact with the ordinary, real, tangible, social world about them.

Insight is important in RET. Insight into the workings of addictions, and insight into the client's personal world that may have allowed for the introduction of the drugs or that may have been altered significantly by the drugs, are necessary to long-term sobriety. Individuals who quit drinking but who do not gain insight or alter their personal perspectives often suffer as "dry drunks." They have the same interpersonal and intrapersonal problems that they had while they were drinking. They seem to have learned little from their experiences and therefore are liable under high stress—a divorce, for example—to relapse back into drinking after many years of "white-knuckled sobriety." It is of great importance for clients not only to know about, but to be able to trust their thinking about drugs. RET is well designed to help clients understand how their upsets tend to happen, how their beliefs support or undermine their sobriety, and how their interaction with others can be enlisted as an aid to reinforce sobriety. RET also supports the view that we cannot change others—only ourselves. Therefore, clients would do well to consider what kinds of friends they want, especially if their friends are drinking or using.

RET does not stress complex assessment or diagnosis or historical reconstruction of problems. If clients are so ill or developmentally delayed that they cannot quickly learn to take responsibility for their actions, they would probably do better to find another form of treatment—a more behavioral, milieu-oriented approach, perhaps. RET's nonhistorical, nonassessment techniques alleviate some difficulties in interaction with clients and create some others that must be better understood. First, RET allows the counselor to move very quickly toward helping clients assume responsibility for their lives by examining the belief structures that keep them bogged down in self-defeating feelings and actions, and by designing new ways of thinking and doing. On the down side, however, RET may allow the counselor to underestimate the importance of concurrent problems (a dual diagnosis, for example), the existence of cultural or sexual differences that may sabotage therapy if not addressed (such as homosexuality), and the far-reaching nature of internal dynamics of unfinished business with the past (Corey, 1991).

Finally, in our view, chemical dependence counselors should work to develop a st*rategic* RET approach for early treatment, one that emphasizes a clear understanding of how addictions affect cognition (and as a result the formation of irrational beliefs), the development of a firm working alliance, and a respect for the subtleties in the relationships among drug dependence, relapse, and unfinished business with the past. Strategic RET pays special attention to the counselor's understanding of how both client's and counselor's social and economic class, ethnic status, sexual orientation, physical limitations, and age may exacerbate the drug-abuse cycle. When these interlocking conditions are examined in detail with the client, RET is deepened and its applicability is broadened. Thus therapists can avoid the one-size-fits-all application of RET that is, unfortunately, sometimes cited as a reason to dismiss the therapy's strengths along with its weaknesses.

GESTALT THERAPY IN CHEMICAL DEPENDENCE TREATMENT

Because of their shared existential backgrounds and compatible strengths, we suggest that Gestalt therapy and RET be used as partners in alcohol and other drug treatment. In addition to applying techniques that have a long history of effective use in drug treatment (such as the "empty chair" technique and other forms of confrontational role-playing), Gestalt therapists have made a strong case that personality and identity develop normally only to the extent that individuals take responsibility for their lives. Developed by Fritz Perls in the 1950s, Gestalt therapy provides both experiences and experiments designed to help clients overcome their fear, lack of responsibility, emotional blocks, and unfinished business with others in their past. Because it emphasizes responsibility, the here and now, and supportive confrontation with reality, Gestalt therapy has become a cornerstone of chemical dependence treatment. Although there is no exact equivalent in English, the word *Gestalt* refers to the process through which meaningful wholes arise in our perception. Like all existentialists, Gestalt therapists are concerned with the influence of cognition (cognitive schema or worldview) on our perception and understanding. Identity development is contingent on the reciprocity between our internal (indigenous) processes of making meaning and the ordinary world. Thus, the Gestalt process is a basic human process through which cognitive and emotional schemas are formed and made to function together in reality. When this Gestalt process is thwarted in some way, problems arise in accepting responsibility for actions, being authentic, taking care of interpersonal business, staying present in the here and now, and managing fear. Perls designed his therapy to help clients address these problems. Even though he did not design the therapy for use with drug-abusing clients specifically, the kinds of problems that Gestalt therapy focuses on—including irresponsibility, manipulativeness, distorted attribution of causes, fearfulness, and lack of authenticity—are typically exacerbated by chemical dependence.

Gestalt assessment documents specific blocks to emotional expression and responsibility. These may include, for example, obsessive wants and cognitions, fear of social interaction, or humiliating baggage from the past (all quite usual in drug-related behavior). Unblocked cognitive and emotional expression lead to wholeness and closure. Thwarted expression leads to further blocks in which feelings and thoughts cannot recede naturally into the background as new and interesting events arise. These blocks become obsessions and neuroses; they also, of course, form the typical basis for chemical dependence relapse. Gestalt assessment is designed to help clients discover what their emotional baggage looks like, what it means, and how to divest it of power and meaning so that it can recede naturally back into the background.

Gestalt chemical dependence therapists develop experiences and experiments to help individual clients and group members emotionally confront their drug-related baggage, blocks, and irresponsibility. Until clients have emotional awareness and commitment, however, it is unlikely that they will achieve understanding or insight. In a fashion complementary to the RET approach, therefore, Gestalt therapy emphasizes the emotive component of therapy. A dictum of Gestalt therapy (in distinct contrast to RET, which often seems very intellectual and teacherly as applied by Ellis himself) is that clients do not come to therapy for an explanation; they come for an experience.

From a Gestalt view, drugs impede personality development and self-expression because they weaken our connection with the basic processes through which identity is informed by our perceptual, cognitive, and affective experiences. Those basic processes include the development of internally self-evident or phenomenological reality, emotional closure, and wholeness. Drug use causes distortions of perceptual and emotional fields. Drug use encourages shallow and premature closure on complex emotional experiences. Over time and with habituation, however, a sense of emotional closure becomes more difficult to reach and requires higher drug levels to obtain. Soon, closure is lost and fragmentation begins, even though drug use remains constant or is escalated.

The law of wholeness recognizes a particularly important feature of human life: We attach meanings to things beyond the meaning or value associated with their constituents. Even though drugs can accentuate this sense of wholeness and may actually lead to "oceanic" experiences of wholeness and closure (as Timothy Leary never tired of proclaiming about LSD, for example), it appears that experiences that are not the result of hard personal work and true insight quickly fade into insignificance. People are able to approach these experiences again only by continued exposure to usually higher levels of the drug. Drug-induced insights rarely lead to any important personal development, only to further character disorganization—often tragic disorganization for dual-diagnosis clients.

From a Gestalt perspective, drugs cause the following problems. First, even though drugs encourage novel experiences, over the long run they lead to disorganization of our cognitive and emotional lives. Then, to insulate ourselves from feelings of disorganization, we use greater amounts of the drug. Second, drugs may begin to function as the primary regulator for our emotions; thus, drugs become a necessary component of emotional regulation and self-adjustment. When we try to split the drug away from us, we undergo a neurosis, just as we would if we tried to split off any other part of our emotional life. Third, ego boundaries deteriorate as our self-control fails, because both internal and interpersonal boundaries depend upon self-control for proper regulation. Fourth, since our conceptions of reality are distorted by drugs and by the society of other cognitively impaired drug users, our ability to be fully self-supportive and self-regulating deteriorates. Therefore, our grip on social and objective reality, our intuition, and our natural movement toward healthy experiences is progressively weakened.

From a Gestalt standpoint, drugs distort the organizational basis upon which we develop self-awareness, emotional presence, authenticity, responsibility, and a sense of proportion about our place in the world. Gestalt therapy was designed to help individuals rebuild that organizational base, and its theories and techniques have become widely used in a variety of drug therapy settings for that purpose. Fritz Perls once said that clients may need to lose their minds to gain their sanity. Analogously, drug-dependent clients must lose their drug mind and drug culture before they can gain their sanity and sobriety.

In our experience, newly sober clients are much like people who cannot swim and who are floating around in life rings trying to get to the sides of a swimming pool. While they are trying to stay afloat in their overly socialized and overly personalized life rafts, it often seems as though Gestalt therapists are busily prying these people's fingers away from the sides of the pool. Don't recovering people just hang on that much harder to what they think is their life support—their drug mind and drug culture? Aren't Gestalt experiments dangerous? Clearly, experiments need to be designed that are appropriate to the sobriety level of the clients and the setting. In our experience, counselors do more damage by failing to design experiences and experiments around regaining control over sobriety than by being overly experimental.

Key Concepts of Gestalt Therapy

The ideas and exercises set out in the following sections represent some of those that are central to Gestalt therapy.

Ownership and Being Present   An important feature of Gestalt therapy is ownership of thoughts and feelings. This ownership is reestablished through having clients use "I" statements, rather than the ubiquitous "you" or "people" ("you know," "people believe"). Using "I" statements and working in the "now" focus clients' attention on the direct, immediate, tangible present. Important questions are these: What is going on with me now? How am I experiencing my emotions now? How am I attempting to withdraw right now? What is my awareness at this moment? How am I affecting others right now?

Clients must be taught to own their projections. Ownership is facilitated by helping clients learn to apply beliefs they hold about other people to themselves. If clients say, "I believe others are not to be trusted," they must be challenged to examine their beliefs about their own trustworthiness. What the client usually means this: "I am not to be trusted at this time. Come in and find out why!"

Each of us is afraid to expose who we really are. This fear arises even though we cannot exist socially without exposing who we are to significant others. This fear often reaches the level of paranoia among the chemically dependent. Not only are clients afraid for others to discover how weak and ineffectual they really are, they have lost a significant portion of who they once were through the many denial processes of chemical dependence—a frightening admission for clients to make.

Relearning how to become emotionally vulnerable, to take risks, and to move toward full self-support requires structured Gestalt exercises. Gestalt practitioners (Perls, 1976; Perls, Hefferline, & Goodman, 1951; Polster & Polster, 1973) and Gerald Corey (1991, pp. 248–254) have provided exercises that can be used at each level of individual and group Gestalt therapy. Although these authors should be read in detail, these exercises are set out briefly in the following sections.

Contradiction   Paradoxically, all of us hold what appear to be mutually exclusive points of view, beliefs, and feelings. For example, it is possible to both love and hate another person. Addicted clients both love and hate their drugs of choice, and their love does not go away because they have sobered up. Their love of the drug should not be minimized; it must be lived through. This living through entails owning opposing feelings. Without recognizing and owning contradictions, personal growth is constricted. Without growth, the discrepancy between opposing and paradoxical feelings widens. Gestalt work helps clients recognize their personal paradoxes and moves them toward emotional closure. Conflicting feelings must be accepted and allowed to recede into the emotional background.

The Now   The chemically dependent often avoid living in the present moment and act irresponsibly because they cannot act effectively in the now. They spend their lives ruminating on the past or dreaming about the future. Thus, their actions are reactive, rather than proactive. From a Gestalt point of view, "why" questions keep us searching through the past for explanations. "What" and "how" questions, however, are more likely to help us focus on present issues—what we should make of them and how they should be resolved.

It is not hard to understand, of course, why chemically dependent clients want to avoid the present reality of their drug use, and to live in the past or in some drug-induced dream world. The present may have a silver lining, but that lining is very hard-edged. Reality is tough. Irresponsible people are unpopular. Unfinished business is usually ugly. Others are often unkind, especially those who have been injured by clients' irresponsible drug use.

To counteract clients' tendencies to avoid the present, Perls continually confronted them for not using "I" statements and for talking *about* their feelings rather than *from* their feelings. He challenged clients to live up to their own expectations rather than other people's, and not to wallow in irresponsible thinking and behavior. Perls continually invented new experiments to help clients get in touch with their feelings and to speak from those feelings with authenticity. Counselors are encouraged to exercise their own creativity in designing and implementing strategies that challenge clients to be more creative in their own self-care.

Unfinished Business   Many clients were abused or neglected as children. Because they were not shown how to care for themselves or others, their efforts in those directions are often in adequate (including the care of their own children). Clients also have powerful unmet wants and needs because of the dysfunctional relationships they experienced as children. These unfulfilled desires, inappropriate models, bad relationships, self-neglect, and self-abuse are all part of clients' unfinished business. Feelings that derived from these earlier experiences are not self-mending, even though clients may be resilient. These feelings do not usually recede into the past but become material blocks that affect clients in a daily way. Such feelings have become current problems.

Working on unfinished business does not entail meticulously exploring the many hurts from our past, although we should explore the general pattern and results of those past injuries. Working on unfinished business instead means confronting the emotional blocks (or people) in the present that cause problems in interaction with self and with others. Often, overcoming present emotional blocks requires resurrecting and confronting long-dead parents. Role-playing, use of the empty chair technique, and dream and fantasy reconstruction are all parts of the process by which contemporary but submerged feelings are reified, confronted, and responsibly worked through.

Unfinished business keeps us from interacting authentically with others, because we project an overlay of earlier experiences onto present ones. Then, especially during stressful moments, we react to people as we did to those earlier introjects that we swallowed unexamined as children. Gestalt therapy encourages us to spit those introjects back out. To the extent we can dislodge earlier (usually parental) introjects, we can begin to relate to others as they really are, not as our fear of ghosts makes them appear. Like Boszormenyi-Nagy, Perls found resentment about past hurts to be the most frequent unfinished business. Resentment makes itself known symptomatically through guilt, shame, anger, and unexpressed emotional needs. Stating these resentments in therapy, even to (sometimes especially to) the dead, helps to provide a corrective emotional experience. The heart of the corrective experiences is that, rather than resulting in the same old put-downs, self-expression can elicit a new and reinforcing result—namely, support and insight.

Even though they are the identified patients, drug abusers often have unexpressed resentments against family members for neglecting responsibilities and for not setting clear boundaries early in their drinking or drugging careers. These resentments have to be allowed expression in the present, whether or not they seem appropriate or reasonable. Resentments do not have to be rational to need expression, but neither do resentments have to consume entire sessions. In our experience, expression of clients' resentments—many of which may need to be reexperienced and role-played out before they can be resolved—facilitates clients' responsibility.

Not surprisingly, many clients resent the fact that they are in therapy. They are angry that they have been singled out by fate for addiction and that society somehow failed to restrain them. Let clients express specific instances of resentment, guilt, and shame, demonstrating total acceptance of the feelings that arise; then, supportively confront clients each and every time with their present responsibility for any action or belief that may reinforce these same dysfunctional patterns.

Energy Blocks   Drawing on the thinking of Zen Buddhism which they study in detail, Gestalt psychologists believe that the flow of energy in the body results in the natural incorporation into consciousness of the objects of our attention which then form the basis for ongoing cognitive, emotional, and behavioral action. When this flow of energy is normal, objects of our attention take on appropriate meaning and value. They do not become stuck but emerge into attention and recede back into the background in a natural way, according to the amount of relative attention they actually merit. In the case of psychic injury, however—which is often familial, cultural, or drug-related in origin—the flow of energy is diverted, slowed, or blocked.

These blocks are manifested in the release of nervous tension. The site of nervous release—the tapping foot, the shaking hands, the stammer—may give the observer some idea of the source of the block. Blocks may suggest their own treatment if they are given voice, which involves client and therapist in literally talking to and from that part of the body. Energy diverted must be redirected. Energy slowed must be speeded up. Energy blocked must be undammed. Drug use in and of itself, and the social deterioration that takes place with the abuse, distorts the Gestalt perceptual and cognitive-emotional process, diverting energy from our apprehension of social reality and setting up blocks to the normal expression of our emotional lives. Like Zen teachers, Gestalt therapists often attack these blocks vigorously and creatively by helping the client identify actions in the present that will challenge the block, providing corrective emotional experiences, insight into the nature of the block (satori), and plans for continued corrective behavior. Like the Zen teachers they emulate, Gestalt therapists are, as was Perls, energized by clients' resistances, diversions, and self-defeating irresponsibility (or as Perls termed it, bullshit).

Other Concepts   Numerous other Gestalt views bear consideration. For example, Gestaltists see fear as excitement without a natural channel for expression. Also, Gestaltists believe that we all project our problems onto the world. Therefore, when a client says that "the world is too crowded," the client really means "I am crowding my world too much." "People don't like me" means "I don't like people." Finally, therapy is seen as a phenomenological process, not a product with a clear end point. Therefore, therapy is to the client whatever the therapeutic interactions mean to the client. The therapy process can never be the same for client and counselor, and concerns that are unclear, indeterminate, or unknowable must be resolved *in interaction*.

Because of the necessity for direct, experiential mentoring in Gestalt theory and techniques, it is difficult to imagine using Gestalt techniques effectively without participating in intensive Gestalt training workshops or experiencing Gestalt therapy as a client. We encourage counselors, therefore, to take advantage of whatever Gestalt experiences are available, in addition to reading the works of Perls, Zinker, and the Polsters. Reading and theorizing are important rehearsals but cannot take the place of doing. Experience fosters natural experimentation in both individual and group therapy. Just as important, experience makes clients' blowups instructive and productive.

In outline, the goals of Gestalt therapy are as follows (Corey, 1991; Perls, 1969, 1970, 1972, 1976; Zinker, 1977):

1. Movement toward increasing awareness of self
2. Ownership of personal experience, rather than making others responsible for what we feel, think, and do
3. Satisfaction of wants and needs (especially our sexual wants) without violating the rights of others

4. Awareness through all our senses, including intuition
5. Acceptance of responsibility
6. Movement toward increasing internal, as opposed to external, support
7. Development of proactive attitudes
8. Getting in touch with the obvious and with the now
9. Freeing creative energy and potential in both client and therapist by removing emotional and cognitive blocks
10. Pointing out splits and incongruities among what clients say, feel, and do
11. Sensitizing both therapist and client to the Gestalt process

How does Gestalt therapy proceed with alcoholic and other drug-dependent clients? Let us look at the following case.

◆ GESTALT THERAPY: A CASE HISTORY ◆

Ruth was a 32-year-old graduate student in sociology at the university. She was attractive, rather tall, and plainly dressed. From the Midwest, she was the only child of a conservative home. Her parents, who had married late, were in their early 40s when she was born and were not openly affectionate with each other or with Ruth. She felt a definite lack of warmth and relatedness in her family, particularly from her father, who retired early to his room each night, where he stayed up alone, drinking and listening to baseball games.

Ruth entered therapy because of relationship and alcohol problems. Having rented a room two years earlier in a house also occupied by two other graduate students, Ed and Bill, Ruth drifted into ongoing affairs with both of the somewhat younger men.

Ruth had little experience with drugs before leaving the Midwest. Ed and Bill, however, were both heavy drinkers, used marijuana on weekends, and made episodic use of psychedelic mushrooms between school terms. Over time, Ruth began to use these drugs along with her partners. Several weeks prior to intake, Ruth had sex with both Ed and Bill while under the influence of alcohol, which both attracted and deeply disturbed her. At present, Ruth was alternately drinking to drunkenness each weekend and drying out during the week.

Ordinarily very straitlaced, Ruth had begun to interact sexually with her partners more and more frequently while intoxicated. She reported feeling guilty and humiliated by her behavior and remorseful upon sobering up from the weekends. The week before, she had taken a test in a woman's magazine purporting to measure alcohol problems. She had scored in the alcoholic range. This score, arguments with Ed and Bill, and disturbing dreams about her father tipped the scales toward counseling.

Ruth blamed Ed and Bill for her immediate drinking. She also resented her older than average parents for raising her, as she said, to be a repressed prude who had never even had a boyfriend prior to living with her present partners. She recounted fears of living her life out more or less alone like her neurotic mother, even if she were lucky enough to find a husband.

Ruth indicated that she swore off drinking each Monday but was so depressed and lonely by Friday that she often accompanied Ed and Bill to the bars, where their weekend cycle would begin all over again. She also recounted a deep and chronic history of dysthymia, which she quickly linked to her father's lifelong depression and avoidance.

Ruth was referred to a concurrent outpatient treatment group sponsored by the university counseling center. She made contact with her group soon after our first meeting. We contracted to work on immediate abstinence issues during the first week, which included both alcohol and drug education, and to process her fears of being in group therapy. We also agreed to confront her depression and loneliness. She wanted to examine her sexual issues concerning Ed and Bill, whom she felt contributed to her problems; she felt that she might not be able to discuss those issues during group.

During the first two weeks of abstinence, during which Ruth went through moderate withdrawal symptoms, we focused on her immediate cognitions around alcohol and explored the nature of addictions, their physiology, and relapse pressures. During the second week we began to explore her feelings of resentment toward her parents, anger at Ed and Bill, and frustration with her graduate program. Although rather prim and proper in appearance, below the surface Ruth recounted seething with unexpressed hostility about the gender repression she had experienced all her life. Her story also underscored her radical social views and her highly charged sexual feelings. Ruth viewed her inability to express these views and feelings as the product of a repressive society, even though many students around her undoubtedly shared her views. Only under the influence of alcohol did Ruth feel disinhibited enough to say what she really thought and felt. Unfortunately, expressing herself while intoxicated did little to relieve her pent-up anger, frustration, and blame.

Over time, and as her sobriety became more solid, we focused more and more closely on and confronted more directly Ruth's willingness to blame others and not take responsibility for her drinking and sexual behavior (and, ultimately, therefore, for herself). We designed experiences in our immediate therapy for Ruth to express both her thinking and her feelings about women and men, especially her unfinished business, first, with her alcoholic father, and later, with her mother, who had not protected Ruth from her father's rejection and filled her loneliness and longing, and with whom Ruth was even angrier. We also designed experiments where she expressed herself verbally to others, culminating in her presenting a lecture about those she felt to be perpetrating much of the repression against women, minorities, and the poor at the free-speech platform at the university commons. Discovering that the world, she herself, her parents, and Ed and Bill did not disintegrate under her anger, Ruth began to challenge some of her own irrational beliefs about sex and about men and women's roles and to take more responsibility for her situation. She also began to blame Ed and Bill less for her earlier sexual behavior. Under her pressure, her partners began to use alcohol less and to desist from involving her in their marijuana use. With more time and energy to devote to her studies, Ruth began to realize her potential in her department. She began to teach part time at a nearby college and to expand her social relationships.

Clearly, given her family background of alcoholism, her dysthymia, and her history of blackouts, Ruth could not return to social drinking. She was, under almost any definition, alcoholic. However, drinking allowed Ruth to act out in ways that were, for her, often quite positive. Under the influence Ruth was able to express her complex social and political views, and she had also begun to express herself sexually for the first time. Without a form of therapy that stressed finding creative outlets for these feelings, Ruth would continue to be at high risk for relapse every time she felt emotionally blocked. Therefore, Ruth's therapy focused on helping her learn to be both more supportive and confrontational. This confrontational attitude was directed especially toward her parents and her own alcoholism. Therapy also helped her to own her feelings and express them, to risk being more creative in her outlook on life, and to stop blaming others for her immediate problems. Especially important was Ruth's confrontation of her resentments about not being able to drink and flirt like other people. Finally, Ruth accepted that she liked the attentions of both Ed and Bill and that she was not willing in the foreseeable future to give either one of them up. Although the relationship of these three partners was unconventional, Gestalt therapy makes no judgments about sexual arrangements, as long as they do not clearly hurt other people. As Perls indicated, we are not put on the earth to live up to other people's expectations, sexual or otherwise.

STUDY AND DISCUSSION QUESTIONS

1. Consistent with stages and processes of change, different counseling strategies work best at different times in chemical dependence counseling. Outline the particular characteristics typical of newly detoxified clients, and indicate what techniques might best be used as they move through the following types of therapy:

    a. structured outpatient treatment

    b. structured inpatient treatment

    c. concurrent psychotherapy

2. Define psychological separation, and indicate how the concept may be useful in understanding how individuals separate from drugs.

3. Define and describe the status of dual diagnosis.

4. What risk factors are associated with dual-diagnosis status?

5. What problems does dual-diagnosis status present for assessment, conceptualization, and treatment planning?

6. State what special problems dual-diagnosis status presents for chemical dependence treatment among individuals with the following diagnoses:

    a. schizophrenia

    b. unipolar depression and bipolar disorder

    c. personality disorders

7. What are the ABCs of RET?

8. What strengths (and weaknesses) does RET bring to chemical dependence treatment?

9. What is Gestalt therapy?

10. What strengths and weaknesses does Gestalt therapy bring to chemical dependence treatment? With specific reference to the example of Ruth, why might Gestalt therapy be usefully integrated with RET?

DYSFUNCTIONAL PERSONALITY STYLES AND APPROACHES

Style and Positive Aspect	Behavior/Thoughts in Session	Possible Family History	Predicted Current Relationships	Possible Treatment Approach
Paranoid It is important to watch out for injustice	Suspicious, takes remarks out of context and interprets them to support own frame of reference	Probable history of persecution, active family rejection	Controlling behavior, anticipates exploitation quick to anger, may mistrust friends and family	Always be honest, never defensive; structure ahead of time; don't argue, you'll only lose
Schizoid It is useful to be a loner or independent of others at times	Relationship with therapist fragile, constricted body stance, little emotion shown, problems accepting support	Cold family; received little affection, rewarded for being alone and on own, may be identified patient in otherwise normal family	Loner; few friends, superficial relationships	Be consistent, warm supportive—no pressure; social skills training may be helpful
Schizotypal Ability to see things differently than others see them	Ideas of reference, social anxiety, odd magical beliefs, odd behavior, limited affect, distant, vague	Chaotic family style; family anxious/ambivalent with mixed messages, combination of intrusion/rejection	Loner; no close friends, perhaps an unusual or "different" peer group	Same as above; behavior may be seen as engulfing; important to maintain verbal tracking on single topic
Antisocial It is sometimes necessary to be impulsive and take care of our own needs	Acts out; cannot sustain task, involved in crime, drugs, truancy, physical fights; cruel, maltreats family; tries to "con" therapist	Probable abuse as child; avoidant family forced child to take matters into own hands; little affection in home	Abusive, exploitive relationships; fear of abandonment	Be open, honest, and set clear limits; avoid entanglement; expect client to leave treatment if you get close
Borderline Intensity in relationships is desirable at times	Pushes therapist's "buttons" skillfully; impulsive, intense anger or caring, suicidal gestures	Enmeshed family during early childhood; lack of support for individuation; probable sexual abuse	Serial, intense relationships; may have close friends, relationships may move rapidly between extreme closeness and distance	Confront engulfment and support individuation—that is, do opposite of family; group/systems approaches are useful

Histrionic All could benefit at times with open access to emotions	Seeks reassurance; seductive, concerned with appearance, too much affect; self-centered, vague conversation	Enmeshed, engulfing family, with little support for individuation; possible sexual abuse/seduction; little family expectation for accomplishment; aware of others not of self	Similar to the borderline without the externalized anger; Actions directed inward rather than outward	Encourage individuation; use assertiveness, skills training; consciousness raising; examine history of problem; use cognitive-behavioral and systems interventions
Narcissistic A strong belief in ourselves is necessary for good mental health	Grandiose, self-important, sees self as very unique; sense of entitlement; lacks empathy, oriented toward success and perfection	Received perfect mirroring for accomplishments rather than for self; engulfing family; child enacts family's wishes; anxious/ambivalent caregiver	Focuses on selfish needs, tends to engulf others with needs; is charming to get wishes met, Don Juan type, may pair with borderline.	Interpret behavior; look to past; employ cognitive-behavioral, systems, sensitivity training in a group
Avoidant It is useful to deny to avoid some things	Avoids people, shy; unwilling to become involved; distant, exaggerates risk	Either engulfing family or avoidant family; enacting what the family modeled	Not many friends; easily becomes dependent on them or therapist	Use many behavioral and cognitive techniques, assertiveness training and relaxation training useful
Dependent We all need to depend on others	Dependency on therapist even outside of session; indecision, little sense of self	Engulfing, controlling family; not allowed to make decisions; rewarded for inaction, told what to do	Dependent on friends; drives people away with demands	Reward action, support efforts for self, use paradox, assertiveness techniques
Obsessive-Compulsive Maintaining order and a system is necessary for job success	Perfectionistic and inflexible; focuses on details, making lists, devoted to work; limited affect, money oriented, indecisive	Overattached family that wanted achievement; oriented to perfection, like narcissist, but keenly aware of others with a limited sense of self	Controlling, limited affect, demands perfection from others, hard worker; cries at sad movies	Reflect and provoke feeling, orient to client's personal needs, support development of self-concept, orient to body awareness
Passive-Aggressive All of us are entitled to procrastinate at times	Procrastination; seems to agree with therapist, then undercuts; seems to accept therapist, but then challenges authority	Perhaps obsessive family; individual instead moves away from perfectionism and fights back; a more healthy defense needs to be developed	"Couch potato," skilled at getting back at and at criticizing others; defends by doing nothing; resents suggestions not pleasant on the job	Let them learn the consequences of their behavior; do not do things for them, but confront and interpret and pay special attention to their reactions.

From *Developmental Strategies for Helpers*, by A. E. Ivey, published by Brooks/Cole Publishing. Copyright © 1991 Allen E. Ivey. Reprinted with permission.

6

FAMILY DYNAMICS AND TREATMENT

Family treatment has come of age. There are several dominant, overlapping theoretical approaches to family therapy. Chemical dependence clinicians should familiarize themselves with the classic works of the contextual, systems, and structural treatment theorists, including Boszormenyi-Nagy and Spark (1973), Boszormenyi-Nagy and Krasner (1986), Bowen (1978), Haley (1973, 1984), Minuchin (1974), Satir (1972, 1976), and Satir, Stachowiak, and Taschman (1975). Even though family therapy has made great strides, our experience indicates that therapy with severely dysfunctional substance-abusing families is much more complex, difficult, and indecisive of outcome than classical descriptions would suggest.

Estes and Heinemann (1977), Kaufman (1992), and the U.S. Department of Health and Human Services (1993) gathered the following daunting statistics about chemically dependent families: Approximately 90% of mothers in addicted homes are pathologically enmeshed with their children regardless of whether the identified patient is a spouse or child. Following an opposite and equally dysfunctional path, men's relationships with their wives and children in addicted homes are characterized by great emotional distance. Not surprisingly, therefore, approximately 70% of alcoholic men are still living at home with their mothers or other female relatives at age 22, and 50% are still doing so at age 30. High levels of enmeshment and economic dependence are also indicated by the fact that women are four times more likely to stay in a marriage with an alcoholic husband than men are likely to stay with an alcoholic wife. Also, a woman's standard of living typically falls dramatically after she divorces an alcoholic husband, whereas a man's standard of living usually rises after he divorces an alcoholic wife. Finally, confirming the family disease component of addictions (which does not, of course, diminish the great importance of genetic transmission but, rather, reinforces it), more than 50% of all addicted people had parents who were addicted (60% among alcoholics); 50% of adult children of alcoholics (ACOAs) become alcoholics (versus 10% of non-ACOAs); and approximately 50% of ACOAs marry chemically dependent partners (versus 13% of non-ACOAs). Clearly, children of chemically dependent parents are at great risk for a variety of chemical dependence and other psychological problems (Buelow, 1995; U.S. Dept. of Health and Human Services, 1993).

FAMILY CHEMICAL DEPENDENCE THERAPY

Even though empirical data on family dysfunctions in chemically dependent homes is plentiful, the literature evaluating and comparing the efficacy of therapy techniques for alcoholic and drug-addicted families is small (Buelow, 1994b; Cawthra, Borrego, & Emrick, 1991; Kaufman, 1992). Even so, family chemical dependence therapy has great rewards not only for families, but for well-trained family therapists as well. Therapists derive rewards from their role in a social revolution within a previously closed system, one in which the future of an entire group may take a different and more productive course. Not only do individuals get better, but future generations are deeply affected in a positive way. Compared with treatment for the identified patient alone, family treatment has been found to double the identified patient's success in both initial treatment compliance and long-term abstinence (Kaufman, 1992).

Family treatment, which is a specialized form of group therapy, is complex not only because the family unit may be quite large, but because the members are of different generations; have different values, attachments, and grudges; and possess greatly different levels of resilience and emotional health. Therapists do not get to handpick family members. Not only may other family members have drug problems that are on different trajectories (Steinglass, 1980), but family members may have personality disorders that greatly complicate the therapeutic process.

The family is also the most difficult of therapy groups in which to quickly create new problem-solving capacity because the family generally has a long and successful history of protecting itself by sabotaging outside influence. Family members have deeply embedded agendas in dealing with one another and with society at large. These agendas are often covert (Boszormenyi-Nagy & Krasner, 1986). In addition, family members' manipulations of one another not only have general psychological aims (such as power) and aims of creating drug-enabling structures (such as co-dependence in others), these manipulations also encompass tangible financial, spatial, sexual, and occupational payoffs that must be addressed in therapy.

Criteria for Success

As we find when we assess process research generally, evaluations of family treatment are often indeterminate. Some members appear to be better, whereas some may indicate that they feel unchanged or worse. How are we to evaluate such a diverse overall social unit? Clearly, different people get better differently in different settings—a fact that is often baffling for beginning therapists. What will count as summative data for improved family functioning: self-reports by individual family members? Outside evaluation of group process by experts? Further, how long does improvement last before we legitimately strike our tents and declare our work a success? A month? A year? Ten years? Although self-reports of improvement ("we believe our family is better") and objective assessment of specific family characteristics (such as the duration of the identified patient's sobriety) are important, they often lack much of the rich detail found in more ethnographic, natural-history research approaches to family process (Steinglass, 1980; Vaillant, 1983).

Whatever type of evaluation is used, our view is that family chemical dependence treatment should be judged successful only when three general criteria have been met. First, the family has developed and fully accepted sobriety values as a part of their active daily life. Second, the family has developed new and more effective (and verifiable) problem-solving mechanisms and behaviors to deal with individual and group threats of enabling, codependency or dysfunctional dependency, relapse dynamics, sexuality, and power. Third, drinking and drugging behavior has been accepted as a primary psychiatric as well as behavioral concern, one that will not mysteriously disappear if the family system and attendant interaction improves. Unless these three criteria are met, family chemical dependence treatment is rarely a long-term success.

Family chemical dependence treatment must focus effectively and explicitly on the development of knowledge, values, and problem-solving skills that are self-renewing. For example, a willingness to allow more open communication within the family means that democracy must be more highly valued on the one hand (the values domain), but also that techniques are learned to assure that everyone has a fair say in daily affairs (the action domain). By *fair,* we mean that each member's opinion is given a weight that is appropriate for the member's age and level of cognitive and emotional development.

To achieve continued development, values must be activated and supported by action. Conflict management is a learned skill that will deteriorate if family participants do not accept and value interpersonal democracy—that is, basic equity in views and feelings. Action is reinforced in turn by the development of new values that support action. Values clarification leads to the development of new social, interpersonal skills; at the same time, skill development leads to changes in values. Never underestimate the importance of supervised action in the here and now of therapy.

FAMILY DYSFUNCTION

The family (and especially the extended family) possesses great power to heal its members when they are hurt, troubled, or inadequate. The family also has the power, the time, and the resources to continually reinforce emotional problems and deviance. The family exerts its power through its many voices, its formative influence over social and sexual role development, and its enforcement of behavioral rules, particularly those concerning the use of alcohol and other drugs. Families are the bane and the blessing of our existence. They can exert a powerful negative influence on therapy by encouraging members' movement toward socially disapproved and deviant roles and values. Fortunately, adequate family treatment and family-supported individual treatment can move members quickly toward mental and emotional health; families can thus also be powerful forces for positive change. Understanding how to provide meaningful care requires, first, that we recognize the effects that members' chemical dependence has on the family as a functioning unit and, second, that we understand the reciprocal influence of the family on children's likelihood of abusing and becoming dependent on drugs.

Among late adolescents, 50% today routinely describe their families as dysfunctional (Buelow, 1990). Although resilient (hardy) individuals often survive dysfunctional family backgrounds to live relatively normative lives, a significant and growing number do not. Substance use and abuse play a significant role in a majority of family problems. Boyer (1989) and the U.S. Dept. of Health and Human Services (1993) reported that one-third of all American families have an immediate member with an alcohol or other drug problem, and drugs are implicated in 50% to 90% of cases of domestic violence, including a majority of physical and sexual crimes against children in the home. Drugs also play an important part in violent and inappropriate sexual behavior between siblings and among other children who may reside in a blended home. Alcohol and drug abuse plays a central role in the organization (or, more aptly perhaps, disorganization) of the family in as many as half of families seen in family therapy. In many severely dysfunctional chemically dependent families, criminal activities, drug abuse, child sexual exploitation, and prostitution have been socialized into the family over generations and have become ways of life for entire kin groups (Buelow, 1994b). Children of drug-abusive homes or adult children of alcoholics or addicts have at least four times the risk of developing a substance abuse problem themselves. Because members of drug-abusive homes tend to marry others like themselves, these already bad odds are greatly magnified. In short, most dysfunctional individual behavior originates in a dysfunctional family.

Families that have a chemically dependent member are often found to be dysfunctional in a variety of other ways as well, even when family members do not actively support drug abuse. Cawthra, Borrego, and Emrick (1991) pointed out that in such families, other family members tend to be emotionally uninvolved with the drug-abusing client and, often, with one another as well. They are inconsistent in communications about the drug use behavior and usually completely uneducated about the disease theory (or any other substantive theory) of drug dependence. They also have no clear concern about relapse dynamics, and they communicate poorly. Neglect of spouses and children is common in dysfunctional, chemically dependent families, and punishment, rather than reward, forms the basis of family behavioral control. Chemically dependent families also have been noted to have rigid rules, to be chaotic, to show poor cohesion and adaptability over time, and to have disturbed boundaries among members (Preli, Protinsky, & Cross, 1990; Sexias & Youcha, 1985; Steinglass, 1980). The roles other family members take on to cope with chemical dependence in the family often represent attempts to replace the drug-abusing member (Ziter, 1989). Children often take over parental roles and responsibilities (parentification), separate from the family early (or run away from home), or are scapegoated by the family (Buelow, 1990; Potter & Williams, 1991). Typical scapegoating involves blaming specific children for the problems, usually children who oppose family problems by acting out.

Even though alcohol and other drug *use* among family members may be a symptom of other family dysfunction, chemical *dependence* is not. Unfortunately, the symptomatic view of drug use is often improperly generalized to chemical dependence in the popular self-help literature on family systems. Clearly, drug dependence must be treated as a primary, concurrent problem. Even though peer-supported drug *abuse* among children and adolescents often stems from family modeling, chemical dependence develops from the addictive potential of the drug itself, in combination with the specific psychological and physiological features of the drug-dependent family member. Treating family dysfunction, therefore, may or may not impact the member's drug use. The more the family is dysfunctional in ways besides drug dependence, and the longer the dependence cycle has been in action, the more difficult the job of assessing the interrelationships between the family dysfunction and chemical dependence. Developing a genogram—an in-depth structural outline of the family's historical association with drugs and psychiatric problems—is of important assistance in assessing the etiology of chemical dependence problems and in beginning the family's education about chemical dependence.

Family systems therapy that does not pay specific attention to drug-dependent members, as well as to the drug itself, is not likely to be effective over the long run (Cawthra, Borrego, & Emrick, 1991). Chemically dependent clients must be treated not only as symptomatic members of a larger group, but as individuals with a drug problem. The converse is also true: We cannot provide highly professional care for chemical dependence without attending to family functioning and enmeshment. Family therapists must be taught how to intervene and work effectively with specific members' denial dynamics. Family therapists should also know how and when to refer clients (individual family members as well as the identified patient) to structured and concurrent treatment. Chemically dependent clients may also need specific treatment for concurrent psychiatric problems as well, many of which do not have their etiological roots in family dysfunction but in family genetics (such as schizophrenia or bipolar disorder; Buelow & Hebert, 1995). To work more effectively with chemically dependent family members, therapists should understand the complex nature of dual diagnosis and the relapse dynamics that are likely to result. Unfortunately, few graduate programs in marriage and family counseling require specific substantive training in chemical dependence treatment.

Enabling and Denial

Successful treatment of chemically dependent families is an extension of structured intervention techniques. Interventions are successful when they undermine family members' enabling and denial of the addiction syndrome. Treatment differs from intervention in several ways, however. First, whereas intervention is not aimed at resolving family conflict, and possibly even accelerates conflict, longer-term family therapy continues the developmental process by teaching individuals to communicate more effectively and to resolve conflicts. Second, whereas interventions are usually focused in the here and now on giving the identified patient an accurate picture of the effects of his or her drinking or drugging on other family members, longer-term family treatment allows individuals to express their historical resentments, angers, drug abuse triggers, and addiction fears. Third, family members must be allowed time to focus away from the identified patient so they can discuss their own propensity to use alcohol or other drugs to deal with their feelings of anger, alienation, sorrow, grief, and hatred. Fourth, therapy allows the family to move away from the almost exclusively cognitive focus of the first few weeks of treatment and into more affective and experiential techniques designed to decrease enabling and flight from affect—including, for example, psychodrama and family sculpting.

Enabling is a process in which the emotions, cognitions, and behaviors of other family members or peers protect the drug abuser from the consequences of drug use. Enabling stems from attempts to adapt to drug use, rather than to confront and oppose it. Examples include buying alcohol for the dependent family member; paying fines or bail; driving the abuser after he or she has lost a driver's license and continues to drink; comforting the abuser for losses; intervening with others; explaining, or explaining away, problems; altering plans or feelings to help compensate for drug-induced deficiencies; or denying the effects on others of the abuser's behavior. Examples of nonenabling behavior include going on with one's life, setting up a professional intervention, forming a bottom line and sticking to it, not denying the effect of the drug use on you and others, and finding and using therapeutic supports.

Adaptation and Community Standards

A family can be said to be dysfunctional, first, when it can no longer adapt successfully to current stress and, second, when the adaptations it makes are considered inappropriate or abnormal by the family's community. The first definition is formative and functional; that is, it is based on the family's ability to react appropriately and meaningfully (to support itself economically, for example). The second definition is summative and authoritative; that is, it is based on ethical and legal standards of the community at large. Of course, some families that do not meet community ethical expectations—those headed by single mothers or involving a homosexual or polygamous union, for example—are successful adaptations even though others in the community would consider them dysfunctional. These minority families get the family job done, even though their relationships are atypical. In most states, alternative family styles are protected by law unless it can be shown that they endanger children. So far no research has found that children from families with alternative lifestyles are disadvantaged.

In contrast, many families that look like they fit our European, African, Native, or Asian American definitions of family in fact may be adaptationally dysfunctional. These families look as if they are making it, but they are not. Families that have been able to hide their chemical dependency problems fall into this latter group. Their ability to adapt and to help their children develop has been eroded or blocked.

Understanding what adaptational skills a family must have requires a deep understanding of the ethnic background from which the family's values have developed. It is particularly important to understand the potential dissonance between a family's ethnically based value system and the value system of the wider culture surrounding the family, as well as the ways that dissonance may be or is being played out in treatment. Even though each ethnic group has somewhat different central concerns, each family can adapt completely to only a limited number of values. For our purposes, how families adapt to values regarding alcohol and drug use and abuse is the central concern. To understand a family's values specifically, you must not only gain information from observing family interaction, but also ask family members how treatment is affecting and is being affected by their values. Do not assume that, because family members are cooperating, they must agree with your values about treatment. When in doubt, and at regular intervals, ask.

Family Structure

Family structure is made up of consistently recurring interactions concerning rules, roles, interpersonal boundaries, communication, power, and responsibilities. Each of these patterned interactions among family members can further the family's stability and resiliency as a social unit, or instead inhibit the family's adaptability. In dysfunctional families, rules are enforced in a rigid, authoritarian manner, or inconsistently but harshly. Functional families, in contrast, consistently show age-appropriate democracy in the development of rules. Rules are applied consistently and in an authoritative manner ("do as I say *and* do"), as opposed to an authoritarian one ("do as I say, regardless of what I do") (Bloom, 1985; Maltzman & Schweiger, 1991). After all, we are training young people to live in a democratic society, where responsibility, fairness, and consistency are cardinal virtues regardless of cultural background.

Family role expectations must be appropriate to children's age, gender, and level of psychosocial development. Children must be taught to follow socially structured roles in a flexible and creative way. Over-identification with particular family roles, even those that are positive at specific ages (for example, the role of helping parents with siblings), may preclude family members' shifting to new roles as new interpersonal demands arise (Nardi, 1981; Potter & Williams, 1991). Poor role definition often leads to boundary problems because interpersonal rules, a significant component of role performance, are not consistently followed.

Boundaries among family members in functional families are sanctioned (specified) by the community, and are both affectively and cognitively grounded. Usually such boundaries make good sense both emotionally and rationally (an example is the incest taboo). In more functional families, children's physical and emotional space is not invaded, and children's rights and powers within the family are appropriate to children's developmental level and are arbitrated by parents. As rights accrue, so do responsibilities, so that children learn to work for the good of the family as a whole, not only in their own self-interest. Rules, roles, and boundaries cannot be maintained unless communication among family members is clear, effective, and continual (Bloom, 1985; Boszormenyi-Nagy & Spark, 1973; Boszormenyi-Nagy & Krasner, 1986; Buelow, 1990; Hoffman, 1984). Communication includes not only what is spoken between family members, but what is not spoken, what should be spoken, what is consciously and unconsciously withheld from others, and what is meant by what is said.

Assessing Family Functioning

A large literature documents the etiology of family dysfunction in our society, and a variety of instruments have been developed to measure family dysfunction. These instruments include the Family Environment Scale (FES; Moos & Moos, 1981), the Family Concept Q Sort (FCQ; Van Der Veen, 1965), the Family Adaptability and Cohesion Evaluation Schedule (FACES; Olson, Bell, & Portner, 1978), the Family Assessment Measure (FAM; Skinner, Steinhauer, & Santa-Barbara, 1983), and the Family Function Inventory (Bloom, 1985). For all these measures, family assessment includes at least three primary dimensions: relationship, including pride in the family, belonging, conflict resolution, communication, and interpersonal boundary definition; personal growth, including individuation within the family, gratification from social interaction, family idealization or how much the family is prized, and the ability to disengage and reengage constructively; and system maintenance or structure, including control, hierarchy, rigidity of rules, level of involvement (enmeshment concerns), and governance. Governance ranges on a continuum from the positive side, democratic and authoritative, to the more negative side, totalitarian and authoritarian. In their allocation of political power, families also range between stasis on the one end and adaptiveness on the other. Families that are static do not make room for children's growing needs for individuation and control. Let us look more closely at each of these important areas.

Relationship   In more functional families, conflict is effectively regulated through face-to-face interaction among family members. Families with high levels of conflict usually have low commitment to family goals (or completely lack shared goals). Although moderate levels of late adolescent conflictual independence are important to continued psychological separation, high levels of conflict within the family are destructive to interdependence and symptomatic of major dysfunction. Drinking and drugging not only engenders family conflict, but immediately lowers impulse control among members so that outbursts are more frequent and more violent.

Interpersonal boundaries must be clear and cooperatively maintained if families are to function well. Boundary conflicts can arise, and boundaries can become permeable to inappropriate intimacies, when children do not play family roles appropriate to their ages. In dysfunctional families, there is no regular graduation to roles vacated by older children, so younger children conflict with older siblings for scarce resources, including social position. Children may also end up taking care of their parents in what is termed parentification. Parentification further erodes personal boundaries and impedes role development in both the family and the wider community. Parentification also leads to psychological and physical incest (Buelow, 1994b). Because of its erosive effect on impulse control, chemical dependence complicates this already depressing picture.

Personal Growth   Personal growth includes the many contingent processes by which children move through age-appropriate developmental periods into and through adulthood. The periods that appear most critical to identity development include, first, the phase of early infant attachment and exploration (Bowlby, 1973; Mahler, Pine, & Bergman, 1975); second, the consolidation of ego and superego during childhood (Freud's oedipal stage); third, late adolescent psychological separation from parents and individuation (Blos, 1979; Erickson, 1963; Gavazzi & Sabatelli, 1990; Hoffman, 1984); and, fourth, early adulthood and the formation of marriage attachments (Hazan & Shaver, 1987; Shaver & Clark, 1994).

Children's later individuation is negatively affected when primary caregivers fail to provide support for exploration, closeness, and warmth (Ainsworth, 1989). Children who are abused, neglected, or emotionally unsupported are insecure, overly dependent, compulsively self-reliant, or anxiously ambivalent in their attachments to others (Bowlby, 1973). They often see others as inaccessible and unresponsive to their needs (Bartholomew & Horowitz, 1991), and their ability to develop both emotional autonomy and interdependence is constricted or absent. Such children are frequently unable to trust and often stuck in their psychosocial development at the stages of trust versus mistrust and autonomy versus shame and doubt.

Structure   Dysfunctional families are frequently both overly controlled on the one hand and highly disorganized on the other. Parents are inflexible with children, yet laissez-faire in their application of rules. This arbitrary structure undermines commitment to larger family goals, esprit de corps, and family idealization (Bloom, 1985). Children may know that they do not want to raise their children as they were raised, but without support and guidance they may fall into the same web of over-control, arbitrary and severe punishment, and emotional neglect. Dysfunctional parenting is authoritarian (based on coercion) rather than authoritative (based on information and respect). The discouragement of opposing views and voices acts to further block dissent at a time when children should be developing emotional autonomy. Lack of autonomy leads either to dysfunctional dependence (codependence) or counterdependence (compulsive self-reliance). Rather than face their children's growing needs for autonomy and control, parents often become more perfectionistic and behaviorally punitive, while at the same time more emotionally disengaged. Such parents do not meet children's or spouses' emotional needs. Even though severely dysfunctional families often remain intact for long periods, moving back and forth between codependence and fragmentation, children's idealization and commitment to the family are low. At the same time, conflict is usually high, communication is distorted, and impulses are out of control.

Using the following example, we will look at the development of important components of family relationships, including boundaries, enmeshment, parentification, conflict, and alliances; and structure, including rules and roles.

◆ DIMENSIONS OF FAMILY DYSFUNCTION: A CASE HISTORY ◆

Bob and Ann married while they were sophomores in college, and Ann went to work as a secretary to help support the family while Bob completed his engineering degree. From the middle class, Ann's family thought she had married a bit beneath her, even though Bob was bright and ambitious.

Ann's parents were demanding, judgmental, and overly controlling of their only child. Ann grew up as a popular overachiever. Her family was not warm, however, and even though she made friends easily, she was lonely a good deal of the time as a child. Ann recalled depending on her friends for courage and self-esteem.

Bob's large family farmed, cut timber, and raised cattle on leased land. He had four brothers and two sisters who were very close. All of the men and many of the women in his family hunted, fished, and drank heavily. They had many social gatherings that were boisterous and, sometimes, argumentative. Bob's father died of a heart attack soon after Bob's marriage, and Bob's brothers continued to run the family farm together.

After graduation, Bob landed an excellent engineering job in a large southern city with a major aerospace company. He worked hard, was well liked, and advanced rapidly in the company. Bob's son was born the year of his graduation, and three girls were born at two-year intervals. Bob worked hard and played hard. After work he usually spent an hour drinking beer with other engineers at a local bar, where they discussed design and manufacturing problems. Bob often worked on weekends whether or not his section was behind on a project, and he unwound at night with television and mixed drinks.

Wrapped up with the children, Ann did not work outside the home. She devoted·her energy to her children and to her husband. She controlled the home and the children with a strong hand, and the children filled the loneliness that Ann had felt as a teenager. Although she was at a loss to explain why, Ann was not as close to Bob as she was to the children. She frequently found herself defending them, especially her son, Kyle, from Bob's

often lengthy criticisms, rude jokes, and impulsive physical antics. Bob was especially critical of his young son's communication and often made fun of a minor speech defect for
which Kyle was undergoing speech therapy.

Escalating each year along with his job advancement and compulsive overwork, Bob's
drinking led to more abusive criticism of both Ann and the children. It also led to health
problems, marital squabbles, and depression. When pressed about his health and drinking
problems, Bob admitted he felt that he would die as a young man like his father and that
abstaining from alcohol wouldn't buy him any more time. Unable to exert much control
over Bob or his drinking, Ann devoted more and more time to the children, wrapping herself up in their school lives and their problems with their father. Jean, the oldest girl, fought
her mother's intrusiveness and became closer and closer to her father and more distant
from her mother, whom she accused of meddling. She was the only child to whom Bob
paid special attention. When he had had too much to drink, Bob would obey her com-
mands as though she were an authority on all subjects.

At 38, Bob suffered his first heart attack, the result of alcoholic cardiomyopathy. Although he was told he was lucky to have survived the attack and that it was either caused
or greatly exacerbated by his drinking, Bob refused to acknowledge the contribution of alcohol to his health problems, blaming them on genetics. Usually depressed and unso-
ciable, Bob was asked to handle less and less important concerns at work. His work staff
gradually ebbed away, and he was shifted to the bookkeeping side of his engineering section. Bob's self-esteem suffered greatly. He blamed the company for abandoning him and
continued to work long hours. At night and on weekends, Bob drank himself to sleep in
front of the television.

Bob's interaction with his now teenage children was verbally combative. Ann found
herself constantly intervening between Bob and the children. During parental fights, Ann's
son began to come to her aid and even to threaten his father. Bob's favorite daughter,
Jean, often came to his aid, took care of him, cleaned up after him, and often stayed up
watching television, sometimes drinking with him. She also competed with Ann over care
of the younger children and argued with her over every facet of running the household.

Referred by their church pastor, Ann and the younger children began to go to Al-Anon
meetings. Although she came to better understand Bob's alcoholism, Ann could never
launch an effective intervention with her husband, who threatened her with separation if
she tried. With four teenage children and no job experience, Ann could look forward only
to poverty if she left. As long as she could hold on, she could keep her lifestyle, educate
her children, and try to put away some money in case Bob did separate from her or die.

Seven years later, after the children had all finished college or married, Ann gave Bob
an ultimatum: Get treatment or get out. To the great surprise of many who knew him well,
Bob sought help for the first time in his life.

After a 30-day inpatient therapy program, Bob made great progress in developing a
solid sobriety program. The center utilized a 12-step Alcoholics Anonymous format as part
of its formal group structure, as well as hosting community AA groups. Individuals worked
their way through the 12 steps of AA within their treatment groups.

After detoxification, Bob struggled for more than a week with his denial, blaming genetics for his health problems as he had all along. However, family week helped Bob make a
break with the past. Facing his family every day (and his boss on several occasions) over
the difficulties he was causing himself and others, Bob finally accepted responsibility for
his drinking. The final blow was a confrontation with his daughter, Jean, who had accepted

that she also had a problem with alcohol. She refused to bail Bob out. Kyle confronted his father over his abusiveness. Ann continued to hold to her bottom line that she would separate immediately if Bob began drinking again.

After inpatient therapy, Bob and Ann began couples therapy, which allowed them to recover some of the feelings that had brought them together in the first place. Although Bob never recovered his high status within his company, he kept his job and became a useful member of the engineering staff. Ultimately Ann was able to return to college herself. She received psychotherapy during the two years necessary to complete her degree. Ann realized that much of her lack of assertiveness in confronting Bob resulted from the relationship she had with her critical and domineering parents. Much of her treatment revolved around her parental issues. She also paid for her children to receive individual professional counseling and encouraged them to continue with their self-help ACOA groups.

Even though Bob and Ann differed significantly in social class and religious values, Bob's descent into alcoholism was the primary contributor to the relentless decline in the couple's ability to communicate, to resolve conflicts, to adapt to their children's changing needs, and to sustain emotional growth. Bob's growing dependence on alcohol also exacerbated preexisting but remediable problems in his personality. He became even more rigid and authoritarian. In keeping with her background, but also in reaction to Bob, Ann became more judgmental, enmeshed with her children for her emotional needs, angry at life, and codependent on Bob's problems for her own power base in the family. Personality characteristics that were only moderately problematic in adolescence were greatly distorted by years of negative, fruitless conflict. Ann discovered very early, for example, that Bob was more easily manipulated when he was drinking than when he was sober and irritable. Therefore, an important incentive to help him remain sober was absent, and Ann felt encouraged when Bob was drinking to exercise her often repressed need for control.

As their relationship eroded, Bob and Ann made allies among their children, becoming further and further enmeshed with them as the illness grew. Their daughter Jean took on a mothering role with her father in a process of parentification, including defending Bob while attacking her mother's inadequacy; Ann reacted by withdrawing. In response to Jean's caretaking, Bob gave his daughter complete freedom, while at the same time making even stricter demands on the other children, especially his son. Kyle, allied with his mother, defended her against Bob and Jean and rescued her emotionally. Even brighter than his father in math, Kyle achieved quick academic success, which insulated Ann from feeling as though she had been a total failure with her children.

As Jean and Kyle were elevated as equals to their parents, the intergenerational boundaries were crossed, and the children began to parent their parents. This lack of boundaries led to emotional enmeshment and, between Jean and her father, an emotionally sexualized although nonphysical relationship. Alliances with their children flourished as communication between Bob and Ann deteriorated. Through the use of their children, the parents were able to triangulate one another—that is, set the children up as a buffer against emotional interaction. The children began to play out a fixed and dysfunctional interpersonal script.

As these distorted interactions became the rule of the day, the parents' emotional growth stopped. Walled away from each other, with their children's allegiances split, parental roles became pathologically distorted, and their identity as parents was lost. As they began to lose their sense of identity, personality fragmentation accelerated.

Family Systems Theory

This case history clarifies several important problems that might arise in defining Bob and Ann's problems primarily in terms of systemic faults rather than chemical dependence. First, many family systems therapists might see Bob's drinking as a symptom of prior or present family dysfunction. In our view, however, causation was the other way around: Bob inherited a predisposition to alcoholism and became alcoholic because he drank. Alcoholism is the primary diagnosis. Bob's addicted drinking caused much of the family dysfunction. The family and marital problems that Bob and Ann developed certainly did not go away on their own after Bob received treatment, but until he reached a high-quality sobriety, these problems would never have gone away, no matter how much therapy the family received.

Some family therapists seem overly intent on the concept of homeostasis, or system equilibrium. Such therapists are likely to believe that the various symptoms (Jean's and Kyle's acting-out, for example) stem from the family's attempts to recover its balance. Unlike our bodies, however, families do not have a specific temperature or balance point at which they function optimally. Families are always out of simple equilibrium because they always are (or should be) changing to meet each member's evolving level of psychosexual development. A nuclear family is not itself an organism, although the analogy is a useful heuristic (but an oversimplification). Individuals are held in interpersonal proximity by thoughts, feelings, and behaviors, not by nerve, sinew, and bone. Unlike an individual, the family has no central processor or intrinsic central focus.

Our view is that notions of family balance or equilibrium, although they may be useful heuristics, are not analytic. Based on the assumption of equilibrium or a state of fine balance, family systems therapists are likely to believe that changes in one person or in one area within the system will inevitably affect everyone else. This truism can be verified in some respects, but it is clear that each person in the system is affected to greater or lesser degrees and with vastly different consequences. Our assessment difficulty with families is to determine exactly how each person is actually affected and to develop a treatment plan that will address these widely differing effects. An assessment of all individuals within the family, as well as the family as a whole, for example, requires a very detailed understanding of how power is actually allocated and exercised within the group and through the agency of specific individuals. A knowledge of one does not substitute for knowledge of the other.

EARLY, MIDDLE, AND LATE STAGE FAMILY TREATMENT

Therapy with drug-abusing individuals within families, then, can proceed either with the family together, with the abusive individual, or with the nonabusive members. Deciding with whom to work is critical and is the topic we will examine next.

Early Abusive Stage

Families in the early stage of alcohol and other drug abuse usually have one or more members who are abusing drugs, but the family continues to value sobriety and to be connected to other families who value sobriety. Many parents value sobriety because chemical dependence was a major destructive force in their own families of origin; they have made a pact with their partners not to re-create what they experienced as children in chemically dependent homes, and they stick to that pact. As having been ill with a particular virus protects one from coming down with that illness again, such parents may be to a certain degree inoculated against a replay of their experiences in their families of origin. Many ACOAs, however, do not view alcohol or other drug use itself as their family's central problem. They often believe that drug experimentation and use is normal, that drug overuse is a product of a marriage that is troubled, and that drug dependence is a form of chronic marital instability in which alcohol and other drugs play a contributing but not determining role. Unfortunately, growing up in a chemically dependent home does not provide enough protection against drug use for many (if not most) ACOAs.

Individual therapists see many couples and families in the early stages of chemical dependence dysfunction. With little training in alcohol and drug treatment, therapists are likely to help the partners work on better communication and conflict management, but often miss not only the rising level of drug use, but also the importance of underlying values and behaviors that do not support sobriety.

Individuals from dysfunctional and chemically dependent families most often marry people from similar social backgrounds. They seem to know one another immediately. Even though their backgrounds are very similar, however, their personalities are often complementary opposites: Dominants find submissives, exploiters find codependents, drug abusers find enablers (Kaufman, 1992). Marriages, therefore, are likely to be authoritarian, conflictual, and self-defeating. Although therapy must focus on alcohol and drug use as its central concern, it must also concurrently address basic personality differences and lack of identity development in both partners.

More functional families who have sought treatment in the early stages of chemical dependence are often able to develop self-interventions for their problems. Because they have normative role models in their own families of origin, they often know what they should be doing, but they need help working out how to do it. They need support and fundamental education about drugs, communication, conflict management, and tough love. Often, one or several members of the family must be referred to structured treatment. Family therapy should focus on reinforcing the identified patient's structured group work and AA, NA, or Rational Recovery support groups as well.

Assuming that the identified patient has been properly referred to structured treatment, the first step is to identify how drugs fit into the family's problems and to develop a plan for abstinence as a family. Family members are usually able to identify quickly what drugs have done to and for them. Second, members should explore their varying levels of commitment to the family (family idealization) and their willingness to commit to specific abstinence behaviors, new roles, and behavioral rules. Third, the counselor should help the family design, discuss, and commit to a contract that incorporates these commitments. Each family member and the family as a whole must have a clearly articulated action plan and bottom line about what they will do if other family members fail to take the contract seriously. Fourth, communication and conflict management should be guided during sessions and practiced at home during specific periods. The homework carried out during the week should be explored during subsequent therapy sessions. Fifth, codependence, enabling, relapse dynamics, dysfunctional roles, denial, and compensatory behaviors should be discussed and experientially worked through. Working through must involve each member of the family. Any family member, no matter how seemingly distant from the lines of power, can effectively sabotage a treatment plan established without unanimity and understanding.

In the early stages of family drug treatment, denial of drug abuse is relatively weak, but blame of others is strong. Compensatory mechanisms (such as the pursuit of sexual affairs when stress is high and alcohol is denied) frequently come into play. Systems problems are initially unclear in the early stages; members have difficulty thinking about the family as a functioning unit and want to pursue their own self-interest. The level of family idealization may be relatively high, but so may be levels of manipulation of other members. Children's compensatory dysfunctional role affiliations (heroic, disengaged, drug-using, scapegoated, or oppositional and defiant, for example) are becoming more fixed and stereotypic, but children remain able to grow and develop. In short, family members have resources and continue to use them in the early stage of chemical dependence dysfunction, but resources go more and more unused. Concurrent, structured outpatient treatment continues to have important therapeutic effects that facilitate family work. Education and guidance are usually successful if initial resistance (often sandbagging or dead weight) and sabotaging are dealt with constructively. A variety of family techniques are successful. However, the power of the drug and the power of individuals using the drugs should never be underestimated; therefore, the focus of therapy should never stray far or for long from the specific realities of drug use.

As the family begins to get better, members will repress their newly won understanding of the power that drugs hold for them. Perversely, the very act of getting better will lead to a suspicion that drugs were not the problem in the first place; that suspicion must be dealt with up front and frequently. Remember that every family will regress in subtle (or not so subtle) ways at some stage of treatment. Family members will lapse and relapse not only when they appear to be getting worse, but when they are clearly getting better.

Families who receive treatment during the early stages of chemical dependence have a relatively good prognosis. Our experience indicates that family recovery, like that of individuals, is subject to the thirds rule: About one-third of families reach a high quality of continued sobriety and development relatively quickly. A further one-third have members who lapse and relapse occasionally but know how to recover their direction, sometimes go back into structured treatment, and usually succeed as a group, even though members may drift into the middle, dependent stage of drug use. A final one-third of families do not reach a high-quality sobriety and do not recover, even though some individual members discontinue drug use. Drinking, polydrug use, and physical and sexual abuse of children become endemic in the family. Even though members divorce the family, they usually form other families with continued problems and severe dysfunctions.

Middle Dependent Stage

The middle dependent stage is characterized by the permeation of alcohol and other drugs into many (quickly becoming most) facets of daily family life. The family has become the primary enabling mechanism for the individual's continued self-esteem and drug use ("I must be OK; my family is still here! At least we're all in this together"). The active development of emotional dependence in spouses and children is necessary for continued dominance by the drug-dependent member. Compensatory family roles (scapegoats for the drug use, for example) become more rigid. Deviation from continually more rigid dysfunctional rules and roles is more often severely (physically, psychologically, or sexually) punished. Individual emotional development is becoming frozen. Systems problems have become deeply embedded, and continued distortions become necessary to maintain power over others. Both denial and blame are strong. More resilient children may have (successfully) walled themselves off from addicted family members, while more system-dependent members heroically attempt to save the family by parenting other family members, including the parents, or sacrificing themselves in some way for the good of the whole.

Although some middle-stage families come into treatment on their own, many are guided into the treatment system by the legal system (driving under the influence—DUIs), by employers (employee assistance programs—EAPs), or as a result of hospitalization due to chronic alcohol problems (often cirrhosis) and other drug-related concerns, including psychiatric and neurological symptoms.

Treatment for families in the dependent stage progresses very slowly or not at all unless those who are drug dependent have committed themselves to a structured treatment program. Although family treatment can form the basis for a successful intervention, treatment that includes drug-using family members should not be continued indefinitely unless the identified patient or patients are maintaining present and verifiable sobriety. Many families, of course, come into long-term family treatment following treatment of individual family members not only to resolve immediate lapse and relapse concerns, but to address dysfunctions that may not be directly attributable to chemical dependence.

Added to the techniques we discussed for early abusive stage families, working with middle dependent stage families often involves working with problems of grief and loss concerning both drugs and family idealization, as well as providing help with gaining employment, reestablishing normative social interaction with other families, uncovering deeply buried relapse triggers, redirecting dependence on the dysfunctional system toward self-responsibility, and confronting covert compensatory mechanisms and power alliances among members. Because blame is very powerful, and feelings of entitlement are often grandly inflated, family members want to be compensated for their prior struggles. Conflict, distancing, and the encouragement of relapse are often used to press for compensation. The family must decide what can be compensated and what cannot. Even though only high-quality continued sobriety can compensate for past drug dependence over the long run, specific compensations can be made and debts can be paid if they are recognized as just by the entire family unit.

As we find in working with clients who have personality disorders, strong affect should be accepted but used in the service of developing rational plans and behavioral contracts. For example, you might respond to the expression of strong emotion as follows: "If you feel so strongly about this, what are you willing to do to change the situation?" Working through feelings (usually, bad ones) involves not only facilitating catharsis, as a first step, but also helping clients learn to use emotions in the service of understanding (self-exploration) and action (motivation).

Ceremonial reentry into the family after structured inpatient treatment can serve a positive, supportive aim. Symbolic activities (reexchange of marriage vows, for example) should be preceded, however, by express verbal acceptance that lapses and relapses are common and that intensive family therapy will follow release. Because most structured programs include a concurrent family treatment week, each member should be aware of the potential conflicts that may arise when the identified patient returns home. There is usually a brief honeymoon because everyone is on their best behavior. But after several weeks the family members begin to seethe with many interpersonal problems similar to those they had before the identified patient received treatment. Because of their newly learned willingness to own up to problems with one another, family therapy often makes some of its greatest gains during the post-euphoria doldrums. Members want to look forward, even though they may be looking through rose-colored glasses, and interaction is painful enough to make changes appear preferable to stasis, as in fact they are.

Late Deteriorative Stage

Families that are in the late deteriorative stage of chemical dependence are often fragmented or self-absorbed. Addicted members are physically and emotionally ill. Both parents and children may strongly defend behavior that compensates for the drug dysfunction (with children supporting their parents financially, for example), or members may have scapegoated and ejected some members from the family. Without strategic intervention, the addicted individuals and the family itself will die of their illness. Dysfunctional dependencies, exploitation, and enabling are deeply entrenched. Family members who have escaped may have already developed dysfunctional support systems of their own, while being drawn back to the family they have left like moths to a flame.

Interventions among families in the deteriorative stage most often occur because the group comes to the attention of a social service agency due to child abuse or neglect, criminal activity, or illness. Members are often hospitalized due to severe drug-related psychiatric and health problems. Typical alcohol-related illnesses include liver dysfunction (cirrhosis), delirium tremens (DTs), and heart problems (alcoholic cardiomyopathy); intravenous drug-related health problems can include hepatitis and acquired immune deficiency syndrome (AIDS). Medical facilities often refer chemically dependent patients to in-house facilities for concurrent psychiatric treatment until they are ready for chemical dependence therapy.

Clearly, families with members in the late stages of addictions are faced with enormous difficulties, whether or not the identified patient recovers. Medical, legal, and economic stresses are often insurmountable over the short run. Private therapists working with families in this stage should take a consultative and educative role, teaching the family the fundamental facts of chemical dependence, encouraging the involvement of the family with the identified patient while he or she is in treatment and especially during any formal periods when family members are brought into the treatment facility to encourage, support, and confront the client. Therapists working independently with the family should build close ties with treatment center and other psychiatric personnel when that is feasible and make themselves available when possible to visit the center or hospital with the family.

FAMILY WEEK IN STRUCTURED TREATMENT

Family week within structured outpatient or inpatient treatment is a time for emotional support and confrontation within the family. This time can be a very real agency for change and should begin the client's psychic reentry into the family. Usually taking place during the third week of 30-day inpatient structured treatment, and during the fourth or fifth week of intensive outpatient treatment, family week focuses on both the practical and the symbolic acceptance of the client back into a changed and reinvigorated family system—a family that should be making concurrent treatment progress. This reentry entails supportive confrontation of clients about the effects of their denial and the family's enabling, how family members intend to change their enabling behaviors, and how family members intend to deal with lapses. The family's bottom lines concerning relapse should be a central focus of discussion. Although threats should be avoided, bottom lines should be explored in detail.

Family week is a time of emotional sharing and necessary catharsis. The emotional level rarely needs to be raised artificially. At least two therapists, and sometimes more, should be available to the group at all times. Depending on the center's policy, entire families usually meet all morning for one week. Some families may also meet for a debriefing during the afternoon without the identified patient as well. The family treatment group may be composed of as many as three families, or about 12 group members, who begin therapy together so that families can learn from one another's experiences but not be dominated by "old-timers." Clients undergoing the stress of family week often bring their family issues back into their afternoon individual treatment group. Although clients should be given group support and allowed time for appropriate synthesis, they must be shown how to focus on their immediate stress and relapse issues, rather than focusing on family issues that might better be taken back to their family group sessions. This is a complex set of reciprocal counseling concerns, and group leaders must exercise discretion about which topics should be referred back and which should be explored in greater detail.

Preparation and Ground Rules

Clients' readiness for family week is usually discussed at a meeting attended by their counselors, the clinical supervisor, and the director and therapists of the family program. Clients who may be excluded from the routine family week rotation are those with special problems and needs, including dual-diagnosis clients who are not experiencing good medication regulation; clients who may have left against medical advice at some point during their treatment; clients who have failed a drug screen; particularly difficult, disruptive, and manipulative clients (especially those with narcissistic or antisocial personality disorders); families who are clearly disintegrating or in which the client is facing incarceration subsequent to treatment. These clients with special needs often meet with their families and older children without other family groups present and with at least two therapists to facilitate the interaction.

Prior to family week, family members should meet with the therapist or therapists who will lead the group. During this time members are reminded of important ground rules. First, confidentiality issues are explained. Since more than one family may be present, complete confidentiality cannot be assured, and members need to be periodically reminded of this fact. Groups may contract with one another to keep what is said in the treatment room, but such contracts have little legal force. Also, if incest or other child abuse issues are central to a family's therapy, the family may need to meet with a therapist (and a representative of child protective services) alone. The family should always be made aware that the treatment center has a legal obligation to report child abuse to social services. In most cases, however, reports have already been made prior to family week. Children who are too young to understand the meaning and value of this emotion-laden time should not be included in the early cathartic period of family therapy sessions. Everyone, however, may attend sessions in which the family is on a positive course and in the process of emotional reunion. Who will be included should be discussed in full with the family's therapists and the therapists' supervisors.

Second, no bombshells should be dropped for manipulative purposes. Family week is not the time for the spouse to inform the client that the house has been sold, the divorce has taken effect, and that he or she has lost visitation rights with the children. Unilateral decisions of this nature should be discussed with the client during a couple's meeting that is supervised by someone on the staff who is close to the client and who is expert in crisis intervention. Family week is a time to try to bring the family back together, not provide legal distance. Families must also be encouraged to persist when the going gets rough. The family should not withdraw except to walk around outside and cool off.

Third, the family should be given reading material reinforcing the ground rules, especially describing how to establish therapeutic group norms, including owning feelings through use of "I" statements, nonabusively confronting, not enabling or rescuing, and giving support. Many centers provide self-help reading materials and preliminary guidance or therapy to help ready the spouse for family week.

Anger, Pain, and Learning

Families learn much during family week. They are able to observe the strengths and weaknesses of other families struggling with similar problems. They also observe their therapists' role modeling, including authenticity, supportive confrontation, and unconditional acceptance. Further, through role-playing, direct engagement, and other creative activities such as family sculpting, members are taught to interact more directly and to resolve conflicts more concretely. Finally, family members are allowed sufficient time to express their anger, loneliness, and pain, while at the same time being encouraged to accept these feelings and to forge a new sense of solidarity and purpose.

Family treatment can be volatile. Rage, pain, and blame will be expressed that cannot be deflected and should not be minimized but confronted head on. Families will feel grief and mourn losses. Family members must be encouraged and shown how to express their feelings without acting out physically and without using feelings as armor against change. Family members must learn to accept feelings as important information, to learn from them, and to move on. Families who have stuck together during interventions with the identified client usually have an excellent prognosis for coming through family week intact. They are then ready to continue therapy with a family treatment specialist outside the treatment center or as a part of extended center care. It is important for both the identified patient and other family members to sum up where they are in their treatment programs. The family members should be encouraged not only to express themselves emotionally, but to state their treatment and sobriety goals. Families who don't know where they want to go usually go nowhere. Members must be reminded to focus on how their interaction skills will help them reach their intended goals. For example, how is the family going to adjust itself to the client's sobriety? What current difficulties with sobriety can the family identify? What is family problem solving actually going to look like? How is role rigidity going to be tackled? How are alliances going to be broken down? How is triangulation to be avoided when someone wants power? All of these questions should be the subject of ongoing family counseling that uses family week as an initial model for constructive and sober family interaction.

In conclusion, nothing can help prepare therapists to work in the drug counseling field as quickly as working as a cotherapist during family week. This experience is crucial to understanding how both group and individual treatment must be focused so that clients can gain the skills to effectively reenter their families. Although we have not explored in detail the many constructs used by family treatment specialists, the reader should personally evaluate the family literature to better understand and use these concepts, including (1) multidirected partiality (joining, alliances, and triangulations); (2) entitlements; (3) invisible loyalties; (4) structural, systems, and transactional analysis; (5) family genograms; (6) relapse dynamics; and (7) personal boundaries and parentification.

STUDY AND DISCUSSION QUESTIONS

1. What data about families might lead one to believe that family treatment is critical if treated clients are to remain abstinent?

2. Family chemical dependence treatment can be judged successful when three general criteria are met. What are those criteria, and why are they so critical?

3. Outline the cognitive, affective, behavioral, and structural problems that lead to family dysfunction in general and chemical dependence dysfunction in particular.

4. Define parentification and evaluate its importance.

5. What is family structure actually composed of?

6. Consistent with your particular theory of family therapy (contextual, for example), outline the steps you might use in confronting an entire family about its drug use.

7. Outline the progression of a family through the early to late deteriorative stages of chemical dependence, and suggest how you might function as a therapist entering the system during each major stage.

8. What is family week, and how might you help a family make the most of it?

9. Review and discuss the following family treatment outline.

Treatment Focus Timeline

a. *Weeks 1–2*: Work on weakening denial system through supportive confrontation, educate about dependence cycle, contract for nonescalation of conflict.

b. *Weeks 1–4*: Address enabling, educate about dependence cycle, teach regulation of conflict skills, develop further behavioral contracting as necessary to deescalate conflict.

c. *Weeks 1–6:* Work to reformulate relationships with drug-using friends, peers, and more remote family members.

d. *Weeks 3–6*: Consider new structural and emotional problems arising in the family as the client struggles to remain sober and in the here and now, especially those that appear to stem from the client's sobriety; continue to monitor conflict management scheme exercises in session.

e. *Weeks 4–8:* Excavate and examine in detail the emotional and cognitive-behavioral triggers each family member uses, set up self-monitoring of self-defeating ideation and behaviors.

f. *Weeks 4–8*: Work on esteem around family unit, continue to monitor conflict management and communication in session.

g. *Weeks 4–8*: Try family sculpting or other experiential techniques, move from predominantly cognitive to include some affective techniques, make a firm recommendation whether to refer the client (or clients) to structured treatment if that decision has not already been made.

h. *Weeks 8–16*: Move from more educative, consultative role to more involved role if and only if the client has developed sound sobriety.

Critical Assessment Decisions

a. Assess whether identified client is currently drinking and whether earlier intervention has been successful enough to elicit real change among members.

b. Assess the involvement of each family member and group as a whole with drug dependent behavior and loyalties (alliances).

c. Assess the strengths and weaknesses of the marriage bond, the degree of dependence or codependence of the spouse, the level of conflict and the mechanisms holding conflict in place (such as long-held resentments).

d. Assess the degree to which children are using drugs, roles they play in the family, abuse and incest.

e. Assess the degree to which individual psychopathology, especially more primitive types of personality disorders, schizophrenia, and manic depression, are holding the patterns static.

f. Assess family and member goals and the extent to which they are shared.

g. Assess the family's ability to resist peer and extended family influences at each generational level.

Treatment Decisions

a. Decide whether, how, and with whom individuals with severe pathology will be treated.

b. Decide whether you will work individually with any of the family members concurrent with family therapy.

c. Decide the level of confidentiality that will be maintained in working with individuals within the group if they triangulate you and level with the co-therapist who may be working with members.

Planning Decisions

a. Plan how to enter the system: as ally, as consultant?

b. Plan deescalation tactics and ground rules.

c. Plan for identified clients' slips and changes in impulse control among family members.

d. Plan for an end to the honeymoon phase.

7

CHILDREN AND ADULT CHILDREN
OF ALCOHOLICS AND OTHER
DRUG ABUSERS

It is estimated that the COA/ACOA risk group comprises approximately 30 million people, 7 million of whom are under the age of 18 (U.S. Dept. of Health and Human Services, 1993). It is also estimated that another 12.5% of all Americans (one in eight) are children of problem drinkers. About one in every three children, therefore, lives in a family where alcohol and other drug abuse is a serious problem. Taking into consideration the wide variety of emotional problems that flow from these addicted and problem homes and the toll they take, the most important risk is reflected in the fact that ACOAs are approximately four times more likely than non-ACOAs to become alcoholic. Between 40% and 50% of alcoholics have an alcoholic parent (Potter & Williams, 1991; Henderson, Albright, Kalichman, & Dugoni, 1994; U.S. Dept. of Health and Human Services, 1993; Roush & DeBlassie, 1989; Schuckit, 1985). The Children of Alcoholics Screening Test (CAST) is provided in Worksheet 7.1 at the end of this chapter, and the reader is encouraged to review the items in order to better understand significant diagnostic features.

Guided by the recovery of family members in Al-Anon, ACOA groups began to meet independently to share their common concerns long before they became an important treatment and research population among academic psychologists (Haaken, 1993). Anecdotal evidence from clinicians who facilitated ACOA groups during the 1970s indicated that both children and adult children of alcoholic and drug-abusing homes were at high risk for a wide range of emotional and behavioral problems (Black, 1981; Cermak & Brown, 1982; Wegscheider, 1981). Research was begun that compared COAs/ACOAs with groups of normal controls from normative families in which alcohol dysfunction did not exist. Although some researchers found no significant differences between COA/ACOAs and controls in such areas as personality (Calder & Kostyniuk, 1989) and self-reported problem solving and suicidal ideation (Wright & Heppner, 1991), others found significant differences in a variety of areas. As we previously indicated, the most critical concern—due principally to genetic predisposition—is that ACOAs are approximately four times more likely to develop alcoholism than non-ACOAs (Barnes & Welte, 1990; Cotton, 1978; U.S. Dept. of Health and Human Services, 1993; Schuckit, 1985). Further, COA/ACOAs have been found to be more anxious and depressed, to have lower self-esteem than those from normative homes (Bensen & Heller, 1987; Black, Buckey, & Wilder-Padilla, 1986), and to adjust less well in college (Buelow, 1990, 1995).

Although the weight of evidence indicates that ACOAs are at heightened risk for social and emotional problems, the more narrow question of whether ACOAs' psychiatric risks are greater than those who come from dysfunctional but non-alcoholic homes (DFs) has only recently been investigated. This question is especially important because ACOAs and DFs could be included in the same treatment and self-help groups if these populations do not differ in important ways. As we found in prior comparisons, the results depend on what characteristics are being measured, on the size and randomness of the sample, and on the treatment status of the sample. For example, although Hadley, Holloway, and Mallinckrodt (1993) found no differences between ACOAs and DFs in object relations deficits, self-expression, or emotional distress among a clinical sample, Buelow (1995) found that ACOAs from a non-clinical sample scored significantly higher than individuals from otherwise dysfunctional homes (DFs) on measures of alcoholism (Michigan Alcoholism Screening Test or MAST) and dysfunctional family role affiliation, and lower on measures of college adjustment and family functioning. Garbarino and Strange (1993) also found significant differences between ACOAs and DFs in family functioning and college adjustment. Apparently, even though their problems often differ in kind, the problems that ACOAs and DFs have in common occur at similar intensity.

What conclusions can be drawn from these research findings? First, there is little doubt among researchers and clinicians that ACOAs and children from dysfunctional families are at higher risk than those from normative and intact homes for personal and emotional, marital, academic, and career adjustment problems. Although ACOAs' personalities and temperaments (which have highly significant genetic determinants) do not appear to differ greatly from others, ACOAs have a greater variety of interpersonal deficits in communication, adult role development, ability to have their emotional needs met, and conflict resolution. Second, ACOAs clearly differ in significant ways from those who indicate their families are dysfunctional in other ways besides chemical dependence. Among college students, for example, ACOAs appear to have more social problems; they tend to play out the dysfunctional roles they played in their families with their college peers more often; and they tend to have riskier physical and interpersonal results when they drink or use other drugs than their DF counterparts do. By the time ACOAs and DFs present themselves for treatment intervention, however, their levels of distress and lack of family support may be roughly equivalent (Hadley, Holloway, & Mallinckrodt, 1993). Their distress may come from significantly different psychodynamic sources, however, and this difference may affect therapy in a variety of ways. These potential differences in clinical outcome need further empirical exploration.

TREATMENT CONCERNS

ACOAs are clearly a population at risk. The problems ACOAs face, however, are not always manifested early in life. Black, Buckey, and Wilder-Padilla (1986) pointed out that many ACOAs do not experience difficulties until they are in their late 30s, and their marriages and relationships with their children have deteriorated due to role dysfunction, faulty communication, conflict mismanagement, and lack of identity development. Contrary to Burk and Sher's (1990) belief that early identification and development of preemptive programs may harm ACOAs because of potential negative stereotyping, we believe that early identification and education are crucial. The theoretical risk entailed in alerting people to potential harm is vastly outweighed by the potential advantages of that knowledge. Historically, ACOAs have more often suffered from their ignorance than their knowledge. So far, we have never experienced a situation where a client entered therapy because of emotional problems stemming from being *labeled* an ACOA; all have entered therapy because of problems associated with *being* an ACOA!

Even though many ACOAs have no clearly demonstrable psychopathology that requires psychotherapy, we should not hastily dismiss the potential problems this group may suffer. Rather, we should be sensitized to the fact that ACOAs developed useful self-help groups independently of the therapy and research communities. We should be wary, therefore, of researchers' attempts to impose goals on this complex group without direct input from them. Further, given that a majority of prisoners in our jails come from families with long histories of alcohol and other drug dependence dysfunction, we would do well not to minimize the nonpsychiatric but nevertheless negative personal and social consequences that early identification might positively affect.

Fortunately, many people who come from substance-abusing families appear to be resilient in the face of their environmental stress. In fact, many have increased resistance to interpersonal stress because a side effect of their family problems was stress-inoculation training. Children adapt to stress through a variety of means, including affiliation with accepted family roles such as hero or scapegoat (Black, 1981; Nardi, 1981; Potter & Williams, 1991); developing cognitive coping strategies (Werner, 1986); and maximizing the protection of the most functional parent or surrogate parent (Roosa, Tein, Groppenbacher, Michaels, & Dumka, 1993). Finally, on an optimistic note, Moos and Moos (1984) found that many families that were successfully treated for alcohol and drug dependence functioned as well as nonalcoholic families and that in some areas, such as depth of problem solving, they functioned better.

Many psychiatric compensations for abuse and neglect within dysfunctional families, however, negatively affect clients' quality of life. Some compensatory family roles, for example, are a mixed blessing. Although they allow children to connect with their parents in acceptable ways (rescuing the chemically dependent parent, for example), they return to haunt adults later in life when they should be parenting their children, not rescuing them from potential problems (Black, 1981; Buelow, 1994b; Potter & Williams, 1991). Unfortunately, hero children who parent their parents usually over-parent their spouses and children. Mascots, who psychologically separate early in life from their parents, are often compulsively self-reliant or dismissive of emotionally close relationships. In the absence of large-scale cohort longitudinal research on nonclinical ACOAs, however, we must be content with in-depth clinical findings to guide our conceptualization and treatment.

As with other dual-diagnosis clients who need concurrent treatment, ACOAs who are also drug-dependent often present with more complex social and emotional problems, are frequently less able to utilize their families as resources due to parental drug abuse or enmeshment, are stuck in stereotyped dysfunctional role behavior with peers and partners, and often carry heavy loads of guilt and shame for perpetuating what they see as their family's disease.

A majority of ACOAs will drink or use other drugs at some time in their lives. Despite their firsthand experience of the ill effects of drug use (which does not necessarily confer an understanding of the associated risks), many are drawn into drug use by a combination of factors. These include, for example, normal age-related drug experimentation; drinking or drugging parents who encourage their children to drink or drug along with them; and membership in peer groups in which other drug use is expected. Like others who are at high risk for alcohol dependency, ACOAs do not appear to differ from their peers early in their drinking careers. Like their alcoholic parents before them, their drinking begins as an innocuous social experiment. Having direct experience with their parents' difficulties with alcohol and other drugs, however, they may be suspicious and watch for warning signs of aberrant behavior. There are usually few clear red flags. In fact, many may notice that they can drink more than their peers with fewer ill effects; they have inherited a greater than normal processing capacity. Naive ACOAs may see this capacity as a positive indication that they will have no problems drinking, even though it actually places them at higher risk because addiction factors can develop in the absence of symptoms. Most do not seem psychologically or behaviorally different than their peers during the early stages of social drinking or drug use. In fact, with the exception that ACOAs may have greater processing capacity and therefore appear more resilient to drug use, they usually display few noticeable differences from their non-ACOA peers (Milam & Ketcham, 1983).

With time, however, ACOAs who are susceptible to the addictive effects of alcohol first may experience more difficulty refraining from drinking greater quantities during any given drinking episode. They also may show more irritability when they do not drink. These small personality changes, however, are easily attributable to other influences, especially social and emotional stressors. Second, they may feel fewer incentives to discontinue drinking because their social anxiety may be lowered by alcohol. ACOAs often have difficulty refraining from using alcohol and other drugs as social lubricants. Their greater tendency to use drugs to reduce stress and increase sociability results both from a continuation of family coping patterns and from a defensive reaction to the press of interpersonal problems that stem from family dysfunction. Early on, then, ACOAs may become involved with alcohol and other drugs more quickly due to lack of family intervention, while at the same time experiencing fewer clearly negative physical effects.

As we have indicated, about 50% of chemically dependent clients who come into treatment are ACOAs. A majority believed as children that they would not take the same path as their chemically dependent parents. Because many could see the results of the addiction cycle, they had clear intentions not to become hooked themselves. Because of their family addiction history, therefore, ACOAs are frequently more self-reproachful about their chemical dependence than other clients; self-hatred runs high. Like their parents before them, many continue to believe that their addictive drinking is the result of their family dysfunction, not a combination of drugs, biological predisposition, and family and peer exposure.

We have found the following problems to be the typical focus of treatment in working with ACOAs who drink or use other drugs. First, because their parents had chemical dependence problems, ACOAs feel more guilty that they fell into the drug trap in the first place and are more greatly shamed when they relapse after treatment. Second, ACOAs learned dysfunctional self-control and social control strategies from their chemically dependent parents, and their background leads them to find either drugging or drug-enabling partners. Third, drugging ACOAs have less family and general social support than others, while at the same time possessing many avoidant, exploitative, passive-aggressive, and inadequate interpersonal characteristics, which undermine what little social support they do find. Fourth, ACOAs are more likely to be in reduced economic circumstances and single-parent homes due to their own and their parents' drug use. Fifth, ACOAs are more likely to be without the support of social and ceremonial institutions like the church and to have fewer supportive family rituals (special outings and holidays, for example) that could serve to produce higher levels of family and self-idealization. Sixth, ACOAs are more likely to be neglectful and avoidant with their own children while they are preoccupied with their parents and spouses. Finally, ACOAs are more likely to compete with their siblings and spouses over what they perceive to be scarce emotional resources and, therefore, cooperate less effectively to get what they need from others (Buelow, 1990).

As a result of this legacy of dysfunction, ACOAs have great difficulty in the following important areas: (1) forming supportive adult attachment relationships with peers, partners, and parents, tending instead to pseudomutuality; (2) reaching functional emotional self-regulation (connecting and coordinating thinking and feeling), that is not related to drug use; (3) developing and maintaining cognitive coping strategies (rational, nonmagical thinking); (4) clearly perceiving and identifying feelings (alexithymia); and (5) developing and maintaining psychological separation from parents or authority introjects, tending instead to pseudoindividuation. These characteristic problems not only have debilitating effects on clients' relationships with their immediate families, partners, and peers and keep clients from seeking treatment; these problems also raise specific barriers within individual and group therapy relationships that must be fully explored and worked through. We will discuss the issues of attachment, psychological separation, codependence, and treatment in following sections.

ATTACHMENT AND INDIVIDUATION AMONG ACOAS

Present theories of adult attachment (Bartholomew & Horowitz, 1991; Collins & Read, 1990; Hazan & Shaver, 1987) and late adolescent psychological separation (Armsden & Greenberg, 1987; Hoffman, 1984) stem from developmental and observational research describing the emergence of parent-infant bonding processes (Ainsworth, 1989; Ainsworth & Bowlby, 1991; Blos, 1979; Bowlby, 1969, 1980). Mirroring research by Harry Harlow and other primate behaviorists, absence or ambivalence of the primary caregiver during early infant bonding was found to affect infants' later attachment and exploration behavior negatively and sometimes catastrophically. Without sufficiently positive attachment, later exploration and individuation processes are diminished. Early attachment problems that are typical to neglectful and abusive families with parental chemical dependence impede late adolescent psychological separation (Buelow, Kazelskis, McIntosh, & McClain, 1997; Hoffman, 1984).

Based on their observational research, Bowlby (1969), Ainsworth, Blehar, Waters, and Wall (1978), and Ainsworth (1989) found that infants attach to primary caregivers, according to how caregivers meet their infants' needs, in at least three styles: secure, anxious-ambivalent, and avoidant. Infants are thought to develop positive working models, or cognitive schemas, if their early socialization needs are met. These working models are then used to meet relational needs. Bowlby (1973) identified two important working models through which later attachment is affected: one model of others as either positive or negative caregivers, and one model of self as either positive or negative in value. In the first model, the child internalizes the primary attachment figure as one who is or is not accessible for support and protection. In the second model, the child internalizes an idea of the self as one to whom others are or are not likely to respond in a positive way. According to Ainsworth (1989) and Bowlby (1980), these early working models are retained and continue to condition relationships throughout life. They also condition the counseling relationship and may weaken the necessary therapeutic alliance.

Bowlby contended that an individual's working models of the self and others are self-perpetuating and persist throughout development (Bowlby, 1973). Furthermore, Bowlby found that individuals interpret their experiences in ways consistent with their working models and, thus, successively validate and firmly establish these models throughout life (Bowlby, 1973).

> Working models once developed, have their own means of self-regulation that tend to maintain the current direction of development. For example, cognitive and behavioral structures determine what is perceived and what is ignored, how a situation is construed, and what plan of action is likely to be constructed to deal with it. Internal working models, moreover, determine what sorts of person and situation are sought after and what sorts are shunned. In this way an individual comes to influence the selection of his/ her own environment; and so the wheel comes full circle. (pp. 368–369)

Like other family dysfunction, alcohol and other drug abuse and dependence early in children's attachment development strike at the heart of their relationship formation throughout life, particularly true when the chemically dependent parent is the primary caregiver. Due to the fragmenting effects of drug use, parents are inconsistent in their emotional, behavioral, and cognitive relationship with their infant children, who are in the process of developing attachment and autonomy. Although ameliorated somewhat by care from the nondependent parent and others, infants whose mothers and fathers are neglectful become anxious about the protection of others and unsure about whether or not they deserve such protection and care. Such children become anxious in the face of their parents' absence (even though they may be ambivalent about their parents when they do return) or become compulsively self-reliant. In moderately neglectful cases, children reach partial autonomy that at different times may look either enmeshed or ambivalent. They often display a fragmented view of self and others because they have not internalized a consistent, integrated representation of the parent. Thus, they tend to be self-critical, prone to guilt, and overly controlling in relationships. These deficits are fertile ground for the development of relationships based on alcohol and other drugs—relationships that provide a sense of belonging, sexual partnership, recreation, and insulation from the family of origin (Buclow, McClain, & McIntosh, 1996).

A further feature of parental neglect is introjective depression (Jarmas & Kozak, 1992), which stems from the incorporation of an inadequate parental model during infancy and which is represented by ambivalence, hostility, perfectionism, and self-deprecation. Children who have been severely neglected or abused often display anaclitic depression (Jarmas & Kozak, 1992). They may fail to internalize a stable internal object representation of the parent, which creates a lifelong emotional vulnerability to potential loss of significant others and a fear of abandonment. This fear of loss or actual loss may send the more unstable of these individuals into profound and suicidal depressions. Borderline personality disorders, which may stem from these backgrounds, are characterized by unstable and inadequate internal representations and identity confusion. Although Jarmas and Kozak (1992) found that parental inconsistency accounted for a large majority of the variance in depression (and in the development of depressive subtypes), paralleling Protinsky and Shiltz (1990) they also found that family conflict and a lack of cohesion, expressiveness, organization, and communication were significant contributors.

In summary, ACOAs in treatment have often had severely disturbed attachment relationships that must be explored and worked through in individual and group treatment. Dependent personality styles must work on developing and asserting necessary interpersonal and intrapersonal boundaries. Dismissive or compulsively self-reliant types must be taught the value of interdependence and helped to practice closer interaction in group therapy. Such clients must be shown that relaxing their hypervigilance and rigid emotional boundaries will not cause catastrophic encroachment from others.

Disturbed attachment patterns often account for clients' unsteady progress in group. Confrontational group interactions often trigger fears of encroachment (absorption due to poor boundaries) on the one hand and fears of abandonment by the group on the other. Although a majority of clients begin to remedy developmental identity problems through group support and confrontation, those who continue to destructively cycle in their borderline and antisocial traits should be referred to individual treatment or into a treatment group specifically designed for the rehabilitation of more difficult, characterologically dysfunctional clients. Clearly, assessment by a psychiatrist who can help monitor the situation is called for if a client has a history of or begins to use suicidal gestures as a means of defending against group process.

Although individuation is a lifelong process (beginning with early attempts to develop autonomy from the primary caregiver among infants, and ending, perhaps, in separation from family at death), psychological separation is the primary developmental concern of late adolescence. Separation is profoundly influenced by early attachment relationships, continuing family functioning, and the development of peer relationships (Hoffman, 1984). ACOAs often display pseudoindividuation, which is reflected in their profound difficulties with achieving proper psychological distance from their parents. Although these teenagers technically move away from parents toward involvement with peers or partners, they have not resolved their abandonment and encroachment conflicts with parents. These problems are extended into other intimate relationships. Although these young adults appear to have physically separated from their parents, they continue to be emotionally enmeshed with them or quickly become dependent on a surrogate parent, often a sexual partner.

Family therapy is the treatment modality of choice for helping ACOAs tackle enmeshment concerns. With their parents present, children can work to increase their power, establish their boundaries, and define their developing roles in the family. In the absence of supportive family members, ACOA therapy groups can provide a surrogate family within which struggles for autonomy, self-control, power, and role development can be processed. Through its emphasis on intimacy, genuineness, and the here and now, the group can provide the continual interaction necessary to jump-start psychological separation and identity development.

TREATING ACOAS FROM SEVERELY DYSFUNCTIONAL FAMILIES

As we have indicated, children from severely chemically dependent and alcoholic homes are at high risk for a wide range of developmental problems, including deficits in identity exploration, psychological separation, and adult role assimilation (Burk & Sher, 1988; Cleveland, 1981; Grotevant & Cooper, 1985; Vannicelli, 1987). Problems in adult role assimilation that are typical to ACOA families have consistently been identified by clinicians as interfering with normal transition to adulthood and subsequent relationship building (Black, Buckey, & Wilder-Padilla, 1986; Harris & MacQuiddy, 1991; Perkins, 1989; Wegscheider, 1981). Based on clinical experience with adult children of alcoholics, these authors have theorized that this interference results in slowed identity development because children internalize and emulate roles that are either overly enmeshed with parents (appeasement types and helper types), disengaged from parents (avoidant or missing types and separation or mascot types), or oppositional to parental expectations (opposition or scapegoat types). Under these adverse conditions, neither interdependence nor strivings for normal conflictual independence find support (Erikson & Perkins, 1989).

Empirical research (Buelow, 1990, 1995; Potter & Williams, 1991) has found evidence for the existence of dysfunctional roles much like those that Black (1981) and Wegscheider (1981) originally described. This research has also found that these roles exist in a hierarchy from very low to moderately high ego development, that individuals may play dominant and subsidiary roles, and that dysfunctional roles consist of normal family role behaviors distorted by family pathology.

ROLE DEVELOPMENT AMONG ACOAS

Unlike factors that clearly support resilience among ACOAs, such as cognitive coping strategies, dysfunctional roles are thought to be particularly complex. Like the Trojan horse, they appear to be adaptive and compensatory while children reside in the family, but become serious liabilities in later social interaction because of their rigidity (Black, 1981; Cleveland, 1981; Harris & MacQuiddy, 1991; Perkins, 1989; Wegscheider, 1981). The primary adaptive feature of roles appears to be that they provide a sense of consistency and identity within an inconsistent and identity-damaging system. Roles may also be compensatory in that they are attempts to gain power and control within a system that is characterized by competition for scarce emotional resources.

The most clearly negative intrapsychic outcome of dysfunctional role development is that roles may be rigidly played to such an extent that family role and identity become fused. This over-assimilation, or role stereotypy, may interrupt children's ability to take on new roles in changing social relationships. The inability to develop a wide repertoire of roles clearly undermines well-being by limiting behavioral, emotional, and cognitive flexibility (Thoits, 1985). Stereotyped roles, passed on through generations, may serve as the most important nongenetic factor in extending the cycle of abuse and exploitation through generations. Let us examine the following case history and its relationship to treatment.

◆ DYSFUNCTIONAL ROLE DEVELOPMENT: A CASE HISTORY ◆

Dee was a 33-year-old, white woman in her senior year in college. She was on financial aid and had stopped visits with her family of origin. She was doing well in school despite her dyslexia. She attended both Alcoholics Anonymous and Narcotics Anonymous, and she wanted group counseling because of relationship difficulties with her female partner. Dee's parents and grandparents had moved from the Midwest to the Northwest, together with her two siblings, a brother and sister, and her two maternal aunts. Soon after their arrival in Seattle when Dee was less than 5 years old, Dee's father left town to avoid criminal prosecution for drug activities. Dee's aunts engaged in prostitution to help support the family, all of whom lived together in a "crash pad" for two years. After moving into more stable physical circumstances at the age of 6, Dee and her younger sister and brother were shifted from their mother to their aunts depending on money and circumstances. When Dee was 8 years old, her mother remarried. Dee's mother was alcohol and drug dependent at that time and physically abusive to the children. Dee remembered that her sister's and her own sexual experience began with her grandfather while they were living in the crash pad. She also remembered sexual activity with other male members of the household from the time she was around 6 years old. She remembered one of her aunt's attempts to protect her, and she established a strong bond with this aunt.

Dee recalled being in constant competition with her sister and, later, her brother for physical necessities and emotional support from her parents. After her mother remarried, Dee recalled her stepfather initiating sex with her in exchange for gifts from him when she was 10 years old. Dee described her stepfather as weak and manipulable. Dee remembered being afraid as a teen that her stepfather would commit suicide because of his emotional and drug problems. She recalled eating huge portions of food to please him when he cooked and later purging the food. She recalled teaching her brother and sister to play in silence when her mother was home because of her explosive personality. At the age of 14, Dee quit school and began supporting herself and her siblings through prostitution. At the age of 18, Dee's biological father returned to Seattle; Dee fell in love with her father and began living with him as his wife. They continued this relationship for more than a year, after which he abruptly left Seattle again to avoid drug prosecution. During this time, Dee, already an alcoholic, became addicted to heroin. After several drug-related arrests, Dee was jailed. Dee earned her high school equivalency degree in jail, stopped using drugs, and began to plan a different life for herself. These plans were thwarted at times because of alcohol relapse. However, Dee worked, managed to continue in college, and was on track to earn a degree, despite her difficulties.

Dee's story is typical of her ACOA treatment group in several important ways. First, the family had a long, involved history of drug abuse and dependence. Second, child abuse and neglect were institutionalized behaviors that channeled the children's emotional energies toward the gratification of adults. Third, continual competition with adults and siblings for scarce physical and emotional resources made role changes very risky; children were expected to play specific roles in the family and were punished when they did not.

For example, Dee, the eldest, played an appeasement or helper role. She was held responsible for her brother and sister from an early age; she acted as a parent and undertook to support them financially. Dee was also viewed, and viewed herself, as a second wife by both her biological father and stepfather, who vied for her attention. Dee's status in the family derived from her helping, codependent role and her sexual relationships with males in the parental generation. As a teenager, the few attempts Dee made to leave the family system were crushed or manipulated. Dee married as an older teenager and moved with her husband to another town where she remained, even though her marriage failed. She continued to provide a safe haven and, episodically, financial support for her brother and sister.

In therapy, Dee worked on several central issues. First, she felt compelled to enter any relationship extended to her, even though she could predict it would not be good for her. Second, once in relationships, she could not express conflicting views. All of the independence she seemed to develop during periods in which she lived alone collapsed in interaction. Although she was aware that her avoidant sister and her oppositional brother exploited her much as her parents had, she felt unable to resist them. In the group, Dee did a great deal of caretaking and fixing for other members. At first her efforts were welcomed; later, because she continually interfered with other members' processing, these efforts were rejected. Even though she was often hurt by the lack of acceptance of her helping, she would not withdraw but kept trying to "fix" the relationship with the person who rejected her help. Her help had a frantic, controlling quality to it. Early interventions with Dee were directed at helping her examine each incident in which she intervened to help another group member. Over time, Dee came to accept that it was other members' right to withdraw from her and that she didn't need to "catch" them if they withdrew. Further, as Dee was given effective support to withdraw (avoid) and to sit with her hurt feelings until they dissipated, she came to accept that others did not need to fix things for her because she was needy. Finally, Dee was engaged in playing boundary games with other group members where she was encouraged to role-play by either walking away or actively opposing interaction. Group members were encouraged with Dee's permission to invade her physical or emotional space by, for example, asking her to solve their problems, interrupting her, or sitting too close to her. Over time, Dee was able to move from accepting others' control to avoiding, and, finally, actively opposing it. As she did so, she became less controlling herself.

In families like Dee's, where substance dependence has been entrenched for many generations, structural, economic, and affective relationships take on a competitive structure that leads to alteration of traditional intergenerational role boundaries. Often the family accepts intrafamily sexual relationships or incest. Competition develops out of the relative scarcity of material and emotional rewards. Surplus cash and many necessities are converted into drugs.

Not only were all group members in constant competition with other family members for tangible rewards of money, school clothes, and drugs; but they also were in competition for emotional rewards for which they bartered time, affection, sex, money, drugs, or subservience. The covert rule, as a client once phrased it, is this: "In my family you have to pay for what you get; if you don't pay one way, you pay another way." Paradoxically, the overt rule is, often, "We don't take anything from anybody" or "We don't take anything off of anybody." Competition is usually carried over into love and peer relationships, undermining cooperation and trust. Drug-abusing and dependent parents usually do not have positive time to share with their children, because the parents' emotional lives are fragmented by their drug use, criminal activities, or codependent emotional status. Within this system, children learn quickly how to compete for what they need within the family and are sometimes actively pitted against one another by the parents as a means of social control. Younger, less able, and less competitive children are more likely to adopt avoidant roles.

Patterns of Severe Dysfunction

Our experience with severely dysfunctional and sexually abusive ACOA families (Buelow, 1994b) has shown that they tend to be similar in their patterns of chemical dependence and sexual abuse.

Chemical Dependence   Chemically dependent and dysfunctional families intermarry with other families with chemical dependence histories. Thus, chemical dependence problems often can be traced many generations into the past. ACOAs often described intense efforts by family members, however, to minimize the importance of chemical dependence as a problem. Their deep-seated denial system successfully isolates members from knowledge about or use of treatment alternatives. Treatment is often equated with personal failure, and clients often worry that their present treatment is a sign of weakness or giving in to social pressure.

Sexual Abuse   Incest and child sexual abuse are commonly found to be institutionalized within the family. In some cases incest operates at the level of a sexual preference. Parents may also have an economic incentive to prostitute their children. Physical, sexual, and psychological abuse of children is supported by rigidly held family beliefs which include male superiority, physical and sexual punishment, total subservience of children to the wishes of adults, avoidance of telling family secrets, family superiority or specialness, tight control of feelings, and contempt for outside social interference. These very dysfunctional families exhibit high levels of conflict, hierarchical distance, authoritarian rules, lack of democracy, high external locus of control, and low levels of shared family activities.

Research and clinical contact indicates that severely dysfunctional families like the ones just described are often starkly isolated from the general culture, while at the same time enmeshed within a subculture of drug-using relatives and peers. This subculture may include past wives or husbands who rarely drop completely out of the family system, lovers, retainers, children, stepchildren, stepparents, surrogate parents, distant or fictive relatives, drug suppliers, and cronies, many of whom are drug abusive or dependent. This subculture is typified by rejection of ordinary social norms about the meaning of, and restraints on, substance use and sexual abuse. These families often adopt both overt and covert rules that insulate them from scrutiny by educational, religious, legal, and child protection agencies. For example, family members typically believe that their family is special, that external rules do not apply, and that only the head of the household is a fit judge of what is right and wrong.

Changing Dysfunctional Role Stereotypy

Although clinicians have outlined many of the role dysfunctions ACOAs suffer (Black, 1981), few have described specific strategies for remediation. Perkins (1989) suggested the following techniques to help alter rigid family role behaviors among adolescents: family sculpting, writing journals and letters to family members, negotiating alternatives to behaviors that set off role conflict, trading or changing roles within family therapy sessions, and replaying role conflicts within sessions. Many of these techniques, however, require the family's active participation. Unfortunately, many ACOAs cannot count on this participation.

Our clinical experience supports a role development strategy within which these specific techniques for overcoming role stereotypy should be organized (Buelow, 1994b). This strategy is suggested by the hierarchical, developmental nature of the dysfunctional roles themselves. Older children, who have been in the dysfunctional environment longest, may appear on the surface to be the most successful (heroes), but are often the most crippled by dysfunctional roles by the time they reach middle age. Appeasement or helper types are often the first-born. Normal helping or pleasing behavior on the part of the child is gradually distorted into appeasement role-playing, in which the child takes over parental functions (parentification) and boundaries between the child and adults are eroded. This distorted role is especially likely for a child who is female and when sexual abuse has become institutionalized.

Second-born children often receive fewer payoffs than first-borns. Males are especially likely to rebel against parents (or against the caretaking sibling) and become oppositional or defiant and antisocial. Although both avoidant and oppositional behaviors are normal in children, family dysfunction rigidifies these normal expressions of developing autonomy. Second- or third-born children who are female are more likely to become avoidant children with varying degrees of learned helplessness.

Youngest children, especially males, may separate from the family early and become separation or mascot types. Their separation behavior stems from several sources. First, by the time the third or fourth child is born, the family has often fragmented to the point that children can avoid parental control. Their peers become the primary reference group. Second, parents may be so separated that by default young children are allowed more autonomy and, therefore, expressiveness. The youngest child is often the only member, for example, who is allowed to joke, to act childish, or to express how badly off the family really is. A mascot may act as a safety valve by expressing other family members' emotions (Harris & MacQuiddy, 1991; Minuchin, 1974). Third, mascots may be more autonomous because they have observed the effects their parents have on their siblings; the mascots have therefore developed more effective coping strategies. Further, incomplete immersion in the family's dysfunction may produce stress-inoculation effects. Although the causes are not completely clear, separation or mascot types have usually reached a higher level of psychological separation and ego development than other dysfunctional role types. Unfortunately, very early psychological separation can diminish mascots' abilities to enjoy intimacy in personal relationships (Buelow, 1990; Harris & MacQuiddy, 1991).

Based on treatment observation, dysfunctional role types may be ranked from highest to lowest degree of psychological separation as follows: separation types, avoidant types, opposition types, and, finally, appeasement types. Appeasement types frequently appear to have the lowest internal locus of control, even though their self-esteem seems intact because of their compulsive striving to care for others. Unfortunately, caring for others does not directly increase children's self-care. Also, their self-esteem is based not on who they are, but on what they do for their parents or siblings. Appeasement types appear to learn as teenagers that they can never do enough to feel adequate; dysfunctional codependence and depression result. There is an old ACOA joke that a codependent is someone who, on the verge of death, sees someone else's life flash before his or her eyes.

Each family role type has templates or generative structures for role types that are close in developmental level, particularly true if there were siblings in the home who played more developed roles. Thus, helper types can play avoidant roles; they sometimes play oppositional roles, but they rarely play separation roles. Oppositional types are able to play avoidant roles, and sometimes play separation roles; they rarely play appeasement or helper roles. Separation types more often play oppositional roles, rarely play avoidant roles, and almost never play appeasement or helper roles.

During both individual and group therapy, clients should be encouraged to play roles directly above them in the developmental schema through role-playing, role-swapping, and writing and enacting scripts. After many interactive trials, clients can be coached to move successfully through the hierarchy of roles toward more independent, separation role-playing. Unlike conventional therapy, this strategy takes into consideration the difficulty ACOAs have in reaching immediately for separation behaviors. They must first learn avoidant and oppositional roles (especially anger expression and management) that are developmentally prior to the separation role. To be internalized, independent role behaviors must coalesce into a coherent set of behaviors set in an interpretive framework; these behaviors cannot simply be adopted as discrete actions. Integration takes time. When these behaviors are not integrated into interpersonal roles, they do not appear to be acted on over the long run.

In conclusion, children from severely chemically dependent and sexually abusive families play dysfunctional roles that have been successfully integrated into their personalities. Changing these roles requires time, patience, and emotional support. New roles must be developed while older role behaviors diminish. Treatment strategies that pay special attention to the stereotypic and compensatory nature of dysfunctional roles are more likely to produce long-term developmental change.

CODEPENDENCE

Dysfunctional dependence on others for self-esteem and efficacy, often called codependence in the chemical dependence literature, stems from a lack of identity development, individuation, and social role flexibility (Potter-Efron & Potter-Efron, 1989; Rothberg, 1986). The term *codependence* was coined within Al-Anon and

ACOA groups to describe the dependent, enabling, enmeshed, and stereotyped behaviors of the spouse or child of a chemically dependent person in response to the personality and behavioral changes brought on by an addiction. Even though the term has been overused in the popular psychology literature and often misapplied as well, we believe that the basic construct is useful (with caveats). Reasons to give weight to the codependency idea include the following. First, the idea of codependency was developed outside the psychological mainstream, which gives it ethnographic authenticity. Second, people make very clear compensatory responses to the chemical dependence of significant others that parallel those people make to a variety of physical and emotional illnesses. Unfortunately, the term *codependency* (a category description) has been used to explain and rationalize a variety of often competing individual behaviors among dependent persons without a clear theoretical or empirical basis (Schaef, 1986; Wegscheider-Cruse, 1985).

Although many ACOA group participants are women, and more women than men are socialized into dependent and codependent roles, we now know that many men play enabling and codependent roles as well. In fact, men with apparently dismissive attachment styles can show codependent traits when they are involved in intimate relationships: Their ego structures become melded with a powerful relationship partner, and they cycle between feelings of enmeshment and abandonment. For a thoughtful discussion of the political and feminist issues that have arisen (and continue to arise) from the codependence literature, we suggest the reader begin with Janice Haaken's (1993) work.

It became clear to Al-Anon members who shared their war stories that chemical dependence in one partner caused direct emotional and behavioral changes to occur in the other. Dysfunctional dependence was noted not only in the spouse, but among children in the family. These dependencies are now seen not only as compensatory (and sometimes exploitative, as well), but also as a way of protecting the family's interpersonal relationships from risky change. Protecting and enabling the drug user's behavior however, furthers chemical dependence, which further threatens family relationships, in turn requiring heightened levels of enabling, control, and system repair.

Clinical experience confirms that chemical dependence enhances the dysfunctional dependence of spouses and children through a variety of control mechanisms, including family isolation and a distorted system of rewards and punishments. Also, individuals with a family history of chemical dependence often select spouses *because* they recognize signs of codependence in them. Characteristics that appear to attract drug abusers (and batterers as well) include compulsive parenting and fixing problems, a history of enabling parental drinking and drugging, openness to physical and sexual aggression (usually such individuals were coerced and battered as children), dependence on others for rules and roles, susceptibility to suggestion, and an external locus of control (Barnett & Fagan, 1993; Buelow, 1990).

The development of dysfunctional dependence or codependence, so common among ACOAs, dramatically increases their chances of selecting chemically dependent mates with whom they can continue not only their dependence, but also their passive-aggressive control. Codependence makes possible many secondary gains, which must be addressed in treatment. Children's success in family management through playing enabling roles, for example, dramatically increases the odds they will play dysfunctionally dependent roles in peer relationships and, especially, in marriage.

Codependence is signaled by the following activities: caretaking younger siblings; parenting parents when they are drunk or having mental problems; acting as a surrogate spouse to one or both parents (which often includes psychological and sexual enmeshment); maintaining secrecy from outsiders about family social, sexual, and chemical dependence patterns; and maintaining continuing isolation from others in the community. Mendenhall (1989) called such individuals "self-centered but other-focused" because of their compulsion to maintain an external locus of control.

Although we ordinarily associate codependence with the spouse of an alcohol or other drug abuser, dysfunctional dependence can arise in anyone whose social interactions are significantly and importantly affected by a chemically dependent person or another dependent or codependent. Like other forms of dysfunctional dependence, codependence in chemically dependent homes can be attributed to the following factors: direct pressures to enable parental drug use, denial of autonomy and democracy to children in the family, dysfunctional feedback and communication within the group, and an intergenerational legacy of blame and entitlements. Under these conditions, children are often rewarded for giving emotional pleasure to parents while subjugating their own desires. These rewards create distorted pleasure in self-denial, as well as destructive feelings of entitlement concerning debts that have accrued to the child and that can never be repaid by the chemically dependent parent or partner. Self-denial and overemphasis on parents stifles exploration and the development of normal boundaries. Children become confused about the limits of personal, emotional, and sexual space, and they seem gullible and easily manipulated.

Denying emotional autonomy distorts children's identity development. Messages interpreted as saying "I love you when you're good to me" lead children to attempt chronically to please not only their parents, but significant others as well. It is painful but common to hear ACOA clients stoutly deny the obvious reality that they were not loved, but rather manipulated. Working with ACOAs who have been emotionally and sexually exploited has convinced us that many alcoholic or other drug-abusing parents have become incapable of forming loving, nonexploitative relationships with their children or with anyone else. Teaching such deficient parents to recontact others, especially their children, meaningfully and democratically is a long and difficult journey of reeducation and reparenting.

Codependent communication can be thought of as any signal, interaction, or exchange that serves to meet the individual's dependency needs. Failure to communicate effectively as children sets the stage for faulty communications throughout life. Of course, those who communicate less effectively have fewer of their interpersonal needs met and tend to meet others' needs through deviant means. Communication can be complementary (equal but opposite, as in a dance when one partner matches movements to the other) or noncomplementary (with confrontational behaviors running head on into one another). When complementarity is demanded at all times, individuals learn to manage conflict (and confrontation) by matching the steps of their partners' dance—typical codependent behavior. If the partner is angry, the codependent becomes passive. If the partner is passive, the codependent may become more aggressive. This complementary control leads to a pattern of cyclical passive-aggressiveness. Over-aggressiveness (moving the battle beyond the dance) is often met with triangulation (pulling someone else into the dance—children, lovers) as a way of softening and resocializing the confrontation.

Phases of Codependence Treatment

Potter-Efron and Potter-Efron (1989, p. 161) noted that

> Co-dependent individuals, because they live in chronic highly stressful situations, often have difficulty recognizing or expressing a full range of feelings. Recognizing feelings may produce a strong desire to live differently, but since co-dependents often believe they are caught in an unalterable family trap, it becomes more efficient to deny or minimize feelings. Also, free expression of affect is only possible in a safe environment. When co-dependents attempt to express their feelings within an alcoholic family they may be met with ridicule, disinterest, or violence. Eventually these persons learn to "stuff" their feelings in order to keep the peace.

These authors approach codependency treatment from the standpoint of goals that apply at different points within therapy, including the following:

1. *Behavioral goals*: Attending treatment and Al-Anon, and practicing self-care, detachment, and interdependence.
2. *Cognitive goals*: Understanding the disease concept of alcoholism, codependence, individuation, mutuality, and boundaries.
3. *Spiritual goals*: Replacing hopelessness, shame, and disrespect with appropriate hope and belonging, and developing a sense of commitment to a higher power.
4. *Affective goals*: Identifying, sharing, and being responsible for feelings accurately and in a timely way.

Paralleling Potter-Efron and Potter-Efron's (1989) goal-directed therapy, Mendenhall (1989) pointed out a variety of important therapy goals, including developing a more internal locus of control, restoring self-trust, taking proper responsibility, recognizing emotional indigency, reconnecting feelings with experience, owning personal needs, learning moderation, recognizing the importance of flashbacks, unraveling confusion, restoring multiple patterns of relationships, and drawing up a bill of personal rights. Mendenhall (1989) also outlined six stages of recovery that include developmental periods of undoing, of gathering and sorting data, of relinquishing maladaptive behaviors, of consolidating learning, of finding baseline wants and values, and, finally, of achieving a new and firm grip on the realities of peace and serenity.

Harper (1990) suggested that couples treatment with recovering and codependent partners goes through a polarization phase, a rejoining phase, and a regeneration phase. In the polarization phase, couples are widely divided and alienated. In rejoining, couples are helped to develop a new vision of the relationship (renewed family idealization). During the regeneration phase, the partners, acting through insight and responsibility, not only retake old ground, but reactualize and reinvent the relationship. Each of these stages requires developing new patterns of communication, conflict resolution, family roles, and sexual interdependence. Paralleling Harper (1990), Boyer (1989) and Ziter (1989) wrote of four management levels, including clustering (reengagement), conflict, individuation, and connection.

Family Therapy and Codependence

In conclusion, even though many codependents find their way into individual therapy, dysfunctional dependencies are best treated in family therapy. Spousal dependence is held in place not only by the chemically dependent family member, but often by other members of the family who profit from controlling and dominating the codependent member and the chemically dependent member by turns. Many chemically dependent clients establish a high-quality sobriety, only to find that their codependent family members begin to develop subtle strategies to regain lost control over family affairs.

Codependence usually begins in childhood through the agencies of physical abuse, emotional neglect, psychosexual exploitation, and denial of rights to independent identity development. Where physical abuse is common, clients often anesthetize themselves not only to physical pain, but to rage and hatred, which diminishes the client's ability to experience the physical pleasures of life. Clients who have suffered emotional neglect over- or under-attach to others; they frequently also display a lack of coordination between thinking and feeling, and an inability to identify at any given moment what they feel (alexithymia). Such clients must be taught to identify feelings through a variety of immediate and homework exercises that emphasize, for example, naming feelings, noticing shifts in feeling, and developing a sensate (as opposed to purely thinking) focus, for example. Family group therapy can aid in the coordination of thoughts and feelings through observing other members accurately identify and express feelings, and through confrontation about avoidance of affect.

Clients who have been sexually exploited or abused, or who have been involved in incest often shut down their sexual expressiveness, rejecting sexual gratification or learning to use it to manipulate others. Even though such clients may be sexually promiscuous and exploitative, their gratification is often through domination and control, not through sexuality itself. These clients must learn how to give up cognitive and emotional control within a safe and supportive interpersonal therapy context. That learning can be transferred to other social relationships only through supportively structured practice in session and at home.

Finally, codependence treatment involves helping clients over the long term (and, sometimes, over a lifetime) to develop a firmer sense of self, greater personal power, and individuation from parents and partners. Codependence treatment, therefore, is less a technical process than an existential one in which responsibility, insight, and commitment become central themes. Without addressing these themes over and over again, codependents will not only remain enmeshed with dysfunctional people, but will be ensnared in a continuing cycle of self-victimization and avoidance of responsibility.

Children in all cultures pass through a succession of family and social roles that ordinarily engender a sense of consistency, trust, and status within the family and community. Normal transition through family role expectations nurtures a sense of identity, because roles act as cognitive, emotional, and behavioral templates against which children and young adults compare themselves as they strive for autonomy and psychological separation. Fulfilling important role expectations while at the same time "finding oneself"—establishing identity, power, and autonomy within the social group—are essential steps toward reaching adulthood in all cultures. Unfortunately, dysfunctional families are characterized by their relative inability to prepare adolescents for the competing expectations of adult roles (Boszormenyi-Nagy & Spark, 1973; Thornton & Nardi, 1980).

STUDY AND DISCUSSION QUESTIONS

1. What are COAs and ACOAs exactly, and why do they form such an important risk and intervention group?

2. Given the potential ramifications of identifying people with their potential problems (so that the person becomes a problem), why does it make sense to provide preintervention education and services to COAs and ACOAs?

3. What are the major legacies of dysfunction that have been found to be common among ACOAs?

4. Define and briefly discuss the importance of role stereotypy.

5. Describe typical family roles often found in dysfunctional and chemically dependent families, and explain how they might come about.

6. How might one go about treating family and social role dysfunction?

7. Define and briefly explain the importance of the concept codependence.

8. What are the important assessment indicators of codependence?

9. What are the phases and activities typical to codependence treatment or other dysfunctional dependence treatment?

CHILDREN OF ALCOHOLICS SCREENING TEST (CAST)

Please check (√) the answer below that best describes your feelings, behavior, and experiences related to a parent's alcohol use. Take your time and be as accurate as possible. Answer all 30 questions by either checking "Yes" or "No."

Sex: Male _____   Female _____   Age: _____

Yes   No

___ ___   1. Have you ever thought that one of your parents had a drinking problem?

___ ___   2. Have you ever lost sleep because of a parent's drinking?

___ ___   3. Did you ever encourage one of your parents to quit drinking?

___ ___   4. Did you ever feel alone, scared, nervous, angry, or frustrated because a parent was not able to stop drinking?

___ ___   5. Did you ever argue or fight with a parent when he or she was drinking?

___ ___   6. Did you ever threaten to run away from home because of a parent's drinking?

___ ___   7. Has a parent ever yelled at or hit you or other family members when drinking?

___ ___   8. Have you ever heard your parents fight when one of them was drunk?

___ ___   9. Did you ever protect another family member from a parent who was drinking?

___ ___   10. Did you ever feel like hiding or emptying a parent's bottle of liquor?

___ ___   11. Do many of your thoughts revolve around a problem drinking parent or difficulties that arise because of his or her drinking?

___ ___   12. Did you ever wish that a parent would stop drinking?

___ ___   13. Did you ever feel responsible for and guilty about a parent's drinking?

___ ___   14. Did you ever fear that your parents would get a divorce due to alcohol misuse?

___ ___   15. have you ever withdrawn from and avoided outside activities and friends because of embarrassment and shame over a parent's drinking problem?

___ ___   16. Did you ever feel caught in the middle of an argument or fight between a problem drinking parent and your other parent?

___ ___   17. Did you ever feel that you made a parent drink alcohol?

___ ___   18. Have you ever felt that a problem drinking parent did not really love you?

___ ___   19. Did you ever resent a parent's drinking?

___ ___   20. Have you ever worried about a parent's health because of his or her alcohol use?

___ ___   21. Have you ever been blamed for a parent's drinking?

Source: From "The Children of Alcoholics Screening Test: A Validity Study," by J. W. Jones, 1983, *Bulletin of the Society of Psychologists in Addictive Processes, 2*(3), 155–163. Copyright © 1983. Reprinted with permission of the author.

Yes   No

___ ___ 22. Did you ever think that your father was an alcoholic?

___ ___ 23. Did you ever wish that your home could be more like the homes of your friends who did not have a parent with a drinking problem?

___ ___ 24. Did a parent ever make promises to you that he or she did not keep because of drinking?

___ ___ 25. Did you ever think your mother was an alcoholic?

___ ___ 26. Did you ever wish that you could talk to someone who could understand and help the alcohol related problems in your family?

___ ___ 27. Did you ever fight with your brothers and sisters about a parent's drinking?

___ ___ 28. Did you ever stay away from home to avoid the drinking parent or your other parent's reaction to the drinking?

___ ___ 29. Have you ever felt sick, cried, or had a "knot" in your stomach after worrying about a parent's drinking?

___ ___ 30. Did you ever take over any chores and duties at home that were usually done by a parent before he or she developed a drinking problem?

CHILDREN OF ALCOHOLICS LIFE-EVENTS SCHEDULE

With ratings of good (G), bad (B), or neutral (N) in parentheses.

1. Your family got together with relatives (aunts, uncles, grandparents) for good times. (G)
2. Household routines got done smoothly (like your dinner on time, regular bedtime, your clothes got washed). (G)
3. You had chores to do around the house (like making meals or cleaning your room). (N)
4. People in your family physically hit each other hard to hurt each other (parents, brothers or sisters). (B)
5. Your Mom and Dad told you about their problems or worries. (N)
6. Your relatives (aunts, uncles, grandparents) said bad things about your parent(s). (B)
7. Mom or Dad fought or argued with your relatives (aunts, uncles, grandparents). (B)
8. People in your neighborhood said bad things about your parent(s). (B)
9. Your parent(s) acted badly in front of your friends (yelled at them, criticized them or was drunk in front of them). (B)
10. You saw Mom or Dad drunk. (B)
11. Mom or Dad forgot important things that she or he promised to do (such as take you on a trip, take you to nice places or come to your school activities). (B)
12. Mom and Dad argued in front of you. (B)
13. Your friends talked about your Mom's or Dad's drinking. (B)
14. You stayed one or more nights away from the house without your Mom or Dad. (N)
15. Mom hit you (slapped, kicked, hit with fist or something hard). (B)
16. Dad or Mom was drunk in public (your school, in your neighborhood). (B)
17. Dad or Mom was very sick, had the shakes (hands shook). (B)
18. Dad or Mom spent one or more nights away from home when he or she should home. (B)
19. You took care of Mom or Dad when he or she was drunk. (B)
20. Mom or Dad got drunk on holidays, birthdays, or family gatherings. (B)
21. Mom or Dad criticized things you've done well. (B)
22. Your family talked about Mom's or Dad's drinking. (N)
23. Dad hit you (slapped, kicked, hit with fist or something hard). (B)
24. Mom said bad things about Dad. (B)
25. You and your Mom or Dad went to bars looking for your Mom or Dad. (B)

26. You spent time with Mom or Dad in a bar. (B)

27. You got toys, clothes and other things you like. (G)

28. Mom or Dad screamed, shouted and broke things. (B)

29. Dad said bad things about Mom. (B)

30. Dad spent time with you (playing games, working together, camping, etc.). (G)

31. Mom spent time with you. (G)

32. Dad attended school functions (plays, open houses, athletic games). (G)

33. Mom attended functions. (G)

34. Dad indicated how special you are or how much he loves you. (G)

35. Mom indicated how special you are or how much she loves you. (G)

36. Dad did extra nice things for you and your Mom. (G)

37. Mom did extra nice things for you and your Dad. (G)

38. Your Mom encouraged you to take part in club or team activities. (G)

39. Your Dad encouraged you to take part in club or team activities. (G)

8

GROUP TREATMENT

Group processes within the family are the guiding forces in socialization. Through rules, roles, and intimate relationships, family groups shape our thinking, our emotions, and our behavior. They also shape our understanding of how we grow and change—the process dimension. Throughout our lives, but especially during adolescent individuation, peer groups also directly influence this shaping process, sometimes in concert with the family, sometimes in opposition to it (Oetting & Beauvais, 1987). Whether an individual has been too loosely controlled by the family (and therefore less affected by group control) or too tightly controlled by the family (and therefore more likely to rebel against it or to depend too heavily on it), peer treatment groups can exert powerful remedial effects by helping the individual learn better adaptive skills. The recapitulation of family dynamics, and the process of publicly working through interactional problems with other group members, give group treatment its power over personal change (Yalom, 1995). As Rogers (1970) indicated, in addition to generalized necessary conditions of empathy, genuineness, and unconditional positive regard, groups also provide safety, intimacy, trust, openness, learning and feedback, support for creative solutions, and expectations that individuals will transfer their learning into other relationships.

Vannicelli (1982) pointed out the importance of group clients' identification with others, the development of self-understanding through observation of others' problems, and guided communication and also further emphasized the normalizing effects of listening to accounts of other people's struggles. Clients discover that their problems are not unique, and neither are they. Other important group curative factors include interpersonal learning (guided practice), group cohesiveness (working together on a common theme), existential factors (insight into the nature of one's being and purpose), universality (ability to generalize away from narcissistic impulses), and catharsis (emotional release in a safe place). Also significant are resocialization, altruism, instillation of hope, imparting of information, role modeling, and the corrective recapitulation of interactional problems within the family of origin (Brown & Yalom, 1977; Yalom, 1995). A corrective emotional experience is a key ingredient in the transfer of learning and the movement from simple (and setting-limited) compliance to full internalization of group values.

215

A variety of personal, strategic, and structural considerations confront counselors as they decide whether and how to work with alcohol and other treatment groups. These include, first, personal considerations—namely, the counselor's personality, experience, and expertise. Have you been specifically trained to facilitate groups? To lead addiction groups? Second, considerations arise from the character of clients: Is the client adolescent? Does the client have a dual diagnosis? Is the client of a different ethnic group? Third, issues arise around the treatment conditions within which therapy will be conducted. Will you be conducting inpatient, outpatient, immediate aftercare, or long-term relapse prevention? Will you be using a 12-step or stage-of-development model? Finally, how will you assess whether the client has moved from situationally limited compliance with the group norms to internalization of those norms? Is the client merely accommodating the group and unlikely to transfer skills from the group into his or her everyday life? How will you assess and plan for the great variety of treatment conditions?

A wide range of treatment experience has confirmed that group therapy is an effective—probably the most effective—chemical dependence treatment strategy when utilized by professionals as part of a structured treatment regimen (Arnold, 1973; Brown & Yalom, 1977; Flores, 1988; Flores & Mahon, 1993; Rugel & Barry, 1990; Vannicelli, 1982). Developed long before Tavistock and other self-exploration groups were retrofitted in the 1960s for use with chemically dependent people, Alcoholics Anonymous had already evolved a particularly effective group support format. AA, NA, and offshoot groups evolved their methods through trial and error. They have proved their effectiveness with many people, though they are certainly not for everyone.

What accounts for the psychological power of groups? Although education and guided practice within the group are very important, we believe that groups' primary power stems from people's innate drive to belong to a social group and to conform to its values as a way of making sense and gaining meaning from our multiple individual experiences (Boszormenyi-Nagy & Spark, 1973; Bowlby, 1988). Without the group, human language and the meanings of which we construct our lives are not possible. We derive our purposes and our values from the group, even as we stray from it into the isolation of addictions and mental illness. Nothing is more debilitating to the client with chemical dependency and mental illness than further isolation from others, although the impulsive and antisocial forces that are a part of their illness often cause that very result.

Of course, although groups do work in the treatment of chemical dependence, some groups work better than others. What conditions are important for chemical dependence group therapy to be productive?

THERAPIST CONSIDERATIONS

To use an old but important cliché, group therapy is both an art and a science. The therapist can approach group work usefully from either perspective, but must learn the importance of both. As an art, the therapy process is original, creative, and often driven by intuition (Zinker, 1977). As a science, therapy requires that we formally check our intuitions against the experience of supervisors, other group leaders, and group members; that we continue to study the group as an "N of one" experiment when that is possible; and that we complete both formative and summative evaluations as a routine part of our group work. Reviewing the group therapy literature, we found (1) that therapist variables (warmth, expertise, trust) were the best predictors of whether a client would stay in treatment; (2) that groups conducted by professional therapists retained more clients than those conducted by paraprofessionals; (3) that therapists especially need to develop expertise in expanding or further limiting self-disclosure concerning group members' questions about therapists' substance use; and (4) that psychodynamic counselors and highly active, aggressive counselors need to "cool their engines" concerning sexuality and confrontation until the client's sobriety has been firmed up by time and group experience.

In our experience, therapists who are most effective with groups tend to like the give and take of group work. They are not overly demanding or perfectionistic. They seem to adjust well to ambiguity and to have a good grasp of who they are and what range of behaviors they expect and can accept from the group. They seem to enjoy either leading the group or following along with it as it does its work, and they are not worried by the transitions between these complementary roles.

Therapists who seem less well suited to group work are not only nervous and confused about their lack of control of group interaction, but also don't seem to improve over time, even with adequate supervision. Some novice counselors are continually paralyzed when they sense the almost infinite number of possible interventions that might be appropriate during every moment of group work. Further, overly structured, demanding, and critical group counselors either develop new skills quickly or burn out from group members' avoidance and antagonism.

Nevertheless, we have seen shy, nervous, and somewhat inappropriate counselors become excellent group therapists over time and with good supervision. What shy or ignorant novices seem to need at heart is a firm commitment to personal growth and a willingness to suffer through mistakes with a sense of humor. As a rule, the group will tell you continually what it needs if you are able to listen. Don't be afraid to ask group members about how they understand ongoing group process. As is true of most counselor education, you often learn more from clients than from anyone else.

In the best of all possible worlds, counselors will have had didactic counselor education and group therapy courses, then chemical dependence treatment courses. Counselors should then demonstrate competence and experiential training with non–chemical dependence groups before launching into supervised group chemical dependence treatment facilitation. Of course, we do not live in the best of all possible worlds. From our perspective, on-the-job training is a suitable place to begin as an addiction therapist. Recovering paraprofessionals, however, should commit themselves to completing the didactic component of their overall training while participating as a cocounselor with a seasoned therapist.

Everyone who looks toward group leadership should certainly read Yalom's classic *Theory and Practice of Group Psychotherapy*. Another effective introduction to the major theories and much of the practical substance of group work is Donigian and Malnati's (1987) *Critical Incidents in Group Therapy*, which contains case work examples by experts in RET, client-centered, and Gestalt group work.

CLIENT CONSIDERATIONS

Clients who present for inpatient and outpatient structured treatment are a diverse group, coming to treatment with a variety of prior self-help and professional intervention experiences. Structured treatment groups are usually ongoing, adding new members ("newbies") as other members (old-timers) cycle out into aftercare relapse prevention groups and concurrent family and individual treatment. Prior to working with groups, inexperienced therapists should undergo closely supervised training at each critical phase of client treatment, including intervention and intake; detoxification (which can teach counselors a great deal about the difficulties of withdrawal and the tendency of some clients to leave against medical advice); regular therapy group; AA or NA 12-step groups, often in the evenings; family groups during family week; and aftercare and long-term relapse prevention groups. Structured groups come in a variety of types. Each has its own characteristic process strengths and weaknesses, with which counselors must gain familiarity through direct, day-to-day involvement.

Group therapy techniques vary depending on whether a group is inpatient or outpatient, structured or not, ongoing (with new members cycling in during a 30-day treatment program as others cycle out into aftercare, for example) or not, predominantly devoted to direct care or treatment aftercare and relapse prevention, and composed of old-timers or short-timers. The composition and aims of structured groups usually reflect the organizational biases and institutional affiliations of the treatment facility context. Most private facilities affiliated with churches, for example, utilize 12-step treatment models but frequently evolve their own group treatment plan. Ongoing structured groups commonly rotate members through a hierarchical sequence of planned interventions (developmental steps, stages, or phases). Inpatient groups usually meet every day of the week for three hours, or twice each day for two hours, morning and afternoon. In daily two-session groups, the morning group may be content-specific (educational), and the afternoon group may be designed to move members through the AA or NA 12 steps.

Time spent gaining an understanding of each new client's needs before he or she is introduced to the group will pay large dividends later on. It is particularly important to know which clients have special needs, especially if these may interfere with group processes. Concurrent psychiatric problems, particularly thought and personality disorders, can make group work very difficult; the contribution of clients with such problems to the group must be continually evaluated by the treatment team. The withdrawal and treatment regimen of all clients who are currently on psychiatric medications (or perhaps should be) should be evaluated by an addictionologist or psychiatric physician (Buelow & Hebert, 1995). Fortunately, the vast majority of clients, even those with severe concurrent problems, are able to work effectively in group settings. Clients with higher levels of sociopathy, however, respond better to coping skills training than to deeper emotional work in which confrontation among members is more typical.

Group leaders in structured outpatient settings are continually confronted with both selection and referral concerns. Even though not selecting a client can sometimes cause hard feelings, expelling a group member later is even more difficult. De-selection after the group has coalesced is certainly painful for therapist and client, but also can be destructive to group process, at least in the short term. Alliances among members are often built very quickly. Some members will feel rejected along with the referred member, whereas some will feel threatened that they may be dropped from group if they express difficulties. These concerns should be discussed in the group in detail and confronted at each difficult juncture in the development of group cohesion.

Group Work with Difficult Clients

Should a very difficult client be included in your group—the group you have worked so exhaustively to bring to a working level of cohesion? If the client is disruptive, should the group be allowed to bridle (or even muzzle) the new member, or should the counselor be responsible for taking the member aside and working with him or her on the issue that seems to be fragmenting the group? Most disruptive to outpatient groups are those who continue to drink or use other drugs (Brown & Yalom, 1977; Vanicelli, 1987). They may lie when confronted about members' suspicions (sandbagging) or may come to group visibly intoxicated or high, even though abstinence is the clearly stated focus of the group. As Brown and Yalom (1977) discovered, such behaviors must be met with a unified front by the group, including the therapist, or the group may be permanently disrupted. Members must be held responsible for conforming to group norms and expectations if the group is to survive and prosper. Individuals who are intoxicated must not be allowed to participate in group until they are sober. Their future participation should focus on moving them into inpatient therapy if they continue to drift into relapse. A member's isolated slip can serve as excellent grist for the mill for the group to process, however, if the lapse remains isolated. The group should be encouraged to explore the relapse dynamic that led to the slip and to work with the member on developing more effective ways to avert future slips. The group must be made part of the process of de-selection of relapsed members and must be helped to understand why the drugging member cannot be allowed in group while he or she is high. Most group members will understand the reasoning behind the decision-making process if it is explained prior to group during members' assessments and a second time during initial meetings of the group.

Clients with borderline, narcissistic, and antisocial personality disorders are difficult to work with in group, especially in outpatient settings. Because their thoughts and feelings are poorly coordinated, these clients demand a great deal of individual attention in group. They often display little empathy with other members or are manipulative and seductive. Because they tend to act out under the stresses of group interaction, these clients are often disruptive to group process. Acting-out may take the form of threats to leave the group, to relapse, or to harm themselves. To protect itself, the group may either isolate the individual or spend inordinate amounts of time on the individual's problems. Neither are acceptable long-term alternatives. Sometimes conflict with difficult members in very new or poorly functioning groups is used to deflect attention from the deficient group process itself. In either case, the focus of the group often moves from the crucial issue of sobriety toward pressuring the counselor to undertake individual treatment with the problem member using a group format. Counselors may find themselves suddenly (and to the novice, inexplicably) doing full-time psychotherapy with particular individuals in group, rather than acting in a facilitative and consultative role.

One solution, of course, is to move low-functioning and personality disordered clients into a more individualized treatment program. Such clients can be reintroduced to long-term group therapy with other personality disordered members when their interpersonal functioning has improved significantly so that they can put their improving social skills into action. A client should be removed from the group, however, only if he or she proves intractable to socialization or resocialization through group process and only after the problem has been discussed thoroughly within the group. It is often possible to use group and individual therapy concurrently to effect necessary immediate behavioral changes, even if deeper change is not forthcoming.

Since many individuals who are in the late middle stages of addiction often appear personality disordered when they enter therapy, how does one assess whether the individual is appropriate for group in the first place? After all, several or many of the client's MMPI subscale scores may be well out of the normal range. Several recommendations are in order.

First, borderline, narcissistic, and antisocial drug users are usually mandated or forced by their families into treatment; they rarely walk in off the street for treatment on their own. Second, although clients are ordinarily emotionally labile, detoxification usually improves their overall stability, even though they tend to be depressed, irritable, or anxious. More disordered clients, in contrast, are often highly impulsive or explosive. Third, there is usually a long paper trail stretching behind personality disordered clients. It is crucial to obtain clients' previous psychiatric records as soon as possible, therefore, whether you are working in a structured setting or privately. Counselors delay completing paperwork only at great professional risk. Finally, dual-diagnosis clients should be concurrently under the care of a consulting psychiatrist to whom they can be referred if their behavior deteriorates while in group treatment.

Although they are not always strictly dual diagnosis, we include as difficult clients those who display poorly controlled sexual drives. Their behavior often includes insistent, thinly disguised sexual joking and seductiveness. Sexual alliances among members often threaten the integrity of the group. If the behavior is directly confronted, the group prospers from resolving this developmental task successfully. Problems inherent in members' developing sexual liaisons need to be discussed beforehand with potential group members, and contracts designed accordingly. The intimacy of group work often engenders sexual feelings, and although the feelings themselves are positive and do not need to be blocked, the potential behaviors that they evoke need to be talked out as a normal part of group process. Therapists themselves may experience sexual feelings toward group members. If fantasies or daydreams about clients intrude into your interaction with them, it is wise to seek supervision. If you find yourself being seductive, or coworkers or family members mention seductiveness in your behavior with or talk about clients, examine the behavior with your supervisor, and debrief the issues with your own therapist if necessary. A professional and ethical booster shot is periodically necessary for all therapists and can prolong the periods between brownouts and burnouts. Sexual interest in clients is a prime symptom of burnout, which many therapists do not immediately recognize.

Gender and age differences, sexual preferences, and cultural, ethnic, and racial concerns are all grist for the group mill. Rather than impeding the development of group solidarity, differences of culture and perspective often intensify it. This intensification follows from the natural curiosity members have about one another's private worlds and helps clients move from investigating cultural diversity to investigating the universality of human experience, particularly the craving, psychological and physical deterioration, and loss of control inherent in chemical dependence among all peoples.

Finally, problems that are difficult in inpatient groups but can be handled in a well-staffed partial hospital setting often become impossible to manage effectively in outpatient groups. For that reason, screening, assessment, consultation with mentors, and knowledge and use of referral resources are crucial.

STAGES OF GROUP ACTION

Chemical dependence group members may be viewed as progressing through a series of developmental stages. Van Wormer (1987) described three phases: first, an early phase of 1 to 6 months during which the primary problem is one of denial versus identity; second, a middle phase of 6 to 12 months during which anger versus acceptance of one's addiction is the primary developmental concern; and, third, an ongoing phase during which problems stem primarily from isolation versus intimacy with others.

In our experience, group members rarely move through developmental stages in a consistent fashion. More often, members advance, then regress, then advance again. Some move slowly through some developmental issue, whereas others appear to bypass that issue altogether. We agree with Lewis, Dana, and Blevins (1994) that development of individuals in group is reflected in the following stages: First, there is movement from strongly narcissistic defenses of the self that include a variety of more primitive mechanisms (avoidance, denial, projection, and regression, for example), to more mature defenses. Second, there is movement from external compliance with group norms toward internalization. This movement indicates that new social and emotional behavior has begun to produce its own intrinsic rewards and, therefore, may become self-sustaining. Third, there is movement from internalization of group norms and accommodation with the specific therapy group toward transfer of these norms, rules, behaviors, and insights into the rest of the client's life (assimilation). Assisting continued movement through each stage of the client's development may require a variety of hierarchically graded clinical strategies.

Stage 1: Early Group Treatment

Working through the early stages of denial, projection, and regression requires supported learning, guided practice and catharsis, help in generalizing away from narcissistic impulses (universality), instillation of hope, and role modeling. At this stage, confrontation should consist of attempts to move the client into an authentic relationship with the therapist and other group members. A majority of clients will look to the therapist for support and guidance at this time. They should receive it without hesitation, even though dependency needs of each member should be examined within the context of the group at appropriate times. However, remember the general maxim: Don't do for clients (or the group) what they can do for themselves. Otherwise you will interfere with the group process and find that you have enabled the group's dependence on you.

McGuire, Taylor, Broome, Blau, and Abbot (1986) also found that members of newly formed groups need more structure (education and planned exercises, for example) to feel productive in the group. Early structure led to fewer miscellaneous comments and dead ends, higher levels of self-disclosure, and more risk taking. Although the comments of the study were directed to facilitators of groups composed of individuals beginning at the same time, this need for early structure is also reflected in newer members of ongoing groups. Structured activities clearly help new members learn the ropes and find meaningful roles to play in the group—not simply recapitulating dysfunctional family roles. Structured activities that demand new members' participation can, in some cases, involve having a particularly trustworthy member act as a new member's sponsor—one who helps them work on their written 12 steps, for example. Structure can also involve using fish-bowl techniques, during which younger members work with one another while they are observed by older members outside the circle who give them supportive feedback after the exercise (McGuire et al., 1986). Gestalt structure can include each member spending a few minutes each session on the hot seat, during which time they work in a structured way to reveal who they are (explaining their place or role in the family, for example, and discussing how that family role might influence their role in the group).

It is very important that new members feel support from the group before they face strong confrontation from more experienced members (McGuire et al., 1986; Rugel & Barry, 1990; Vannicelli, 1982; van Wormer, 1987). Unless they are able to develop a sense of support from, acceptance by, and identification with the group, new members wall themselves off from confrontation and therefore from the group. After that point, these members will work, but only on less threatening concerns. If a group were a chess game, the new member would be sacrificing pawns in order to protect more powerful pieces (more dangerous thoughts, feelings, and behaviors). Hiding or denying important material facts—particularly the power and depth of their addiction—is ego-syntonic or adaptive for clients; such behavior rarely yields to what is perceived as a frontal assault.

The movement from drug abuse to drug dependence is usually characterized by a gradual loss of control over vital life activities and internal processes, particularly the ability to solve problems, structure daily life, effectively resolve conflicts with others, and maintain intrapersonal access to feelings. A structured group approach to treatment can reverse this trend by helping clients regain both a sense of control and actual control over these vital life functions (Milam & Ketcham, 1983; van Wormer, 1987; Vannicelli, 1982). Vannicelli (1982) indicated that therapists need to provide more structure early in treatment because among the chemically dependent, psychiatric discomfort and clients' defenses are more diffuse and therefore more difficult to assess clinically, conceptualize accurately, and treat.

Rugel and Barry (1990) found that structured group treatment had significant effects on members' denial, an especially important component of chemical dependence that must be confronted early in treatment. They found that group acceptance reinforced self-acceptance, which led in turn to a deeper acknowledgment of the deteriorative effects of alcohol. They commented: "'Problems with drinking' become the unacceptable aspect of the self (that is, the rejected self) that cannot be allowed into awareness. . . . The chain of events that must occur if group treatment is [to be] successful in overcoming denial are group acceptance resulting in self-acceptance leading to increased willingness to acknowledge drinking problems—that is, decreased denial" (Rugel & Barry, 1990, p. 47). From their perspective, denial is a way to defend against loss of self-esteem occasioned by negative public and self-valuation. Denial, therefore, may be a necessary step in the recovery process, required in order to defend the ego. Rugel and Barry (1990) also found that, although early supportive self-exploration reduced the need to continue to erect denial defenses, catharsis (the venting of powerful emotions of remorse and shame) was positively correlated with denial and reinforced a lack of self-acceptance.

In an experimental comparison of inpatients in a treatment center with a control group who received center treatment but no social skills training, Eriksen, Bjornstad, and Gottestam (1986) found that the social skills training group were abstinent longer, had significantly fewer work absences, and had significantly more sober days after resumption of drinking. Their findings indicate that the development of social skills throughout treatment is an important component of group development and long-term relapse prevention. Deficits in social skills encourage interpersonal stress, which in turn predicts relapse (Marlatt, 1978).

Self-disclosure is learned most quickly and effectively within a group environment that provides sufficient structure (McGuire et al., 1986; Vannicelli, 1982). Lack of structure early in group development (as one might expect in laissez-faire and heavily client-centered groups, for example) apparently operates against process involvement. Probably, the higher risks of self-disclosure, lessened cohesion early in the group, and delays in learning caused by lack of practice and lack of task focus in unstructured groups are responsible for less effective group process in these situations.

Key Issues   Vannicelli (1982) pointed out six key issues that must be dealt with early in group treatment. First, leaders must be prepared to respond to questions from the group about their own drinking or other drug use history. As a leader, whether you are explicit about your past use or not, you must process the group's underlying fears that you will not understand or accept group members. You must own your level of expertise and confront directly members' concerns that you may not understand their situations.

Second, leaders must exert active outreach to keep members in group and encourage them to return to group after slips or relapses. Each leader must decide independently whether he or she is providing a resource or simply rescuing clients.

Third, the relationships (structural and therapeutic, for example) between your group and concurrent AA or educational groups must be made explicit. Otherwise, members will be ambivalent about which model to follow. Therapy groups stress process and, later, confrontation, both of which may be foreign after the supportive focus of self-help groups like AA and NA (Brown & Yalom, 1977). You should discuss with potential members, before they join the group, how AA and group therapy complement each other and how they differ; continue to discuss these issues during the first several sessions. It is also important to debrief the problems that can develop in the group when members socialize with other therapy group members and build subgroup alliances. Members whose experience has been limited to psychoeducational groups must be encouraged to explore the positive side of group therapy, especially as it differs from more comfortable self-help experiences.

Fourth, issues of confidentiality must be discussed and freely agreed on. This is particularly difficult for some therapists who work with clients mandated into treatment as a condition of employment by an employer who may, even with the best intentions, make unreasonable demands for information. You must, of course, have written consent from your client before you discuss the case, even though you are pressured by an employer, EAP, or governmental agency. Will you talk with clients' families about group members' lapses, absences from group, or other risks? Can confidentiality be maintained in a group? If it cannot be maintained in a rigid way, can it be treated as a developing group norm?

Fifth, contracts with members concerning such matters as what to do if they become suicidal (behavior control hierarchy and contract), what will happen if members come to group inebriated (bottom line), and how referrals will be handled must be agreed on in detail and in advance, and then regularly reinforced by discussion. What will you do with a member who says he is not drinking when you have reliable contradictory information from his family? It will happen sooner or later! Setting limits is critical. Each group member must understand and accept group norms around abstinence in particular. Even if group information about a member's abstinence is incorrect, the member must handle the problem appropriately, rather than behaving impulsively or attacking the group.

Group members and the leader must make contracts concerning group norms and enforce those contracts. If the contract is for total abstinence and a member comes to group inebriated, the member must be asked to leave and come back sober to the next meeting, when the slip or relapse can be more reasonably addressed. In such circumstances, it is also important to meet with the client and the client's family as soon as possible, to process the dynamics that are leading to relapse thoroughly. Continued refusals to acknowledge drug use when it is clearly present, lack of clear intent to stop using as manifested in continual crooked thinking, and frequent disruptions to group (or slips during outpatient work) must be met with tough love. The member may be referred to a more highly structured setting. If the group is already within an inpatient setting, these issues need to be thoroughly addressed by intervention staff and the client's treatment team.

Sixth and finally, you must know how to handle war stories. Members often talk about drug use or prior therapy as a defense against actual work. These stories often serve the same purpose they do in dysfunctional families. By acting out problems for the group rather than resolving them, the member relieves pressures that are building among members without affecting the status quo. How will you recognize these pressures and allow them more proactive release?

Stage 2: The Middle Stage

The second or middle stage is one of movement from acceptance of group norms to the internalization of those norms. This movement requires continued Stage 1 activities coupled with growing confrontation between members and pressure to develop deeper insight and self-supportive behavior. The counselor should help the group develop deeper levels of cohesiveness to combat the fragmentation that can result from more direct confrontation. Cohesion deepens when therapists support members as they confront common intrapersonal and interpersonal themes, including concerns for one another's effects on the group.

Van Wormer (1987) described the middle stage of group recovery as involving anger versus acceptance. Clients often find it frustrating, and sometimes infuriating, to admit that they have become not only habituated to a drug, but physically and psychologically subservient to it despite their best intentions, so that they require other people's intervention and support to succeed in maintaining abstinence. It is particularly important at this stage that clients internalize their identity as recovering persons and as productive members of the group. This identity as a recovering person instead of an addict is reinforced by emotional bonding within the group. Acceptance of the ongoing relationship between the addictive disease and the recovering self is signaled by the development of more normative means of emotional regulation and an acceptance of such powerful emotions as anger, guilt, and shame.

Development of insight into the nature of one's life without drugs should become a central focus in the middle stage of recovery. Misguided rescuing by other group members may be a sign of developing altruism and, therefore, a positive sign, even though the rescuing should be processed (and restricted) by the group. During this stage clients also give up much of their defensiveness and denial. Their ongoing change accelerates the processing of corrective emotional experiences—usually the recapitulation of deficits in clients' families of origin and the exploration of personal losses typical to drug addiction.

Developing healthy communication requires guided practice in managing group confrontation and conflict. Conflict management requires learning to listen actively, to reflect feelings accurately, and to summarize thoughts and feelings effectively. These skills can be taught through Gestalt interaction techniques, in which members are shown how to role-play being effective (and ineffective) cotherapists.

After several weeks of hard work, group members are more likely to profit from heightened levels of confrontation about staying in the "there and then" as opposed to the here and now, as well as confrontation about continuing their illogical thinking, reliance on irrational and magical beliefs, and lack of authenticity. Whereas members previously needed high levels of emotional support, in the middle stage they usually begin to gravitate toward higher and higher levels of self-support and authenticity in their conflictual interactions with one another and with the group facilitator. As communication in group becomes more direct, deeper insights are likely to follow. Toward the end of this stage the therapist spends noticeably less time as an educator and intervener and more time as a facilitator.

As therapy matures, supportive therapy gives way to more cognitively oriented therapy. Clients must achieve insight coupled with new behavioral and cognitive strategies, including guided practice, if they are to maintain their therapeutic gains. Without cognitive restructuring, clients rarely achieve emotional restructuring, and therefore return to drugs for emotional regulation. Interestingly, Gralf, Whitehead, and LeCompte (1986) found that, although supportive-insight groups and cognitive-behavioral groups tended to show the same levels of progress immediately after treatment, cognitive groups fared significantly better on a variety of measures (depression, for example) at four-month follow-up. This research indicates that supportive treatment without cognitive restructuring and behavioral modeling quickly leads to relapse for many clients.

The middle stage of group treatment builds upon early support and cognitive restructuring, and is an invitation to clients to develop deeper cognitive and emotional skills. Important activities include assertiveness training (Orosz, 1982), stress management (Brody, 1982), family role exploration (Buelow, 1994b; Harris & MacQuiddy, 1991), and anger and anxiety management (Suinn & Deffenbacher, 1988). Highly structured programs that teach stress reduction and anger management are not sufficient to overcome clients' relapse dynamics, however, if they are taught in isolation from the existential concerns of loneliness, boredom, emptiness, and isolation.

Inability to express anger, to resist social pressure, and to restructure negative internal states reliably predict relapse (Brownell, Marlatt, Lichtenstein, & Wilson, 1986; Marlatt & Gordon, 1985). Resistance to relapse is a matter not only of social skills training, but of renewed identity development. Those with immature ego structures are unable to handle powerful negative emotional states without drugs to buffer the aftershocks. Emotional regulation requires identity integration. Group members who prove to have very low self-efficacy should be referred to concurrent, long-term individual therapy.

Stage 3: Ongoing Treatment

In the final or ongoing stage of group recovery, therapists need to help clients acknowledge the painful realities of their past lives, make what amends are possible, and bridge into present responsibility (van Wormer, 1987). Later, group process should focus on the development of higher levels of intimacy with others, the reduction of rigidity, and the exploration of emotional responses that may trigger relapse. Clients should also be encouraged to explore ongoing self-help organizations more deeply. In the ongoing stage, existential and psychodynamic techniques can be used to great advantage.

Whether chemical dependence came before a character disorder or after it, drug use quickly evolves into the primary system for self-gratification, emotional self-support, and affect regulation (Flores & Mahon, 1993). Flores and Mahon indicated that the leader should move from the here and now to past events that may help group members better understand how they came to be as they are and believe as they do. The group leader must be able to balance between giving group members gratification (which they crave) and frustration (which they need to grow in the relationship). Therapists need to provide frustration, when that is necessary, by withholding approval and support.

If drugs have become a primary defense mechanism, and a means for emotional regulation as well, what chance does group therapy have raising competing self-structures? Fortunately, when group members are sober, their vulnerability to group persuasion and social control is heightened because they come to rely on group process as a vehicle for emotional expression and regulation. The group is in a solid position, then, to press group members to use more adult defenses and regulatory strategies, and to make group members aware when they regress back to earlier defenses. For example, one group member, John, appeared to be seething with anger as the group processed another members' relatively safe issue. "John," I said, "you seem angry." "Do I?" John practically screamed at me. "I don't feel angry! I was concentrating on what was being said!" When the group helped him process the discrepancy between what he was thinking about (attending to the topic) and how he was actually feeling (needing a drink), he burst into laughter along with the rest of the group.

Personal defenses that are successful in the client's family are less effective in group because more mature members directly confront the defensiveness and are less affected than family members by a comember's reprisals. If a member mistakenly behaves as though the group facilitator is like their authoritarian father, for example, the projection is not likely to succeed, even with a novice facilitator, because members have usually worked their way through the problem and are willing to confront their comember. Because these maneuvers fail so starkly in mature groups, even novice cofacilitators need not be defensive when they find themselves under attack.

The ongoing stage is signaled by deepening levels of insight. During corrective emotional experiences, clients reveal early experiences that injured their ability to trust, love, and respect themselves and others. These early negative experiences acted to block emotional growth by encouraging children to erect defenses against emotional involvement. A corrective emotional experience allows clients to express deeply painful injuries without the catastrophic rejection that they were taught to expect if they revealed family secrets.

Although many group members suffered early emotional injuries from their parents, they also continue to suffer remorse for injuries they have inflicted on others as adults. All injuries, whether done to them or by them, should be fully explored. Clients often receive secondary gains (in the form of continued drugging of their feelings) for their shame, grief, and remorse. Continuing self-punishment will ultimately lead them back into drug use. Because drugs were consistently used for emotional regulation, group members require both support and confrontation from the group as they learn to give up the gains derived from self-punishment.

Long-Term Change Processes   Ongoing and mature phases of treatment have been described in detail by a variety of group specialists, including Brown and Yalom (1977), Duffy (1990), Flores (1988), Flores and Mahon (1993), Vannicelli (1982, 1987), and Yalom (1995), as well as specialists in relapse dynamics (Brownell et al., 1986; Marlatt, 1978; Marlatt & Gordon, 1985). Existential and psychodynamic concerns are central to understanding long-term change processes because, ultimately, we must understand not simply the cognitive and environmental (sociological) contribution to sobriety and relapse but the peculiarly psychological aspects of it. For example, why are individuals with faulty early object relations the most vulnerable to drugs and to drug relapse? For what internal processes and drives do drugs substitute? What long-standing psychic injuries are typical to chemical dependence?

Khantzian and Schneider (1986) described a psychodynamic perspective as one that "attempts to examine the forces at work within an individual related to drives, affects, and those psychological structures that are responsible for regulating drives and affects." These authors encouraged therapists during the ongoing phase of chemical dependence treatment to be concerned with how chemical dependence has redirected clients' expression of normal drives (such as sexuality and sociality), affected emotional regulation, and led to the development of new and pathological drive states (such as constant needs for immediate pleasure).

Khantzian and Schneider (1986) pointed out the following train of events. Whether individuals are attracted to drugs because of early deficiencies in ego development, or whether their chemical dependence leads to cumulative ego deficiencies, addicts show an incremental pattern of disturbance in self-regulation over time.

Their limited ability to manage affect is exacerbated by the artificial drives that develop with chemical dependencies—such as the attraction to euphoria and aversion from withdrawal. Internal gratifications and feelings of security become more and more circumscribed. Self-structures are unstable and ineffective for regulation of feelings. Resulting painful experiences, especially anger and aggression, trigger psychological disorganization and fragmentation. Interpersonal relationships, eroded by chemical dependence, become breeding grounds for more painful experiences, which are then emotionally contained by further drug use. In addition to inadequacies in affect regulation and self-care, disturbances in self-efficacy, need satisfaction, and interdependency with others also develop.

Because painful experiences lurk just below the surface, and because interpersonal dependency needs have been distorted or denied, Khantzian and Schneider (1986) suggested that treatment should begin in a structured environment in which narcissistic traits can be contained—one that allows these experiences and dependencies to manifest themselves in a controlled, regulated way. Because groups can produce high levels of interpersonal control, they are well designed to accomplish this long-term emotional containment. About this power of groups, Flores and Mahon (1993, p. 152) wrote:

> It is in the realm of interpersonal relationships that the group becomes a powerful therapeutic force. Utilizing the power of the here-and-now experience in the group, we began examining and gently pushing each group member to understand and look at the others' interpersonal exchanges in the group. We particularly emphasize all conscious or unconscious destructive interpersonal patterns as they emerge among members and with the group leaders. As Anne Alonso said (August 1990; personal communication) "people don't have to talk about their problems in group, they have them." In essence the group becomes among other things, a laboratory on interpersonal relationships. For instance, members who have difficulty with anger will start having difficulty with angry members or their own anger in group. Members who have difficulty trusting women will start having difficulties trusting women in group. Each member's particular idiosyncratic vulnerability will come alive in the here and now of the group.
>
> More than individual therapy, group treatment helps facilitate the process of modification of altering internal object relation distortions while allowing group members to change destructive patterns of interactions with others in their external world. The group can more readily do this because it gives the substance abuser a far wider array of individuals on whom they can depend. By virtue of the number of group members, the group format dilutes the intensity of the feelings that are sure to be activated in any close interpersonal relationship and that have to be worked through if characterological change is to occur. Although this process is likely to be too threatening in a one-to-one relationship, the group provides a safer holding environment that will give substance abusers more "space" while permitting them to deal with the intense hostility and ambivalence they are sure to experience as their need for approval, dependence, and caring surfaces.

Group members clearly act as cotherapists in ongoing groups. This individual responsibility for group process leads to accelerated healing, but it may also increase liabilities. Group members' liabilities include, for example, feeling incompetent, failing to control the group process, trying to rescue the group facilitator when problems arise, and feeling overly responsible for other members' behavior, especially when members leave group against medical advice (AMA).

Leaving Treatment Against Medical Advice   As we find in all nonmandated therapy, group members leave AMA for a variety of reasons. Experience indicates that clients leave both outpatient and inpatient treatment because of a variety of relapse, family, or financial problems. Like clients who receive no treatment aftercare, those who leave AMA have a very poor prognosis for continued sobriety (Ericksen, Bjornstad, & Gottestam, 1986). It is not clear, however, whether partial treatment has any continued positive effects for clients who leave prematurely.

Unless concerns around a member's leaving treatment are processed immediately and thoroughly, the group may unreasonably blame itself or, in an attempt to regain its cohesion, gang up on the facilitator. This blaming process may be exacerbated if a group member has attempted or completed suicide and the group is not guided through the grieving process (Buelow, 1994a). A group that has successfully processed concerns for self-destructive members, however, may become more resilient and responsible. Group leaders who have successfully faced this threat to group integrity and who receive specific support from both peers and employers, also appear to become more resilient and more willing to push the group to work on difficult issues, including self-destructive thoughts and over-responsibility for other members' behavior.

Suicide   Losing a group member to suicide is the greatest possible stressor for a group (Kibel, 1973) and for the therapist, as both a group member and a mental health professional (Brown, 1987; Buelow, 1994a; Chemtob, Hamada, Bauer, Kinney, & Torigoe, 1988a, 1988b; Goldstein & Buongiorno, 1984). Unfortunately, suicides are significantly more common among chemically dependent people, and particularly among late adolescents. Deykin and Buka (1994) reported a suicide incidence for substance-abusing youth approximately ten times that of a normative sample. Paralleling other studies, they also found that thoughts about suicide were especially predictive of suicide attempts when coupled with general depression, thoughts about death in general (attractiveness), and thoughts about the desirability (positive gains) of dying. Significantly, Deykin and Buka (1994) also found that risk of suicide approximately doubled among young males coming from conditions of victimization (physical and sexual abuse), but that women showed no such elevation. Why this significant difference exists was not clear from the data, but our experience in such cases may provide a clue. Apparently drug-abusing young men and women develop very different coping mechanisms: Men tend to use drugs and act out in impulsive ways, whereas women under the influence tend more to seek social support (Buelow & Buelow, 1995).

Treatment centers must continually assess clients for suicidal ideation and provide psychiatric consultation. They must also develop specific response protocols to facilitate the coping of both the surviving family and the treatment group if a client attempts or successfully completes suicide. It is crucial for the therapist to have emotional and professional support during this critical period (Buelow, 1994a; Resnik, 1969).

ALCOHOLICS ANONYMOUS AND
12-STEP GROUP TREATMENT

Alcoholics Anonymous (AA) was begun in the 1930s by two alcoholics, Bill Wilson and Bob Smith, whose discussions and mutual support served to help them remain sober. Supportively working with small groups of interested individuals with alcohol dependence, by 1939 Wilson and Smith's membership had reached about 100 men and women (George, 1990, p. 167). Publication of the book *Alcoholics Anonymous* by the organization in the late 1930s led to the rapid development of alcoholism self-help groups around the United States and the world. Millions of individuals who have worked the AA program have achieved a high-quality sobriety they might not otherwise have achieved.

From early on, as today, AA has the following features: First, it is open to anyone with a sincere interest in curbing his or her alcoholism. Second, members of the AA fellowship listen nonjudgmentally to one another's accounts of their continuing battle with addiction and to each member's views of what helped and what hurt efforts at sobriety. Third, sobriety is fostered by an AA sponsor. Fourth, members must overcome denial of alcoholism to find physical, emotional, and spiritual healing. And, fifth, in accord with Bowman and Jellinek (1941), Jellinek (1960), and the American Medical Association, AA views alcoholism as a complex physical, emotional, cognitive, and spiritual disease. From an AA point of view, one can only partially recover from such a complex illness and can never return to drinking or drugging without activating the multiple addictive forces of the illness. Thus AA members say that they are recovering, rather than recovered or cured.

The 12 Steps

The 12 steps in AA and Narcotics Anonymous (NA) and other AA-styled, 12-step organizations (Gamblers Anonymous, for example) provide a spiritually oriented, but psychologically sophisticated, strategy to combat addiction. Members of AA recover from addiction by following these steps.

1. Admitted we were powerless over alcohol [or other drugs]—that our lives had become unmanageable.
2. Came to believe that a Power greater than ourselves could restore us to sanity.
3. Made a decision to turn our will and our lives over to the care of God as we understood Him.
4. Made a searching and fearless moral inventory of ourselves.
5. Admitted to God, to ourselves, and to another human being the exact nature of our wrongs.
6. Were entirely ready to have God remove all these defects of character.
7. Humbly asked Him to remove our shortcomings.
8. Made a list of all persons we had harmed and became willing to make amends to them all.
9. Made direct amends to such people wherever possible, except when to do so would injure them or others.
10. Continued to take personal inventory and when we were wrong, promptly admitted it.

11. Sought through prayer and meditation to improve our conscious contact with God as we understood Him, praying only for knowledge of His will for us and the power to carry that out.
12. Having had a spiritual awakening as the result of these Steps, we tried to carry this message to alcoholics [or drug abusers] and practice these principles in all our affairs.

Although AA is not advertised as a treatment for alcoholism, and in order to protect members' privacy the organization does not allow research to be conducted under its auspices, both independent research and treatment experience indicate that AA membership and support, sponsors' interventions, and "working the program" by continuing to progress through the 12 steps has helped millions of individuals achieve sobriety and remain sober (Alford, Koehler, & Leonard, 1991; Arnold, 1973; Brown & Peterson, 1991; Chatlos, 1989; McBride, 1991).

Because AA is not a treatment, it should not be compared with structured inpatient (including residential) or outpatient treatments for addictions. When AA and NA participation is concurrent with structured treatment, however, formal and self-help modalities together provide a formidable intervention, support, and relapse prevention regimen. Despite little comparative research, we do not doubt that other self-help groups, like Rational Recovery, that do not have a spiritual focus, can also be an important adjunct to structured therapy. A note of caution, however, needs to be sounded. Brown and Yalom (1977) discovered that individuals with extensive experience in AA must quickly be taught the differences in structure, process, and goals that exist between AA's supportive format and therapy group's exploratory and confrontational format. Otherwise, group members may feel that the group's confrontation, continual feedback, and focus on psychological process are intrusive and counterproductive. (Indeed, without a well-trained group leader, these strategies may very well be destructive.) If these differences are well explored and explained beforehand, however, concurrent AA participants usually adapt very well to insight and process focused groups.

Concerns About 12-Step Programs

Psychologists have expressed a variety of both reasonable and unreasonable concerns about AA's philosophy and perspective. These criticisms include that AA and NA are not treatments; that AA and NA are treatments but do not allow outcome research; that alcoholism and other addictions are not diseases but preferences; that an admission of powerlessness over alcohol may undermine the necessary internal locus of control; and that references to spirituality and a higher power shift emphasis away from individuals' being responsible for themselves and finding their own solutions (Ellis & Velten, 1992; Lewis, Dana, & Blevins, 1994).

To respond to these criticisms, first, of course, AA and NA are not, and do not claim to be, treatments for addictions. Clients should be referred to self-help groups as an adjunct to structured treatment, to provide support against relapse, or when they simply will not use any other mode of intervention or structured treatment. For many alcoholics and other drug-dependent clients who do not find a psychological approach helpful, however, the social and spiritual guidance of AA/NA may be the only intervention they ever receive.

Second, whether one views chemical dependence as a disease or not (and saying that it is one certainly does not imply that it shares every criterion in common with infectious disease processes), it is important to recognize that it is a primary clinical syndrome that, short of death, is not self-limiting and that is not necessarily caused by any other underlying problem. Also, no matter how well chemical dependencies fit classical disease models, addictions are multifaceted. They rarely yield to individual psychological treatments that do not focus specifically and independently on the realities of addiction processes, stages of behavioral change, and relapse dynamics.

Third, it is our experience that an admission of powerlessness in the face of an addiction does not undermine the client's locus of control. Such an admission is a recognition that one can never return to drinking or other drugs without activating the addiction cycle. It is in this sense that individuals see themselves as recovering, never cured. Addictions undermine internal locus of control so successfully (placing control and emotional regulation in the drug), that such fears are relatively trivial for the vast majority of addicted people. Individuals well into the middle, or in the late, deteriorative phases of addictions are, for all practical purposes, powerless in relation to alcohol or other drugs, and their lives have certainly become unmanageable. In our experience, clients who come to believe that a power greater than they are might help restore their sobriety and sanity, whether that power is AA, society in general, or a friendly godlike figure, rarely find their self-efficacy much undermined.

Although the tenets and 12 steps of AA can be flexed around almost any philosophical problem or paradox, we should reiterate that AA is a fellowship. Like any fellowship, AA is not a specific treatment, makes no guarantees, is not perfect, and is not for everyone. If visitors to AA meetings do not prosper there, they are under no obligation to continue. They should definitely search out a different form of support or treatment. Self-help, step-type support groups designed by nonreligious persons, like Rational Recovery, that do not emphasize a higher power are available in many population centers. We have observed that these secular groups support, educate, and serve their members faithfully and well. Also, nonreligious self-help readings are common. Ellis and Velten (1992), for example, provided well thought-out self-help information and a list of resources for those who wish to use their rational-emotive approach to sobriety.

Stages and 12-Step Programs

As we have studied what works and what does not seem to work in this field, we have learned that the 12-step program contains a hierarchy of sound developmental steps designed to help clients move through many of the stages we have already suggested to be important in treatment (Arnold, 1977; Chatlos, 1989). These 12 steps include: first, a recognition, that drugs have made our lives unmanageable (admission of the problem, or direct conflict with the denial system). Second, we come to believe that forces generated outside ourselves (whether generated by the group, or a god, or loved ones), as well as our own commitment and work, are necessary to help us recover (submission or surrender). Third, we subject ourselves, our minds, our emotions, and our spiritual being or consciousness to as complete an exploration as is humanly possible (reconstruction). And, fourth, we admit our problems and transgressions, and attempt to right them by direct action and self-responsibility (restitution and responsibility).

These four developmental themes are common to most forms of counseling or psychotherapy (Boszormenyi-Nagy & Spark, 1973; Corey, 1991; Okun, 1990; Perls, Hefferline, & Goodman, 1951). Without an admission of the problem, therapy cannot begin. Without submission to others' influence and insight, there can be no consistent insight into the self, particularly the social (and socially abusive) self. Without restitution and reconstruction, responsibility for self is stunted and personality change is blocked. Thus, whether one goes through treatment steps or stages is not especially important. What matters is that individuals progress in their self-exploration from narcissism toward awareness of the needs of self and others; from crooked to straight, rational thinking; from concrete to formal thinking; from emotional constriction to reconstruction (fostering emotional depth, breadth, and flexibility); and from drug-induced emotional regulation to self-regulation.

Self-help groups also provide supportive aftercare. In the case of AA and NA, that aftercare can be lifelong. Most AA members who have achieved a high-quality sobriety, however, interact less and less with AA over time and usually turn their attention to resolving problems of living. Members are likely to go back to AA if they suffer problems that reactivate their craving to drink or use. Dangerous relapse indicators include, for example, increasing denial of feelings; overconfidence about recovery; avoidance of intimacy; overreaction to stress; compulsive behavior around work, sex, and food; living in the there and then rather than the here and now; hoarding; daydreaming; avoiding; feeling helpless; lying; using over-the-counter medications; visiting old drinking buddies; and attempting to practice controlled drinking (George, 1990, p. 181). Although controlled drinking may prove productive with some problem drinkers who have not been dependent on alcohol, it is, as we have indicated, unwise for individuals who have ever been addicted or dependent on alcohol or other drugs to experiment (Lewis, Dana, & Blevins, 1994).

Finally, decisions about whether and how to refer clients to step or stage treatment and aftercare groups should depend upon client characteristics, not therapist prejudices. Severely personality disordered and manipulative clients often do poorly in AA or NA, whereas more normative clients with religious or spiritually oriented backgrounds usually profit from such a fellowship. Individuals who are compulsively self-reliant, however, may suffer debilitating anxiety when confronted in a such a group setting. Counselors should encourage their clients to sample a variety of treatment and relapse prevention modalities when practicable, including AA or NA.

Perhaps the most salient aspect of ongoing groups is the cotherapist status of members who have deepening history with the group and who tend to act as guides, role models, and, at times, transference objects for new members. Because the group is often in full process when a new member enters, the member is thrown into a fully functioning, working group, rather than one that has to move through forming, storming, and norming before it can begin work. Although entering a group in full process can accelerate new members' work with the group, it can also be threatening. If it is overly threatening, new members rapidly begin to act like old hands (asking fellow members how they feel, for example), but do not internalize the model to which they are conforming. They often isolate safe emotional domains in which to work, while protecting deeper problem areas (sexuality, for example) within which many relapse triggers may be buried. It is the therapist's responsibility to move the new member gradually into exposure and confrontation with the group. A sensitive reminder to more mature members, who are able to withstand very direct confrontation, of their responsibility to support as well as (supportively) confront new members may be in order.

At the same time that new members are confronting their many-faceted denial systems and crooked thinking, older members may be working on fears of relapse after release from the center, and on problems that have surfaced during family week. Interestingly, new members rarely forget other members' problems and life stories. They often refer back to the problems and solutions of graduated members. We may hear, for example: "Well, for me it's like it was with John, right before he graduated from group. You remember when he said that he was really more bothered about relapse coming from his getting into a fight with his kids than anything to do with his marriage. Well, that's the way it seems to be with me right now; it's the kids that are driving me crazy!"

Finally, groups go through stages of development that often parallel those of individual clients, as they move from lower-level accommodation (accepting new ideas) toward higher-level assimilation (integrating and using new ideas), insight, and responsibility. Individuals learn, first, about themselves, then about others, then about the processes through which they learn about self and others. In a similar growth pattern, groups learn about themselves—who they are and what they are. Then some group members, though certainly not all, begin to understand the group processes that have fostered their individual change.

STUDY AND DISCUSSION QUESTIONS

1. Besides Rogers's (1970) necessary conditions, what other conditions does group therapy provide that are particularly important in chemical dependence treatment?

2. What particular problems may arise in group therapy with chemically abusive or dependent clients that are much less likely in other groups?

3. Outline personal background, training, and interactional considerations specific to chemical dependence therapists as they interact with their group clients.

4. What group norms and expectations should be clearly enforced if a chemical abuse or dependence group is to prosper?

5. Under what circumstances are dual-diagnosis clients most likely to be successfully integrated into a non-dual-diagnosis group?

6. Evaluate Van Wormer's (1987) developmental stages among chemical dependence group members. Do these stages make sense and reflect your experience?

7. Why is structure and education so important early in group chemical dependence therapy?

8. How should you handle issues of therapists' self-disclosure in chemical dependence groups?

9. How should confrontation be handled in chemical dependence groups?

10. Briefly outline the 12-step approach to group treatment, and compare it with a stage approach of your choice.

REFERENCES

ABLE, E. L. (1985). Late sequelae of fetal alcohol syndrome. In U. Rydberg, C. Alling, & J. Engel (Eds.), *Alcohol and the developing brain* (pp. 125–134). Stockholm: Raven.

ABLE, E. L., & RILEY, E. P. (1986). Studies of prenatal alcohol exposure. In J. R. West (Ed.), *Alcohol and brain development* (pp. 105–119). New York: Oxford University Press.

ABRAMS, D. B., & WILSON, G. T. (1979). Effects of alcohol on social anxiety in women: Cognitive versus physiological processes. *Journal of Abnormal Psychology, 88,* 161–173.

ADELMAN, S. A., FLETCHER, K. E., & BAHNASSI, A. (1993). Pharmacotherapeutic management strategies for mentally ill substance abusers. *Journal of Substance Abuse Treatment, 10,* 353–358.

AINSWORTH, M. D. S. (1989). Attachments beyond infancy. *American Psychologist, 44,* 709–716.

AINSWORTH, M. D. S., BLEHAR, M. C., WATERS, E., & WALL, S. (1978). *Patterns of attachment: A psychological study of the strange situation.* Hillsdale, NJ: Erlbaum.

AINSWORTH, M. D. S., & BOWLBY, J. (1991). An ethological approach to personality development. *American Psychologist, 46,* 333–341.

ALDWIN, C. M. (1994). *Stress, coping, and development.* New York: Guilford.

ALFORD, G. S., KOEHLER, R. A., & LEONARD, J. (1991). Alcoholics Anonymous–Narcotics Anonymous model inpatient treatment and chemically dependent adolescents: A two-year outcome study. *Journal of Studies on Alcohol, 52,* 118–126.

ALLEN, J. P., & COLUMBUS, M. (Eds.). (1995). *Assessing alcohol problems: A guide for clinicians and researchers. National Institute on Alcohol Abuse and Alcoholism Treatment Handbook Series 4* (NIH Publication No. 95-3745). Bethesda, MD: National Institute on Alcohol Abuse and Alcoholism.

ALLING, C. (1985). Biochemical maturation of the brain and the concept of vulnerable periods. In U. Rydberg, C. Alling, & J. Engel (Eds.), *Alcohol and the developing brain* (pp. 5–10). Stockholm: Raven.

ALTERMAN, A. I. (1985). Differentiation of alcoholics high and low in childhood hyperactivity. *Drug and Alcohol Dependence, 15,* 111–121.

ALTERMAN, A. I., O'BRIEN, C. P., McLELLAN, A. T., AUGUST, D. S., SNIDER, E. C., DROBA, M., CORNISH, J. W., HALL, C. P., RAPHAELSON, A. H., & SCHRADE, F. X. (1994). Effectiveness and costs of inpatient versus day hospital cocaine rehabilitation. *The Journal of Nervous and Mental Disease, 182,* 157–163.

AMERICAN PSYCHIATRIC ASSOCIATION. (1994). *Diagnostic and statistical manual of mental disorders* (4th ed.). Washington, DC: Author.

AMERICAN SOCIETY OF ADDICTION MEDICINE. (1996). Patient placement criteria for the treatment of substance-related disorders (2nd ed.). Chevy Chase, MD: Author.

ANTHENELLI, R. M., & SCHUCKIT, M. A. (1993). Affective and anxiety disorders and alcohol and drug dependence: Diagnosis and treatment. *Journal of Addictive Diseases, 12*(3), 73–87.

ARMSDEN, G. C., & GREENBERG, M. T. (1987). The inventory of parent and peer attachment: Individual differences and their relationship to psychological well-being in adolescence. *Journal of Youth and Adolescence, 16,* 427–453.

ARNDT, I. O., MCLELLAN, A. T., DOROZYNSKY, L., WOODY, G. E., & O'BRIEN, C. P. (1994). Desipramine treatment for cocaine dependence. *The Journal of Nervous and Mental Disease, 182*, 151–156.

ARNOLD, R. (1973). The use of milieu therapy in alcoholics anonymous. *Journal of Emotional Education, 13*, 103–119.

ARNOLD, R. J. (1977). AA's 12 steps as a guide to ego integrity. *Journal of Contemporary Psychotherapy, 9*, 62–77.

ARONSON, M., & OLEGARD, R. (1985). Fetal alcohol effects in pediatrics and child psychology. In U. Rydberg, C. Alling, & J. Engel (Eds.), *Alcohol and the developing brain* (pp. 135–146). Stockholm: Raven.

ATKINSON, D. R., MORTEN, G., & WING SUE, D. (1989). *Counseling American minorities: A cross-cultural perspective*. Madison, WI: Brown & Benchmark.

BAKER, R. W., MCNEIL, O. V., & SIRYK, B. (1985). Expectation and reality in freshman adjustment to college. *Journal of Counseling Psychology, 32*, 94–103.

BALCERZAK, W. S., & HOFFMAN, N. G. (1985). Dual treatment rationale for psychologically disordered and chemically dependent clients. *Alcoholism Treatment Quarterly, 2*(2), 61–67.

BALIS, S. A. (1987). Illusion and reality: Issues in the treatment of adult children of alcoholics. *Alcoholism Treatment Quarterly, 3*, 67–91.

BARBER, J. G. (1995). Working with resistant drug abusers. *Social Work, 40*, 18–23.

BARLOW, D. H. (1984). Issues, ethics, and examples in the use of time-series methodology in practice. In D. H. Barlow, S. C. Hayes, & R. O. Nelson (Eds.), *The scientist practitioner: Research and accountability in clinical and educational settings* (pp. 273–290). New York: Pergamon Press.

BARLOW, D. H. (1988). *Anxiety and its disorders: The nature and treatment of anxiety and panic*. New York: Guilford.

BARLOW, D. H., & CERNEY, J. A. (1988). *Psychological treatment of panic*. New York: Guilford.

BARNARD, C. P., & SPOENTGEN, P. A. (1986). Children of alcoholics: Characteristics and treatment. *Alcoholism Treatment Quarterly, 3*(4), 47–65.

BARNES, G. M., & WELTE, J. W. (1990). Prediction of adults' drinking patterns from the drinking of their parents. *Journal of Studies on Alcohol, 51*, 523–527.

BARNETT, D. W., & FAGAN, R. W. (1993). Alcohol use in male spouse abusers and their female partners. *Journal of Family Violence, 8*, 1–25.

BARTHOLOMEW, K., & HOROWITZ, L. M. (1991). Attachment styles among young adults: A test of a four category model. *Journal of Personality and Social Psychology, 61*, 226–244.

BAXTER, L. R., SCHWARTZ, J. M., BERGMAN, K. S., SZUBA, M. P., GUZE, B. H., MAZZIOTTA, J. C., ALAZRAKI, A., SELIN, C. E., HWANG-KWANG, F., MUNFORD, P., & PHELPS, M. C. (1992). Caudate glucose metabolic rate changes with both drug and behavior therapy for obsessive-compulsive disorder. *Archives of General Psychiatry, 49*, 681–689.

BEAN-BAYOG, M. (1986). Psychopathology produced by alcoholism. In R. E. Meyer (Ed.), *Psychopathology and addictive disorders* (pp. 334–345). New York: Guilford.

BEAVERS, W. R., & KASLOW, F. W. (1981, April). The anatomy of hope. *Journal of Marital and Family Therapy, 7*(2), 119–126.

BECK, A. T., RUSH, A. J., SHAW, B. F., & EMERY, G. (1979). *Cognitive therapy of depression*. New York: Guilford.

BECK, A. T., WRIGHT, F. D., NEWMAN, C. F., & LIESE, B. S. (1993). *Cognitive therapy of substance abuse*. New York: Guilford.

BECKMAN, L. J. (1975). Women alcoholics: A review of social and psychological studies. *Journal of Studies on Alcohol, 36*, 797–824.

BECKMAN, L. J. (1980). Perceived antecedents and effects of alcohol consumption in women. *Journal of Studies on Alcohol, 41*, 518–530.

BEGUN, A., & ZWEBEN, A. (1990). Assessment and treatment implications of adjustment and coping capacities in children living with alcoholic parents. *Alcoholism Treatment Quarterly, 7*(2), 23–40.

BENSEN, C. S., & HELLER, K. (1987). Factors in the current adjustment of young daughters of alcoholics and problem drinking fathers. *Journal of Abnormal Psychology, 96*, 305–312.

BERKOWITZ, A. D., & PERKINS, H. W. (1986). Problem drinking among college students: A review of recent research. *Journal of American College Health, 35*, 21–28.

BERN, E. (1964). *Games people play*. New York: Ballantine Books.

BLACK, C. (1981). *It will never happen to me*. Denver: MAC.

BLACK, C., BUCKEY, S. F., & WILDER-PADILLA, S. (1986). The interpersonal and emotional consequences of being an adult child of an alcoholic. *The International Journal of the Addictions, 21*, 213–231.

BLANKERTZ, L. E., & CNAAN, R. A. (1993, Summer). Serving the dually diagnosed homeless: Program development and interventions [Special section: Alcohol and drug abuse services for homeless populations]. *Journal of Mental Health Administration, 20* (2), 100–109.

BLOOD, L., & CORNWALL, A. (1994). Pretreatment variables that predict completion of an adolescent substance abuse treatment program. *The Journal of Nervous and Mental Disease, 182,* 14–19.

BLOOM, B. L. (1985). A factor analysis of self-report measures of family functioning. *Family Process, 24,* 225–239.

BLOS, P. (1979). *The adolescent passage.* New York: International University Press.

BLUM, K. (1982). Neurophysiological effects of alcohol. In E. M. Pattison & E. Kaufman (Eds.), *Encyclopedic handbook of alcoholism* (pp. 105–134). New York: Gardner Press.

BLUM, T. C., & ROMAN, P. M. (1985). The social transformation of alcoholism intervention: Comparisons of job attitudes and performance of recovered alcoholics and non-alcoholics. *Journal of Health and Social Behavior, 26,* 365–378.

BOND, N. W. (1986). Fetal alcohol exposure and hyperactivity in rats. In J. R. West (Ed.), *Alcohol and brain development* (pp. 45–70). New York: Oxford University Press.

BORDIN, E. S. (1979). The generalizability of the psychoanalytic concept of the working alliance. *Psychotherapy Theory, Research and Practice, 16,* 252–260.

BOSZORMENYI-NAGY, I., & KRASNER, B. R. (1986). *Between give and take.* New York: Brunner/Mazel.

BOSZORMENYI-NAGY, I., & SPARK, G. M. (1973). *Invisible loyalties.* New York: Harper & Row.

BOWDEN, B. S., & BERG, R. C. (1992). Group treatment with chemically dependent adolescents in residential settings. *Alcoholism Treatment Quarterly, 9,* 39–51.

BOWEN, M. (1978). *Family therapy in clinical practice.* New York: Jason Aronson.

BOWERS, T. G., & AL-REDHA, M. R. (1990). A comparison of outcome with group/marital and standard/individual therapies with alcoholics. *Journal of Studies on Alcohol, 51,* 301–309.

BOWLBY, J. (1969). *Attachment and loss: Vol. 1. Attachment.* New York: Basic Books.

BOWLBY, J. (1973). *Attachment and loss: Vol. 2. Separation, anxiety, and anger.* New York: Basic Books.

BOWLBY, J. (1980). *Attachment and loss: Vol. 3. Loss, sadness, and depression.* New York: Basic Books.

BOWLBY, J. (1988). *A secure base: Parent-child attachment and human development.* New York: Basic Books.

BOWMAN, K. M., & JELLINEK, E. M. (1941). Alcoholic mental disorders. *Quarterly Journal of Studies on Alcoholism, 11,* 312–390.

BOYER, P. A. (1989). A guide to therapy with families with a chemically dependent parent. *Psychotherapy, 26,* 88–95.

BRENNAN, K. A., SHAVER, P. R., & TOBEY, A. E. (1991). Attachment styles, gender, and parental problem drinking. *Journal of Social and Personal Relationships, 8,* 451–466.

BRODY, A. (1982). S.O.B.E.R.: A stress management program for recovering alcoholics. *Social Work with Groups, 5,* 15–24.

BROWN, H. N. (1987). The impact of suicide on therapists in training. *Comprehensive Psychiatry, 28,* 101–112.

BROWN, H. P., & PETERSON, J. H. (1991). Assessing spirituality in addiction treatment and follow-up: Development of the Brown-Peterson Recovery Progress Inventory (B-PRPI). *Alcoholism Treatment Quarterly, 8,* 21–45.

BROWN, S., & YALOM, L. D. (1977). Interactional group therapy with alcoholics. *Journal of Studies on Alcohol, 38,* 426–456.

BROWN, S. A. (1985). Expectancies versus background in the prediction of college drinking patterns. *Journal of Consulting and Clinical Psychology, 53* (1), 123–130.

BROWN, S. A., GOLDMAN, M. S., & CHRISTIANSEN, B. A. (1985). Do alcohol expectancies mediate drinking patterns of adults? *Journal of Consulting and Clinical Psychology, 53* (4), 512–519.

BROWN, S. A., GOLDMAN, M. S., INN, A., & ANDERSON, L. R. (1980). Expectations of reinforcement from alcohol: Their domain and relation to drinking patterns. *Journal of Consulting and Clinical Psychology, 48* (4), 419–426.

BROWN, T. G., SERAGANIAN, P., & TREMBLAY, J. (1993). Alcohol and cocaine abusers 6 months after traditional treatment: Do they fare as well as problem drinkers? *Journal of Substance Abuse Treatment, 10,* 545–552.

BROWN, T. H., CHAPMAN, P. F., KAIRISS, E. W., & KEENAN, C. L. (1988). Long-term synaptic potentiation. *Science, 242,* 724–728.

BROWNELL, K. D., MARLATT, G. A., LICHTENSTEIN, E., & WILSON, G. T. (1986). Understanding and preventing relapse. *American Psychologist, 41,* 765–782.

BUELOW, G. D. (1990). *An analysis of the influence of dysfunctional roles, chemical dependence, and family functioning on college adjustment.* Unpublished doctoral dissertation, University of Oregon.

BUELOW, G. D. (1994a). A suicide in group: A case of functional realignment. *International Journal of Group Psychotherapy, 44,* 153–168.

BUELOW, G. D. (1994b). Treatment of role stereotypy in severely dysfunctional and chemically dependent families. *Journal of Child and Adolescent Substance Abuse, 3,* 13–24.

BUELOW, G. D. (1995). Comparing students from substance abusing and dysfunctional families. *Journal of Counseling and Development, 73,* 327–330.

BUELOW, G. D., BASS, C., & ACKERMAN, C. (1994). Comparing counselors' and non-counselors' family functioning. *Counselor Education and Supervision, 33,* 162–174.

BUELOW, G. D., & HARBIN, J. (1996). The contribution of blackout to alcohol expectations. *Journal of Alcohol and Drug Education, 42,* 25–34 .

BUELOW, G. D., & HEBERT, S. (1995). *A counselor's resource on psychiatric medications: Issues of treatment and referral.* Pacific Grove, CA: Brooks/Cole.

BUELOW, G. D., KAZELSKIS, R., McINTOSH, I., & McCLAIN, M. (1997). *The influence of family functioning, hardiness, and attachment styles on psychological separation.* Manuscript submitted for publication.

BUELOW, G. D., McCLAIN, M., & McINTOSH, I. (1996). A new measure of an important construct: The attachment and object relations inventory. *Journal of Personality Assessment, 66,* 604–623.

BUELOW, S. A., & BUELOW, G. D. (1995). Gender differences in late adolescents' substance abuse and family role development. *Journal of Child and Adolescent Substance Abuse, 4,* 27–38.

BURK, J. P., & SHER, K. J. (1988). The "forgotten children" revisited: Neglected areas of COA research. *Clinical Psychology Review, 8,* 285–302.

BURK, J. P., & SHER, K. J. (1990). Labeling the child of an alcoholic: Negative stereotyping by mental health professionals and peers. *Journal of Studies on Alcohol, 51,* 156–163.

CALDER, P., & KOSTYNIUK, A. (1989). Personality profiles of children of alcoholics. *Professional Psychologist, 20,* 417–418.

CAMPBELL, B. K., WANDER, N., STARK, M. J., & HOLBERT, T. (1995). Treating cigarette smoking in drug-abusing clients. *Journal of Substance Abuse Treatment, 12,* 89–94.

CAREY, K. B. (1995). Heavy drinking contexts and indices of problem drinking among college students. *Journal of Studies on Alcohol, 56,* 287–292.

CAUDILL, B. D., KANTOR, G. K., & UNGERLEIDER, S. (1990). Project impact: A national study of high school substance abuse intervention training. *Journal of Alcohol and Drug Education, 35*(2), 61–74.

CAWTHRA, E., BORREGO, N., & EMRICK, C. D. (1991). Involving family members in the prevention of relapse: An innovative approach. *Alcoholism Treatment Quarterly, 8*(1), 101–111.

CERMAK, T. L., & BROWN, S. (1982). Interactional group therapy with the adult children of alcoholics. *International Journal of Group Psychotherapy, 32,* 375–388.

CHAPMAN, C. (1992). Diagnosing dissociative disorders in alcohol and drug dependent clients. *Alcoholism Treatment Quarterly, 9,* 67–75.

CHAPMAN, R. J. (1988). Cultural bias in alcoholism counseling. *Alcoholism Treatment Quarterly, 5,* 105–113.

CHARNESS, M. E., SIMON, R. P., & GREENBERG, D. A. (1989). Ethanol and the nervous system. *New England Journal of Medicine, 321,* 442–454.

CHASSIN, L., PILLOW, D. R., CURRAN, P. J., MOLINA, B. S. G., & BARRERA, M. (1993). Relation of parental alcoholism to early adolescent substance use: A test of three mediating mechanisms. *Journal of Abnormal Psychology, 102*(1), 3–19.

CHATLOS, J. C. (1989). Adolescent dual diagnosis: A 12-step transformational model. *Journal of Psychoactive Drugs, 21*(2), 189–201.

CHAVKIN, W., PAONE, D., FRIEDMANN, P., & WILETS, I. (1993). Psychiatric histories of drug using mothers: Treatment implications. *Journal of Substance Abuse Treatment, 10,* 445–448.

CHEMTOB, C., HAMADA, R., BAUER, G., KINNY, B., & TORIGOE, R. (1988a). Patients' suicide: Frequency and impact on psychologists. *Professional Psychology: Research and Practice, 19,* 416–420.

CHEMTOB, C., HAMADA, R., BAUER, G., KINNY, B., & TORIGOE, R. (1988b). Patients' suicide: Frequency and impact on psychiatrists. *American Journal of Psychiatry, 145,* 224–228.

CHIAUZZI, E. J., & LILJEGREN, S. (1993). Taboo topics in addiction treatment. *Journal of Substance Abuse Treatment, 10,* 303–316.

CHICK, J., LLOYD, G., & CROMBIE, E. (1985). Counseling problem drinkers in medical wards: A controlled study. *British Medical Journal, 290,* 965–967.

CLARREN, S. K. (1986). Neuropathology in FAS. In J. R. West (Ed.), *Alcohol and Brain Development* (pp. 158–166). New York: Oxford University Press.

CLAYDON, P. (1987). Self-reported alcohol, drug, and eating disorder problems among male and female collegiate children of alcoholics. *Journal of American College Health, 36,* 111–116.

CLEVELAND, M. (1981). Families and adolescent drug abuse: Structural analysis of children's roles. *Family Process, 20,* 295–304.

CLONINGER, C. R., SIGVARDSSON, S., VON KNORRING, A., & BOHMAN, M. (1988). The Swedish studies of the adopted children of alcoholics. *Journal of Studies on Alcohol, 49* (6), 500–509.

COLLINS, B. G. (1993). Reconstruing codependency using self-in-relation theory: A feminist perspective. *Social Work, 38,* 470–476.

COLLINS, N. L., & READ, S. J. (1990). Adult attachment working models and relationship quality in dating couples. *Journal of Personality and Social Psychology, 58,* 644–663.

CONRAD, K. J., HULTMAN, C. I., & LYONS, J. S. (1993). Treatment of the chemically dependent homeless: A synthesis. *Alcoholism Treatment Quarterly, 10,* 235–247.

COOPER, A., & McCORMACK, W. A. (1992). Short-term group treatment for adult children of alcoholics. *Journal of Counseling Psychology, 39,* 350–355.

COREY, G. (1991). *Theory and practice of counseling and psychotherapy* (4th ed.). Pacific Grove, CA: Brooks/Cole.

CORMIER, W. H., & CORMIER, L. S. (1991). *Interviewing strategies for helpers: Fundamental skills and cognitive behavioral interventions* (3rd ed.). Pacific Grove, CA: Brooks/Cole.

CORRIGAN, G. V., WEBB, M. G. T., & UNWIN, A. R. (1986). Alcohol dependence among general medical inpatients. *British Journal of Addiction, 81,* 237–246.

COTTON, N. S. (1978). The familial incidence of alcoholism: A review. *Journal of Studies on Alcohol, 40,* 89–116.

CRAIG, R. J., & OLSON, R. E. (1990). MMPI characteristics of drug abusers with and without histories of suicide attempts. *Journal of Personality Assessment, 55* (3&4), 717–728.

CRAIN, W. (1992). *Theories of development: Concepts and applications.* Englewood Cliffs, NJ: Prentice Hall.

CRAWFORD, R. L., & PHYFER, A. Q. (1988). Adult children of alcoholics: A counseling model. *Journal of College Student Development, 29,* 105–111.

CUNNIEN, A. J. (1986). Alcoholic blackouts: Phenomenology and legal relevance. *Behavioral Sciences and the Law, 4,* 73–85.

CURLEE, J. (1973). Alcoholic blackouts: Some conflicting evidence. *Quarterly Journal of Studies on Alcohol, 34,* 409–413.

CYR, M. G., & WARTMAN, S. A. (1988). The effectiveness of routine screening questions in the detection of alcoholism. *Journal of American Medical Association, 259* (1), 51–54.

DALEY, J. G., SOWERS-HOAG, K. M., & THYER, B. A. (1991). Construct validity of the circumplex model of family functioning. *Journal of Social Service Research, 15,* 131–147.

DEARDORFF, C. M., MELGES, F. T., HOUT, C. N., & SAVAGE, D. J. (1975). Situations related to drinking alcohol. *Journal of Studies on Alcohol, 36,* 1184–1195.

DE CUBAS, M. M., & FIELD, T. (1993). Children of methadone-dependent women: Developmental outcomes. *American Journal of Orthopsychiatry, 63,* 266–276.

DEFFENBACHER, J. L., & SUINN, R. M. (1988). Systematic desensitization and the reduction of anxiety. *Counseling Psychologist, 16,* 9–30.

DELANEY, E. S., PHILLIPS, P., & CHANDLER, C. K. (1989). Leading an Adlerian group for adult children of alcoholics. *Individual Counseling, 45,* 490–499.

DELL, P. F. (1982). Beyond homeostasis: Toward a concept of coherence. *Family Process, 21,* 21–41.

DEYKIN, E. Y., & BUKA, S. L. (1994). Suicidal ideation and attempts among chemically dependent adolescents. *American Journal of Public Health, 84,* 634–639.

DEYKIN, E. Y., BUKA, S. L., & ZEENA, T. H. (1992). Depressive illness among chemically dependent adolescents. *American Journal of Psychiatry, 149,* 1341–1347.

DIAMOND-FRIEDMAN, C. (1990). A multivariant model of alcoholism specific to gay-lesbian populations. *Alcoholism Treatment Quarterly, 7,* 111–117.

DiCLEMENTE, C. C., & PROCHASKA, J. O. (1982). Self-change and therapy change of smoking behavior: A comparison of processes of change in cessation and maintenance. *Addictive Behavior, 7,* 133–142.

DONIGIAN, J., & MALNATI, R. (1987). *Critical incidents in group therapy.* Pacific Grove, CA: Brooks/Cole.

DONOVAN, D. M., & O'LEARY, M. R. (1979). *Cognitive Therapy and Research, 3,* 141–154.

DOWNING, N. E., & WALKER, M. E. (1987). A psychoeducational group for adult children of alcoholics. *Journal of Counseling and Development, 65,* 440–442.

DRAKE, R. E., & WALLACH, M. A. (1989). Substance abuse among the chronic mentally ill. *Hospital and Community Psychiatry, 40,* 1041–1046.

DRYDEN, W., & ELLIS, A. (1988). Rational-emotive therapy. In K. Dobson (Ed.), *Handbook of cognitive-behavioral therapies* (pp. 214–272). New York: Guilford.

DUFFY, T. K. (1990). Psychodrama in beginning recovery: An illustration of goals and methods. *Alcoholism Treatment Quarterly, 7,* 97–109.

DULIT, R. A., FYER, M. R., HAAS, G. L., SULLIVAN, T., & FRANCES, A. J. (1990). Substance use in borderline personality disorder. *American Journal of Psychiatry, 147,* 1002–1007.

ELKIN, M. (1984). *Families under the influence: Changing alcoholic patterns.* New York: Norton.

ELLIS, A. (1962). *Reason and emotion in psychotherapy.* New Jersey: Citadel.

ELLIS, A. (1971). *Growth through reason.* North Hollywood, CA: Wilshire.

ELLIS, A., & GRIEGER, R. (Eds.). (1986). *The Handbook of rational-emotive therapy* (Vols. 1–2). New York: Springer.

ELLIS, A., & HARPER, R. A. (1975). *A new guide to rational living.* North Hollywood, CA: Wilshire.

ELLIS, A., MCINERNEY, J. F., DIGIUSEPPE, R., & YEAGER, R. J. (1988). *Rational-emotive therapy with alcoholics and substance abusers.* New York: Pergamon Press.

ELLIS, A., & VELTEN, E. (1992). *Rational steps to quitting alcohol: When AA doesn't work for you.* Fort Lee, NJ: Barricade.

ELLIS, A., & WHITELY, J. M. (Eds.). (1979). *Theoretical and empirical foundations of rational-emotive therapy.* Pacific Grove, CA: Brooks/Cole.

ELVY, G. A., WELLS, J. E., BAIRD, K. A. (1988). Attempted referral as intervention for problem drinking in the general hospital. *British Journal of Addiction, 83,* 83–89.

EMBREE, B. G., & WHITEHEAD, P. C. (1993). Validity and reliability of self-reported drinking behavior: Dealing with the problem of response bias. *Journal of Studies on Alcohol, 54*(3) 334–344.

ENDLER, N. S., & PARKER, D. A. (1990). Multidimensional assessment of coping: A critical evaluation. *Journal of Personality and Social Psychology, 58,* 844–854.

ENGEL, J. A. (1985). Influence of age and hormones on the stimulatory and sedative effects of ethanol. In U. Rydberg, C. Alling, & J. Engel (Eds.), *Alcohol and the developing brain* (pp. 57–68). Stockholm: Raven.

ERIKSEN, L., BJORNSTAD, S., & GOTTESTAM, K. G. (1986). Social skills training in groups for alcoholics: One-year treatment outcome for groups and individuals. *Addictive Behaviors, 11,* 309–329.

ERIKSON, E. H. (1963). *Childhood and society* (2nd ed.). New York: Norton.

ERIKSON, M. T., & PERKINS, S. E. (1989). System dynamics in alcoholic families [Special issue: Co-dependency—issues in treatment and recovery]. *Alcoholism Treatment Quarterly, 6*(1), 59–74.

ESSMAN, W. B. (1983). *Clinical pharmacology of learning and memory.* New York: SP Medical and Scientific Books.

ESSMAN, W. B., & NAKAJIMA, S. (1973). *Current Biochemical Approaches to Learning and Memory.* New York: Wiley.

ESTES, J., & HEINEMANN, M. E. (1977). *Alcoholism: Development, consequences, and interventions.* St. Louis: C. V. Mosby.

EVANS, K., & SULLIVAN, J. M. (1990). *Dual diagnosis: Counseling the mentally ill substance abuser.* New York: Guilford.

FERSTEIN, M. E., & WHISTON, S. C. (1991). Utilizing RET for effective treatment of adult children of alcoholics. *Journal of Rational-Emotive and Cognitive-Behavior Therapy, 9,* 39–49.

FERTMAN, C. I. (1991). Aftercare for teenagers: Matching services and needs. *Journal of Alcohol and Drug Education, 36,* 1–11.

FERTMAN, C. I., & TOCA, O. A. (1989). A drug and alcohol aftercare service: Linking adolescents, families, and schools. *Journal of Alcohol and Drug Education, 34,* 46–53.

FINKELSTEIN, N., BROWN, K. N., & LATHAM, C. Q. (1981). Alcoholic mothers and guilt: Issues for caregivers. *Alcohol Health and Research World, 6*(1), 45–49.

FISCHER, B. (1988). The process of healing shame. *Alcoholism Treatment Quarterly, 4,* 25–38.

FISHER, L., KOKES, R. F., RANSOM, D. C., PHILLIPS, S. L., & RUDD, P. (1985). Alternative strategies for creating "relational" family data. *Family Process, 24,* 213–224.

FLANNERY, D. J., VAZSONYI, A. T., TORQUATI, J., & FRIDRICH, A. (1994). Ethnic and gender differences in risk for early adolescent substance use. *Journal of Youth and Adolescence, 23,* 195–213.

FLORES, P. J. (1988). *Group psychotherapy with addicted populations.* New York: Haworth.

FLORES, P. J., & MAHON, L. (1993). The treatment of addiction in group psychotherapy. *International Journal of Group Psychotherapy, 43,* 143–156.

FOLKMAN, S., & LAZARUS, R. S. (1985). If it changes it must be a process: A study of emotion and coping during three stages of a college examination. *Journal of Personality and Social Psychology, 48,* 150–170.

FOLKMAN, S., & LAZARUS, R. S. (1988). *Manual for the ways of coping questionnaire.* Palo Alto, CA: Consulting Psychologists Press.

FRIEDMAN, A. S. (1989). Family therapy vs. parent groups: Effects on adolescent drug abusers. *The American Journal of Family Therapy, 17,* 335–347.

FRIEDMAN, A. S., & GLICKMAN, N. W. (1986). Program characteristics for successful treatment of adolescent drug abuse. *The Journal of Nervous and Mental Disease, 174,* 669–679.

FRIEDMAN, A. S., GLICKMAN, N. W., & MORRISSEY, M. R. (1986). Prediction to successful treatment outcome by client characteristics and retention in treatment in adolescent drug treatment programs: A large-scale cross validation study. *Journal of Drug Education, 16,* 149–165.

FRIEDMAN, A. S., GRANICK, S., KREISHER, C., & TERRAS, A. (1993). Matching adolescents who abuse drugs to treatment. *The American Journal on Addictions, 2,* 232–236.

FROMME, K., KIVLAHAN, D. R., & MARLATT, G. A. (1986). Alcohol expectancies, risk identification, and secondary prevention with problem drinkers [Paper presented at annual meeting of the Association for the Advancement of Behavior Therapy (1985, Houston, Texas)]. *Advances in Behavior Research and Therapy, 8,* 237–251.

FROMME, K., & RIVET, K. (1994). Young adults' coping style as a predictor of their alcohol use and response to daily events. *Journal of Youth and Adolescence, 23,* 85–97.

FULLER, M. G., DIAMOND, D. L., JORDAN, M. L., & WALTERS, M. C. (1995). The role of a substance abuse consultation team in a trauma center. *Journal of Studies on Alcohol, 56,* 267–271.

GARBARINO, C., & STRANGE, C. (1993). College adjustment and family environments of students reporting parental alcohol problems. *Journal of College Student Development, 34,* 261–266.

GAVAZZI, S. M., & SABATELLI, R. M. (1990). Family system dynamics, the individual process, and psychosocial development. *Journal of Adolescent Research, 5,* 499–518.

GEORGE, R. L. (1990). *Counseling the chemically dependent.* Englewood Cliffs, NJ: Prentice Hall.

GERRA, G., MARCATO, A., CACCAVARI, R., FONTANESI, B., DELSIGNORE, R., FERTONANI, G., AVANZINI, P., RUSTICHELLI, P., & PASSERI, M. (1995). Clonidine and opiate receptor antagonists in the treatment of heroin addiction. *Journal of Substance Abuse Treatment, 12,* 35–41.

GIANNINI, A. J., LOISELLE, R. H., GRAHAM, B. H., & FOLTS, D. J. (1993). Behavioral response to buspirone in cocaine and phencyclidine withdrawal. *Journal of Substance Abuse Treatment, 10,* 523–527.

GIBSON, J. M., & DONIGIAN, J. (1993). Use of Bowen theory. *Journal of Addictions and Offender Counseling, 14,* 25–35.

GIDEON, W. L., LITTELL, A. S., & MARTIN, D. W. (1980). Evaluation of a training program for certified alcoholism counselors. *Journal of Studies on Alcohol, 41*(1), 8–20.

GIUNTA, C. T., & COMPAS, B. E. (1994). Adult daughters of alcoholics: Are they unique? *Journal of Studies on Alcohol, 55,* 600–606.

GOLD, M. S. (1994). Neurobiology of addiction and recovery: The brain, the drive for the drug, and the 12-step fellowship. *Journal of Substance Abuse Treatment, 11,* 93–97.

GOLDEN, L., & KLEIN, M. S. (1987). Treatment as a habilitative process in adolescent development and chemical dependency. *Alcoholism Treatment Quarterly, 4,* 35–41.

GOLDMAN, M. S., BROWN, S. A., CHRISTIANSEN, B. A., & SMITH, G. T. (1991). Alcoholism and memory: Broadening the scope of alcohol-expectancy research. *Psychological Bulletin, 110,* 137–146.

GOLDSTEIN, L. S., & BUONGIORNO, P. A. (1984). Psychotherapists as suicide survivors. *American Journal of Psychiatry, 38,* 392–398.

GOODWIN, D. W. (1971). Two species of alcoholic "blackout." *American Journal of Psychiatry, 127,* 1665–1670.

GOODWIN, D. W. (1974). Alcoholic blackout and state-dependent learning. *Federation Proceedings, 33,* 1833–1835.

GOODWIN, D. W. (1986). Area review: Heredity and alcoholism. *Annals of Behavioral Medicine, 8,* 3–6.

GOODWIN, D. W. (1989). Biological factors in alcohol use and abuse: Implications for recognizing and preventing alcohol problems in adolescence [Special issue: Psychiatry and the addictions]. *International Review of Psychiatry, 1,* 41–49.

GOODWIN, D. W., CRANE, J. B., & GUZE, S. B. (1969a). Alcoholic "blackouts": A review and clinical study of 100 alcoholics. *American Journal of Psychiatry, 126,* 191–198.

GOODWIN, D. W., CRANE, J. B., & GUZE, S. B. (1969b). Phenomenological aspects of the alcoholic "blackout." *British Journal of Psychiatry, 115,* 1033–1038.

GOODWIN, D. W., HILL, S. Y., POWELL, B., & VIAMONTES, J. (1973). Effect of alcohol on short term memory in alcoholics. *British Journal of Psychiatry, 122,* 93–94.

GOODWIN, D. W., OTHMER, E., HALIKAS, J. A., & FREEMON, F. (1970). Loss of short term memory as a predictor of the alcoholic "blackout." *Nature, 227,* 201–202.

GOODWIN, D. W., POWELL, B., BREMER, D., HOINE, H., & STERN, J. (1969). Alcohol and recall: State-dependent effects in man. *Science, 163,* 1358–1360.

GORSKI, T. T. (1990). The CENAPS model of relapse prevention: Basic principles and procedure. *Journal of Psychoactive Drugs, 22,* 125–133.

GRALF, R. W., WHITEHEAD, G. I., & LeCOMPTE, M. (1986). Group treatment with divorced women using cognitive behavioral and supportive insight methods. *Journal of Counseling Psychology, 33,* 276–281.

GREEN, R. G., KOLEVZON, M. S., & VOSLER, N. R. (1985). The Beavers-Timberlawn model of family competence and the circumplex model of family adaptability and cohesion: Separate, but equal? *Family Process, 24,* 385–398.

GREENWALD, D. J., REZNIKOFF, M., & PLUTCHIK, R. (1994). Suicide risk and violence risk in alcoholics. *The Journal of Nervous and Mental Disease, 182,* 3–8.

GROTEVANT, H. D., & COOPER, C. R. (1985). Patterns of interaction in family relationships and the development of identity exploration in adolescence. *Child Development, 56,* 415–428.

HAACK, M. R., & ALIM, T. N. (1991). Anxiety and the adult child of an alcoholic: A co-morbid problem. *Family and Community Health, 13,* 49–60.

HAAKEN, J. (1990). A critical analysis of the co-dependence construct. *Psychiatry, 53,* 396–406.

HAAKEN, J. (1993). From Al-Anon to ACOA: Codependence and the reconstruction of caregiving. *Signs, 18,* 321–345.

HADLEY, J. A., HOLLOWAY, E. L., & MALLINCKRODT, G. (1993). Common aspects of object relations and self-representations in offspring from disparate dysfunctional families. *Journal of Counseling Psychology, 40,* 348–356.

HAGMAN, G. (1994). Methadone maintenance counseling. *Journal of Substance Abuse Treatment, 11,* 405–413.

HALEY, J. (1973). *Uncommon therapy.* New York: Norton.

HALEY, J. (1984). Marriage or family therapy. *American Journal of Family Therapy, 12*(2), 3–14.

HALL, J. F. (1989). *Learning and memory.* Boston: Allyn & Bacon.

HALL, J. M. (1993). Lesbians and alcohol: Patterns and paradoxes in medical notions and lesbians' beliefs. *Journal of Psychoactive Drugs, 25,* 109–119.

HALLER, D. L., KNISELY, J. S., DAWSON, K. S., & SCHNOLL, S. H. (1993). Perinatal substance abusers. *The Journal of Nervous and Mental Disease, 181,* 509–513.

HAMMAR, R. P. (1986). Alcohol effects on developing neuronal structure. In J. R. West (Ed.), *Alcohol and Brain Development* (pp. 184–203). New York: Oxford University Press.

HARMON, M. A. (1993). Reducing the risk of drug involvement among early adolescents. *Evaluation Review, 17,* 221–239.

HARPER, J. (1990). Recovery for the relationship: A treatment model for couples with a recovering chemically dependent partner. *Alcoholism Treatment Quarterly, 7*(2), 1–21.

HARRIS, S. A., & MacQUIDDY, S. (1991). Childhood roles in group therapy: The lost child and the mascot. *The Journal for Specialist in Group Work, 16,* 223–229.

HARRIS, S. N., MOWBRAY, C. T., & SOLARZ, A. (1994). Physical health, mental health, and substance abuse problems of shelter users. *Health and Social Work, 19,* 37–45.

HAWKS, R. D., BAHR, S. J. & WANG, G. (1994). Adolescent substance use and codependence. *Journal of Studies on Alcohol, 55,* 261–268.

HAZAN, C., & SHAVER, P. (1987). Romantic love conceptualized as an attachment process. *Journal of Personality and Social Psychology, 59,* 270–280.

HELLMAN, R. E., STANTON, M., LEE, J., TYTUN, A., & VACHON, R. (1989). Treatment of homosexual alcoholics in government-funded agencies: Provider training and attitudes. *Hospital and Community Psychiatry, 40,* 1163–1168.

HENDERSON, M. C., ALBRIGHT, J. S., KALICHMAN, S. C., & DUGONI, B. (1994). Personality characteristics of young adult offspring of substance abusers: A study highlighting methodological issues. *Journal of Personality Assessment, 63*, 117–134.

HENNECKE, L. (1984). Stimulus augmenting and field dependence in children of alcoholic fathers. *Journal of Studies on Alcohol, 45*, 486–492.

HERSHENSON, D. B., & POWER, P. W. (1987). *Mental health counseling: Theory and practice.* New York: Pergamon Press.

HESTER, R. K., & MILLER, W. R. (1989). *Handbook of alcoholism treatment approaches: Effective alternatives.* New York: Pergamon Press.

HILL, A., & WILLIAMS, D. (1993). Hazards associated with the use of benzodiazepines in alcohol detoxification. *Journal of Substance Abuse Treatment, 10*, 449–451.

HIRST, M., HAMILTON, M., & MARSHAL, A. (1977). Pharmacology of isoquinoline alkaloids and ethanol interactions. In K. Blum, D. L. Bard, & M. G. Hamilton (Eds.), *Alcohol and the opiates* (pp. 167–187). New York: Academic Press.

HOEGERMAN, G. S., RESNICK, R. J., SCHNOLL, S. H. (1993). Attention deficits in newly abstinent substance abusers: Childhood recollections and attention performance in thirty-nine subjects. *Journal of Addictive Diseases, 12*, 37–53.

HOFFMAN, J. P. (1984). Psychological separation of late adolescents from their parents. *Journal of Counseling Psychotherapy, 31*, 170–178.

HOFFMAN, J. P. (1994). Investigating the age effects of family structure on adolescent marijuana use. *Journal of Youth and Adolescence, 23*, 215–235.

HOLLERAN, P. R., & NOVAK, A. H. (1989). Support choices and abstinence in gay/lesbian and heterosexual alcoholics. *Alcoholism Treatment Quarterly, 6*, 71–83.

HOLMES, T. H., & RAHE, R. H. (1967). The Holmes and Rahe Social Readjustment Scale. *Journal of Psychosomatic Research, 11*, 213–218.

HORNER, A. J. (1979). *Object relations and the developing ego in therapy.* New York: Aronson.

HOROWITZ, M., WILNER, N., & ALVAREZ, W. (1979). Impact of event scale: A measure of subjective stress. *Psychosomatic Medicine, 41*, 209–218.

HSER, Y. (1995). A referral system that matches drug users to treatment programs: Existing research and relevant issues. *The Journal of Drug Issues, 25*(1), 209–224.

HUDSON, C. J. (1981). Brief communication: Tricyclic antidepressants and alcoholic blackouts. *The Journal of Nervous and Mental Disease, 169*(6), 381–382.

ISRAELSTAM, S. (1986). Alcohol and drug problems of gay males and lesbians: Therapy, counseling, and prevention issues. *The Journal of Drug Issues, 16*, 443–461.

ISRAELSTAM, S., & LAMBERT, S. (1989). Homosexuals who indulge in excessive use of alcohol and drugs: Psychosocial factors to be taken into account by community and intervention workers. *Journal of Alcohol and Drug Education, 34*, 54–69.

JACOB, T., & LEONARD, K. (1986). Psychosocial functioning in children of alcoholic fathers, depressed fathers, and control fathers. *Journal of Studies on Alcohol, 47*, 373–380.

JARMAS, A. L., & KOZAK, A. E. (1992). Young adult children of alcoholic fathers: Depressive experiences, coping styles, and family systems. *Journal of Consulting and Clinical Psychology, 60*, 244–251.

JELLINEK, E. M. (1952a). Current notes: Phases of alcohol addiction. *Quarterly Journal of Studies on Alcoholism, 13*, 673–684.

JELLINEK, E. M. (1952b). The emphases of alcohol addiction. *Quarterly Journal of Studies on Alcohol, 13*, 673–684.

JELLINEK, E. M. (1960). *The disease concept of alcoholism.* New Haven, CT: Hillhouse Press.

JOHNSON, C. D., REEVES, K. O., & JACKSON, D. (1983). Alcohol and sex. *Heart and Lung, 12*, 93–97.

JOHNSON, L. K. (1989). How to diagnose and treat chemical dependency in the elderly. *Journal of Gerontological Nursing, 15*(12), 22–26.

JOHNSON, M. E., & PRENTICE, D. G. (1990). Effects of counselor gender and drinking status on the perceptions of the counselor. *Journal of Alcohol and Drug Education, 35*, 38–44.

JOHNSON, N. P., & CHAPPEL, J. N. (1994). Using AA and other 12-step programs more effectively. *Journal of Substance Abuse Treatment, 11*(2), 137–142.

JOHNSON, S. D. (1990). Toward clarifying culture, race, and ethnicity in the context of multicultural counseling. *Journal of Multicultural Counseling and Development, 18*, 41–50.

Jones, J. W. (1983). The Children of Alcoholics Screening Test: A validity study. *Bulletin of the Society of Psychologists in Addictive Behaviors, 2*(3), 155–163.

Julien, R. M. (1995). *A primer of drug action* (7th ed.). New York: W. H. Freeman.

Kaczkowski, V. R., & Zygmond, M. J. (1991). Grief resolution in the recovery of individuals who are addicted to alcohol. *Journal of Mental Health Counseling, 13,* 356–366.

Kadden, R. M., Getter, H., Cooney, N. L., & Litt, M. D. (1989). Matching alcoholics to coping skills or interactional therapies: Posttreatment results. *Journal of Consulting and Clinical Psychology, 57,* 698–704.

Kaplan, M. S. (1979). Patterns of alcoholic beverage use among college students. *Journal of Alcohol and Drug Education, 24*(2), 26–40.

Kapur, N. (1988). *Memory disorders in clinical practice.* London: Butterworths.

Kaufman, E. (1992). Family therapy: A treatment approach with substance abusers. In J. H. Lowinson, P. Ruiz, R. B. Millman, & J. G. Langrod (Eds.), *Substance abuse: A comprehensive textbook* (pp. 520–532). Baltimore: Williams & Wilkins.

Kennedy, B. P., & Minami, M. (1993). The Bech Hill Hospital/Outward Bound adolescent chemical dependency treatment program. *Journal of Substance Abuse Treatment, 10,* 395–406.

Kern, M. F., Kenkel, M. B., Templer, D. I., & Newell, T. G. (1986). Drug preference as a function of arousal and stimulus screening. *The International Journal of the Addictions, 21,* 225–265.

Khan, A. U. (1986). *Clinical disorders of memory.* New York: Plenum.

Khantzian, E. J., & Schneider, R. J. (1986). Treatment implications of a psychodynamic understanding of opioid addicts. In R. E. Meyer (Ed.), *Psychopathology of addictive disorders* (pp. 323–333). New York: Guilford.

Kibel, H. D. (1973). A group member's suicide: Treating collective trauma. *International Journal of Group Psychotherapy, 23,* 42–53.

Kimball, K. E., Healey, J. C., McIntire, W. G., & Smith, D. (1981). Families in alcoholic transaction: The family systems approach to alcoholism in the family and family rehabilitation. *International Journal of Family Psychiatry, 3*(1), 57–67.

King, B. L. (1986). Decision making in the intervention process. *Alcoholism Treatment Quarterly, 3*(3), 5–22.

Kinney, J. (1983). Relapse among alcoholics who are alcoholic counselors. *Journal of the Studies of Alcohol, 44,* 744–748.

Kinney, J. (1991). *Clinical manual of substance abuse.* St. Louis, MO: Mosey Yearbook.

Kirk, D. L., Chapman, T., & Sadler, O. W. (1990). Documenting the effectiveness of adolescent substance abuse treatment using public school archival records. *The High School Journal, 74,* 16–21.

Knapp, J. M., Rosheim, C. L., Meister, E. A., & Kottke, T. E. (1993). Managing tobacco dependence in chemical dependency treatment facilities: A survey of current attitudes and policies. *Journal of Addictive Diseases, 12,* 89–104.

Kofoed, L. (1993). Outpatient vs. inpatient treatment for the chronically mentally ill with substance abuse disorders. In N. S. Miller & B. Stimmel (Eds.), *Comorbidity of addictive and psychiatric disorders* (pp. 123–137). New York: Haworth.

Kolpack, R. M. (1992). Credentialing alcoholism counselors. *Alcoholism Treatment Quarterly, 9*(3–4), 97–112.

Koob, G. F., & Bloom, F. E. (1988). Cellular and molecular mechanisms of drug dependence. *Science, 242,* 715–724.

Kosson, D. S., Steuerwald, B. L., Newman, J. P., & Widom, C. S. (1994). The relation between socialization and antisocial behavior, substance use, and family conflict in college students. *Journal of Personality Assessment, 63,* 473–488.

Kosten, T. A., Ball, S. A., & Rounsaville, B. J. (1994). A sibling study of sensation seeking and opiate addiction. *The Journal of Nervous and Mental Disease, 182,* 284–289.

Kranzler, H. R., Boca, F. D., Korner, P., & Brown, J. (1993). Adverse effects limit the usefulness of fluvoxamine for the treatment of alcoholism. *Journal of Substance Abuse Treatment, 10,* 283–287.

Krestan, J., & Bepko, C. (1990). Codependency: The social reconstruction of female experience. *Smith College Studies in Social Work, 60,* 216–232.

Kus, R. J. (1988). *Alcoholism and non-acceptance of gay self: The critical link.* New York: Haworth.

Lazare, A. (1979). Hypothesis testing in the clinical interview. In A. Lazare (Ed.), *Outpatient psychiatry: diagnosis and treatment.* Baltimore: Williams & Wilkins.

LECCESE, M., & WALDRON, H. B. (1994). Assessing adolescent substance use: A critique of current measurement instruments. *Journal of Substance Abuse Treatment, 11,* 553–563.

LEHMAN, A. F., MYERS, C. P., CORTY, E., & THOMPSON, J. (1994). Severity of substance use disorders among psychiatric inpatients. *The Journal of Nervous and Mental Diseases, 182,* 164–167.

LEIGH, B. C. (1993). Alcohol consumption and sexual activity as reported with a diary technique. *Journal of Abnormal Psychology, 102,* 490–493.

LEIGH, B. C., & STACY, A. W. (1991). On the scope of alcohol expectancy research: Remaining issues of measurement and meaning. *Psychological Bulletin, 110,* 147–154.

LEVY, M. (1993). Psychotherapy with dual diagnosis patients: Working with denial. *Journal of Substance Abuse Treatment, 10,* 499–504.

LEVY, M. S., & MANN, D. W. (1988). The special treatment team: An inpatient approach to the mentally ill alcoholic patient. *Journal of Substance Abuse Treatment, 5,* 219–227.

LEWIS, J. A., DANA, R. Q., & BLEVINS, G A. (1994). *Substance abuse counseling* (2nd ed.). Pacific Grove, CA: Brooks/Cole.

LICKEY, M. E., & GORDON, B. (1983). *Drugs for mental illness.* New York: W. H. Freeman.

LINDSTROM, W. W., & SRNEC, S. (1986). *Proposal for a continuum of services for those who are mentally ill and chemically dependent.* Paper presented at meeting of NASADAD, Cincinnati, OH.

LISMAN, S. A. (1974). Alcoholic "blackout": State dependent learning? *Archives of General Psychiatry, 30,* 46–53.

LOGUE, M. B., SHER, K. J., & FRENSCH, P. A. (1992). Purported characteristics of adult children of alcoholics: A possible "Barnum effect." *Professional Psychology: Research and Practice, 23,* 226–232.

LOVINGER, D. M., WHITE, G., & WEIGHT, F. F. (1989). Ethanol inhibits NMDA-activated ion current in hippocampal neurons. *Science, 243,* 1721–1724.

LUKOFF, D., NUECHTERLEIN, K. H., & VENTURA, J. (1986). Manual for expanded brief psychiatric rating scale (BPRS). *Schizophrenia Bulletin, 12,* 594–602.

LYSAKER, P., BELL, M., BEAM-GOULET, J., & MILSTEIN, R. (1994). Relationship of positive and negative symptoms to cocaine abuse in schizophrenia. *The Journal of Nervous and Mental Disease, 182,* 109–112.

MACHELL, D. F. (1991). Deprivation in American affluence: The theory of stimulus addiction. *Journal of Alcohol and Drug Education, 36,* 42–45.

MADDAHIAN, E., NEWCOMB, M. D., & BENTLER, P. M. (1985). Single and multiple patterns of adolescent substance use: Longitudinal comparisons of four ethnic groups. *Journal of Drug Education, 15,* 311–325.

MADDAHIAN, E., NEWCOMB, M. D., & BENTLER, P. M. (1986). Adolescents' substance use: Impact of ethnicity, income, and availability. *Alcohol and Substance Abuse in Women and Children.* New York: Haworth.

MAHLER, M., PINE, F., & BERGMAN, A. (1975). *The psychological birth of the human infant.* New York: Basic Books.

MAHON, L., & FLORES, P. (1992). Group psychotherapy as the treatment of choice for individuals who grew up with alcoholic parents: A theoretical review. *Alcoholism Treatment Quarterly, 9,* 113–125.

MALTZMAN, I., & SCHWEIGER, A. (1991). Individual and family characteristics of middle class adolescents hospitalized for alcohol and other drug abuse. *British Journal of Addiction, 86,* 1435–1447.

MARLATT, G. A. (1978). Craving for alcohol, loss of control, and relapse: A cognitive-behavioral analysis. In P. E. Nathan, G. A. Marlatt, & T. Loberg (Eds.), *Alcoholism: New directions in behavioral research and treatment* (pp. 271–314). New York: Plenum.

MARLATT, G. A., & GORDON, J. R. (Eds.). (1985). *Relapse prevention.* New York: Guilford.

MARTIN, E. D., & SHER, K. J. (1994, January). Family history of alcoholism, alcohol use disorders and the five-factor model of personality. *Journal of Studies on Alcohol, 55*(1), 81–90.

MATHENY, K., AYCOCK, D., CURLETTE, W., & JUNKER, G. (1993). The coping resources inventory for stress: A measure of perceived resourcefulness. *Journal of Counseling Psychology, 49,* 815–829.

MCBRIDE, J. L. (1991). Assessing the Al-Anon component of Alcoholics Anonymous. *Alcoholism Treatment Quarterly, 8,* 57–65.

MCCARTNEY, J. (1994). Understanding and helping the children of problem drinkers: A systems-psychodynamic perspective. *Journal of Substance Abuse Treatment, 11,* 155–166.

MCCARTY, D., ARGERIOU, M., HUEBNER, R. B., & LUBRAN, B. (1991). Alcoholism, drug abuse, and the homeless. *American Psychologist, 46,* 1139–1148.

MCCONNAUGHY, E. A., DICLEMENTE, C. C., PROCHASKA, J. O., & VELICER, W. F. (1989). Stages of change in psychotherapy: A follow-up report. *Psychotherapy: Theory, Research and Practice, 26,* 494–503.

MCCONNAUGHY, E. A., PROCHASKA, J. O., & VELICER, W. F. (1983). Stages of change in psychotherapy: Measurement and sample profiles. *Psychotherapy: Theory, Research and Practice, 20,* 368–375.

McGOLDRICK, M., & GERSON, R. (1985). *Genograms in family assessment.* New York: Norton.

McGUIRE, J. M., TAYLOR, D. R., BROOME, D. H., BLAU, B. I., & ABBOT, D. W. (1986). Group structuring techniques and their influence on process involvement in a group counseling training group. *Journal of Counseling Psychology, 33,* 270–275.

McLELLAN, A. T., KUSHNER, H., METZGER, D., PETERS, F., ET AL. (1992). The fifth edition of the Addiction Severity Index. *Journal of Substance Abuse Treatment, 9,* 199–213.

McLELLAN, A. T., LUBORSKY, L., O'BRIEN, C. P., WOODY, G. E. (1988). An improved diagnostic instrment for substance abuse patients: The Addiction Severity Index. *Journal of Nervous and Mental Disorders, 168,* 26–33.

MEEK, B., & EDELBERG, J. C. (1990). Assessment and multi-group treatment of adolescent substance abusers. *Residential Treatment for Children and Youth, 8,* 17–38.

MEILMAN, P. W., STONE, J. E., GAYLOR, M. S., & TURCO, J. H. (1990). Alcohol consumption by college undergraduates: Current use and 10-year trends. *Journal of Studies on Alcohol, 51,* 389–395.

MELITO, R. (1985). Adaptation in family systems: A developmental perspective. *Family Process, 24,* 89–100.

MENDENHALL, W. (1989). Co-dependency treatment. *Alcoholism Treatment Quarterly, 6,* 75–110.

MILAM, J. R., & KETCHAM, K. (1983). *Under the influence.* New York: Bantam Books.

MILGRAM, G. G. (1993). Adolescents, alcohol and aggression. *Journal of Studies on Alcohol, 11,* 53–61.

MILLER, N. S. (1993). Comorbidity of psychiatric and alcohol/drug disorders: Interactions and independent status. *Journal of Addictive Diseases, 12*(3), 5–16.

MILLER, N. S., DACKIS, C. A., & GOLD, M. S. (1987). The relationship of addiction, tolerance, and dependence to alcohol and drugs: A neurological approach. *Journal of Substance Abuse Treatment, 4,* 197–207.

MILLER, W. R. (1983). Motivational interviewing with problem drinkers. *Behavioral Psychotherapy, 11,* 147–172.

MILLER, W. R. (1992). The effectiveness of treatment for substance abuse: Reasons for optimism. *Journal of Substance Abuse, 9,* 93–102.

MILLER, W. R., BENEFIELD, R. G., & TONIGAN J. S. (1993). Enhancing motivation for change in problem drinking: A controlled comparison of two therapist styles. *Journal of Consulting and Clinical Psychology, 61,* 455–461.

MILLER, W. R., & HESTER, R. K. (1986). Inpatient alcoholism treatment: Who benefits? *American Psychologist, 41,* 794–805.

MILLER, W. R., & KURTZ, E. (1994, March). Models of alcoholism used in treatment: Contrasting AA and other perspectives with which it is often confused. *Journal of Studies on Alcohol, 55*(2), 159–166.

MINUCHIN, S. (1974). *Families and family therapy.* Cambridge, MA: Harvard University Press.

MONTOYA, I. D., & HAERTZEN, C. (1994). Reduction of psychopathology among individuals participating in non-treatment drug abuse residential studies. *Journal of Addictive Diseases, 13,* 89–97.

MOORE, R. D., BONE, L. R., GELLER, G., MAMON, J. A., STOKES, E. J., & LEVINE, D. M. (1989). Prevalence, detection, and treatment of alcoholism in hospitalized patients. *Journal of American Medical Association, 261,* 403–407.

MOOS, R. H., & MOOS, B. S. (1981). *Family Environment Scale manual* (2nd ed.). Palo Alto, CA: Consulting Psychologists Press.

MOOS, R. H., & MOOS, B. S. (1984). The process of recovery from alcoholism III. Comparing functioning of families of alcoholics and matched control families. *Journal of Studies on Alcohol, 45*(2), 111–118.

MORRIS, J. A., & WISE, R. P. (1992). The identification and treatment of the dual diagnosis patient. *Alcoholism Treatment Quarterly, 9,* 55–63.

MORRISON, J. R., & PENDERY, M. (1973). Suicidal behavior during alcoholic blackouts. *Quarterly Journal of Studies on Alcohol, 35,* 657–659.

MUESER, K. T., YARNOLD, P. R., LEVINSON, D. F., SENGH, H., BELLACK, A. S., KEE, K., MORRISON, R. L., & YADALAM, K. G. (1990). Prevalence of substance abuse in schizophrenia: Demographic and clinical correlates. *Schizophrenia Bulletin, 16,* 31–56.

MULLIGAN, D. H., McCARTY, D., POTTER, D., & KRAKOW, M. (1989). Counselors in public and private alcoholism and drug abuse treatment programs. *Alcoholism Treatment Quarterly, 6*(3–4), 75–89.

NARDI, P. M. (1981). Children of alcoholics: A role theoretical perspective. *Journal of Social Psychology, 115,* 237–245.

NATHAN, P. E. (1986). Some implications of recent biological findings for the behavioral treatment of alcoholism. *The Behavior Therapist, 8,* 159–161.

NEWSOME, R. D., & DITZLER, T. (1993). Assessing alcoholic denial. *The Journal of Nervous and Mental Disease, 181,* 689–694.

NEWTON, M. (1992). Living again. *Journal of Substance Abuse Treatment, 9,* 71–80.

NIGAM, A. K., RAY, R., & TRIPATHI, B. M. (1993). Buprenorphine in opiate withdrawal: A comparison with clonidine. *Journal of Substance Abuse Treatment, 10,* 391–394.

OBERMEIER, G. E., & HENRY, P. B. (1989). Adolescent inpatient treatment. *Practical Approaches in Treating Adolescent Chemical Dependency.* New York: Haworth.

O'CONNELL, D. F. (1988). Managing the borderline patient in addictions treatment settings. *Alcoholism Treatment Quarterly, 5,* 61–71.

O'CONNOR, L. E., BERRY, J. W., INABA, D., WEISS, J., & MORRISON, A. (1994). Shame guilt, and depression in men and women in recovery from addiction. *Journal of Substance Abuse Treatment, 11*(6), 503–510.

OETTING, E. R., & BEAUVAIS, F. (1983). The drug acquisition curve: A method for the analysis and prediction of drug epidemiology. *The International Journal of the Addictions, 18,* 1115–1129.

OETTING, E. R., & BEAUVAIS, F. (1987). Peer cluster theory, socialization characteristics, and adolescent drug use: A path analysis. *Journal of Counseling Psychology, 34,* 205–213.

O'FARREL, T. J. (1989). Marital and family therapy in alcoholism treatment. *Journal of Substance Abuse Treatment, 6,* 23–29.

O'GORMAN, P. (1991). Codependency and women: Unraveling the power behind learned helplessness. *Feminist Perspectives on Addictions.* New York: Springer.

O'KEEFE, J., & NADEL, L. (1978). *The Hippocampus as a Cognitive Map.* Oxford: Clarendon.

OKUN, B. F. (1990). *Seeking connections in psychotherapy.* San Francisco: Jossey-Bass.

OLSON, D. H., BELL, R., & PORTNER, J. (1978). FACES item booklet. St. Paul: University of Minnesota Family Social Science.

OLSON, D. H., RUSSELL, C. S., & SPRENKLE, D. H. (1983). Circumplex model of marital and family systems: VI. Theoretical update. *Family Processes, 22,* 69–83.

ORFORD, J., OPPENHEIMER, E., EGERT, S., HENSMAN, C., & GUTHRIE, S. (1976). The cohesiveness of alcoholism-complicated marriages and its influence on treatment outcome. *British Journal of Psychiatry, 128,* 318–339.

OROSZ, S. B. (1982). Assertiveness in recovery. *Social Work with Groups, 5*(1), 25–31.

OSHER, F. C., & KOFOED, L. L. (1989). Treatment of patients with psychiatric and psychoactive substance abuse disorders. *Hospital and Community Psychiatry, 40,* 1025–1030.

OTTO, M. W., POLLACK, M. H., SACHS, G. S., REITER, S. R., MELTZER-BRODY, S., & ROSENBAUM, J. F. (1993). Discontinuation of benzodiazepine treatment: Efficacy of cognitive-behavioral therapy for patients with panic disorders. *American Journal of Psychiatry, 150,* 1485–1490.

PADGETT, D., STRUENING, E. L., & ANDREWS, H. (1990). Factors affecting the use of medical, mental health, alcohol, and drug treatment services by homeless adults. *Medical Care, 28,* 805–821.

PASCARELLA, E. T., & TERENZINI, P. T. (1980). Predicting freshman persistence and voluntary dropout decisions from a theoretical model. *Journal of Higher Education, 51,* 60–75.

PATON, A. (1989). Alcohol misuse. *British Journal of Hospital Medicine, 42,* 394–400.

PEELE, S. (1992). Alcoholism, politics, and bureaucracy: The consensus against controlled-drinking therapy in America. *Addictive Behaviors, 17,* 49–62.

PENICK, E. C., POWELL, B. J., BINGHAM, S. F., LISKOW, B. I., MILLER, N. S., & READ, M. R. (1987). A comparative study of familial alcoholism. *Journal of Studies on Alcohol, 48*(2), 136–146.

PERKINS, H. W. (1992). Gender patterns in consequences of collegiate alcohol abuse: A 10-year study of trends in an undergraduate population. *Journal of Studies on Alcohol, 53,* 458–462.

PERKINS, S. E. (1989). Altering rigid family role behaviors in families with adolescents. *Alcohol Treatment Quarterly, 6,* 111–120.

PERLS, F. S. (1969). *Ego, hunger, and aggression.* New York: Random House.

PERLS, F. S. (1970). Four lectures. In J. Fagan & I. L. Shepherd (Eds.), *Gestalt therapy now* (pp. 14–39). Palo Alto, CA: Science & Behavior Books.

PERLS, F. S. (1971). *Gestalt therapy verbatim.* New York: Bantam Books.

PERLS, F. S. (1972). *In and out the garbage pail.* New York: Bantam.

PERLS, F. S. (1976). *"The Gestalt approach" and "eyewitness to therapy."* New York: Bantam Books.

PERLS, F. S., HEFFERLINE, R., & GOODMAN, P. (1951). *Gestalt therapy.* New York: Dell.

PETTIGREW, A. G. (1986). Prenatal alcohol exposure and development of sensory systems. In J. R. West (Ed.), *Alcohol and brain development* (pp. 225–274). New York: Oxford University Press.

PHILLIPS, S. C. (1986). Alcohol and histology of the developing cerebellum. In J. R. West (Ed.), *Alcohol and brain development* (pp. 204–224). New York: Oxford University Press.

PISTOLE, M. C. (1989). Attachment in adult romantic relationships: Style of conflict resolutions and relationship satisfaction. *Journal of Social and Personal Relationships, 6,* 508–510.

PISTOLE, M. C. (1993). Attachment relationships: Self-disclosure and trust. *Journal of Mental Health Counseling, 15,* 94–106.

POLCIN, D. L. (1992a). A comprehensive model for adolescent chemical dependency treatment. *Journal of Counseling and Development, 70,* 376.

POLCIN, D. L. (1992b). Issues in the treatment of dual diagnosis clients who have chronic mental illness. *Professional Psychology: Research and Practice, 23,* 30–37.

POLSTER, E., & POLSTER, M. (1973). *Gestalt therapy integrated: Contours of theory and practice.* New York: Brunner/Mazel.

PORKORNEY, A. D., MILLER, B. A., & KAPLAN, H. B. (1972). The brief MAST: A shortened version of the Michigan Alcoholism Screening Test. *American Journal of Psychiatry, 129,* 342–345.

POTTER, A. E., & WILLIAMS, D. E. (1991). Development of a measure examining children's roles in alcoholic families. *Journal of Studies on Alcohol, 52*(1), 70–77.

POTTER-EFRON, P. S., & POTTER-EFRON, R. T. (1991). Anger as a treatment concern with alcoholics and affected family members. *Alcoholism Treatment Quarterly, 8,* 31–46.

POTTER-EFRON, R. T., & POTTER-EFRON, P. S. (1989). Outpatient co-dependency treatment. *Alcoholism Treatment Quarterly, 6*(1), 151–167.

PRELI, R., PROTINSKY, H., & CROSS, L. (1990). Alcoholism and family structure. *Family Therapy, XVII,* 1–8.

PREST, L. A., & PROTINSKY, H. (1993). Family systems theory: A unifying framework for codependence. *The American Journal of Family Therapy, 21,* 352–359.

PROCHASKA, J. O. (1979). *Systems of psychotherapy: A transtheoretical analysis.* Homewood, IL: Dorsey Press.

PROCHASKA, J. O. (1991). Prescribing to the stages and levels of change. *Psychotherapy, 28,* 463–468.

PROCHASKA, J. O., & DICLEMENTE, C. C. (1982). Transtheoretical therapy: Toward a more integrative model of change. *Psychotherapy Theory, Research and Practice, 19,* 276–288.

PROCHASKA, J. O., & DICLEMENTE, C. C. (1986). The transtheoretical approach. In J. C. Norcross (Ed.), *Handbook of eclectic psychotherapy* (pp. 163–200). New York: Brunner/Mazel.

PROCHASKA, J. O., & DICLEMENTE, C. C. (1992). Stages of change in the modification of human behaviors. In M. Hersen, R. M. Eisler, & P. M. Miller (Eds.), *Progress in behavior modification* (pp. 184–214). Sycamore, IL: Sycamore Press.

PROCHASKA, J. O., DICLEMENTE, C. C., & NORCROSS, J. C. (1992). In search of how people change: Applications to addictive behaviors. *American Psychologist, 47,* 1102–1114.

PROCHASKA, J. O., DICLEMENTE, C. C., VELICER, W. F., GINPIL, S. E., & NORCROSS, J. C. (1985). Predicting change in smoking status for self-changers. *Addictive Behaviors, 10,* 395–406.

PROCHASKA, J. O., NORCROSS, J. C., & DICLEMENTE, C. C. (1994). *Changing for good.* New York: William Morrow.

Prochaska, J. O., VELICER, W. F., DICLEMENTE, C. C., & FAVA, J. (1988). Measuring processes of change: Applications to the cessation of smoking. *Journal of Consulting and Clinical Psychology, 56,* 520–528.

PROCHASKA, J. O., VELICER, W. F., ROSSI, J. S., GOLSTEIN, M. G., MARCUS, B. H., RAKOWSKI, W., FIORE, C., HARLOW, L. L., REDDING, C. A., ROSENBLOOM, D., & ROSSI, S. R. (1994). Stages of change and decisional balance for twelve problem behaviors. *Health Psychology, 13,* 39–46.

PROTINSKY, H., & SHILTZ, L. (1990). Adolescent substance use and family cohesion. *Family Therapy, 17,* 173–175.

QUINTANA, S. M., & KERR, J. (1993). Relational needs in late adolescent separation-individuation. *Journal of Counseling and Development, 71,* 349–354.

QUINTANA, S. M., & LAPSLEY, D. K. (1990). Repproachment in late adolescence separation-individuation: A structural equation approach. *Journal of Adolescence, 13,* 371–385.

RASKIN, V. D., & MILLER, N. S. (1993). The epidemiology of the comorbidity of psychiatric and addictive disorders: A critical review. *Journal of Addictive Diseases, 12*(3), 45–57.

RATNER, E. (1988). A model for the treatment of lesbian and gay alcoholic abusers. *Alcoholism Treatment Quarterly, 5,* 25–46.

RAVEIS, V. H., & KANDEL, D. B. (1987). Changes in drug behavior from the middle to the late twenties: Initiation, persistence, and cessation of use. *American Journal of Public Health, 77,* 607–610.

RAWSON, R. A., SHOPTAW, S. J., OBERT, J. L., McCANN, M. J., HASSON, A. L., MARINELLI-CASEY, P. J., BRETHEN, P. R., & LING, W. (1995). An intensive outpatient approach for cocaine abuse treatment. *Journal of Substance Abuse Treatment, 12*(2), 117–127.

RAYBUCK, C. S., & HICKS, G. F. (1994). KIDS CARE: Building resilience in children's environments. *Journal of Alcohol and Drug Education, 39,* 34–45.

REESE, F. L., CHASSIN, L., MOLINA, B. S. G. (1994, March). Alcohol expectancies in early adolescents: Predicting drinking behavior from alcohol expectancies and parental alcoholism. *Journal of Studies on Alcohol,* 276–284.

RESNICK, H. L. (1969). Psychological resynthesis: A clinical approach to the survivors of a death by suicide. In E. S. Schneidman & M. J. Ortega (Eds.), *Aspects of depression,* Boston: Little, Brown.

RICE, K. G. (1992). Separation-individuation and adjustment to college: A longitudinal study. *Journal of Counseling Psychology, 39,* 203–213.

RICHARDSON, J. I. (1981, January). The manipulative patient spells trouble. *Nursing,* 48–52.

RIDGELY, M. S., GOLDMAN, H. H., & WILLENBRING, M. (1990). Barriers to the care of persons with dual diagnoses: Organizational and financing issues. *Schizophrenia Bulletin, 16,* 123–132.

RIDLEY, C. R. (1995). *Overcoming unintentional racism in counseling and therapy: A practitioner's guide to intentional intervention.* Vol. 5 of *Multicultural aspects of counseling series* (series ed. P. Pederson). Thousand Oaks, CA: Sage.

RILEY, E. P., BARRON, S., & HANNIGAN, J. (1986). Response inhibition deficits following prenatal alcohol exposure. In J. R. West (Ed.), *Alcohol and Brain Development* (pp. 71–102). New York: Oxford University Press.

ROGERS, C. R. (1970). *Carl Rogers on encounter groups.* New York: Harper & Row.

ROHRER, G. E., THOMAS, M., & YASENCHAK, A. B. (1992). Client perceptions of the ideal addictions counselor. *International Journal of the Addictions, 27,* 727–733.

ROOSA, M. W., SANDLER, I. N., GEHRING, M., BEALS, J., & CAPPO, L. (1988). The Children of Alcoholics Life-Events Scale: A stress scale for children of alcohol-abusing parents. *Journal of Studies on Alcohol, 49,* 422–429.

ROOSA, M. W., TEIN, J., GROPPENBACHER, N., MICHAELS, M., & DUMKA, L. (1993). Mother's parenting behavior and child mental health in families with a drinking parent. *Journal of Marriage and Family, 55,* 107–118.

ROSETT, H. L., & WEINER, L. (1984). *Alcohol and the Fetus.* New York: Oxford University Press.

ROTHBART, M. K., & AHADI, S. A. (1994). Temperament and the development of personality. *Journal of Abnormal Psychology, 103*(1), 55–66.

ROTHBERG, N. M. (1986). The alcoholic spouse and the dynamics of co-dependency. *Alcoholism Treatment Quarterly, 3*(1), 73–85.

ROUNSAVILLE, B. J., DOLINSKY, Z. S., BABOR, T. F., & MEYER, R. E. (1987). Psychopathology as a predictor of treatment outcome in alcoholics. *Archives of General Psychiatry, 44,* 505–513.

ROUSH, K. L., & DeBLASSIE, R. R. (1989). Structural group counseling for college students of alcoholic parents. *Journal of College Student Development, 30,* 276–277.

RUGEL, R. P., & BARRY, D. (1990). Overpowering denial through the group: A test of acceptance theory. *Small Group Research, 21,* 45–58.

RUYLE, J. (1987). Group therapy with older alcoholics: How it can happen and work. *Alcoholism Treatment Quarterly 4,* 81–95.

RYDBERG, U., ALLING, C., & ENGEL, J. (1985). *Alcohol and the developing brain.* Stockholm: Raven.

SARA, V. R., & THAM, A. (1985). Hormonal regulation of brain growth and the possible effects of alcohol. In U. Rydberg, C. Alling, & J. Engel (Eds.), *Alcohol and the developing brain* (pp. 27–34). Stockholm: Raven.

SATIR, V. (1972). *People making.* Palo Alto, CA: Science & Behavior Books.

SATIR, V. (1976). *Making contact.* Millbrae, CA: Celestial Arts.

SATIR, V., STACHOWIAK, J., & TASCHMAN, H. A. (1975). *Helping families to change.* Prepared and edited by D. W. Tiffany, J. I. Cohen, A. M. Robinson, High Plains Comprehensive Community Mental Health Center, K. C. Ogburn, & Hutchinson Public School System, Hutchinson, Kansas. New York: Aronson.

SCHACHTER, S. (1982). Recidivism and self-cure of smoking and obesity. *American Psychologist, 37,* 436–444.

SCHAEF, A. W. (1986). *Co-dependence: Misunderstood-mistreated.* Minneapolis: Winston.

SCHALL, M., WEEDE, T. J., & MALTMAN, I. (1991). Predictors of alcohol consumption by university students. *Journal of Alcohol and Drug Education, 37,* 72–80.

SCHANDLER, S. L., BRANNOCK, J. C., COHEN, M. J, ANTICK, J., & CAINE, K. (1988). Visuospacial learning in elementary school children with and without a family history of alcoholism. *Journal of Studies on Alcohol, 49*(6), 538–545.

SCHANDLER, S. L., COHEN, M., McARTHUR, D., NALIBOFF, B., & HASSELL, A. (1988). Activation peaking in intoxicated and detoxified alcoholics during visuospacial learning. *Journal of Studies on Alcohol, 49*(2), 126–130.

SCHINKA, J. A., CURTISS, G., & MULLOY, J. M. (1994). Personality variables and self-medication in substance abuse. *Journal of Personality Assessment, 63*(3), 413–422.

SCHLIEBNER, C. T. (1994). Gender-sensitive therapy. *Journal of Substance Abuse Treatment, 11*(6), 511–515.

SCHNEIDER, F. R., & SIRIS, S. G. (1987). A review of psychoactive substance use and abuse in schizophrenia: Patterns of drug choice. *Journal of Nervous and Mental Disease, 175,* 641–652.

SCHNEIDER, S. G., FARBEROW, N. L., & KRUKS, G. N. (1989). Suicidal behavior in adolescent and young gay men. *Suicide and Life-Threatening Behavior, 19,* 381–394.

SCHOPLER, E., & REICHLER, R. J. (1976). *Psychopathology and child development.* New York: Plenum.

SCHUCKIT, M. A. (1978). The disease of alcoholism. *Postgraduate Medicine, 64,* 78–149.

SCHUCKIT, M. A. (1985). Genetics and the risk for alcoholism. *Journal of the American Medical Association, 254,* 2614–2617.

SCHUCKIT, M. A. (1986). Genetic and clinical implications of alcoholism and affective disorder. *American Journal of Psychiatry, 143*(2), 140–147.

SCHUCKIT, M. A. (1994). A clinical model of genetic influences in alcohol dependence. *Journal of Studies on Alcohol, 55,* 5–17.

SCHWARTZ, L. S., LYONS, J. S., STULP, F., HASSAN, T., JACOBI, N., & TAYLOR, J. (1993). Assessment of alcoholism among dually diagnosed psychiatric inpatients. *Journal of Substance Abuse Treatment, 10,* 255–261.

SCOTT, E. M. (1978). Hypnosis with an alleged blackout. *The American Journal of Clinical Hypnosis, 20*(3), 209–212.

SEEFELDT, R. W., & LYON, M. A., (1992). Personality characteristics of adult children of alcoholics. *Journal of Counseling and Development, 70,* 588–593.

SELZER, M. L. (1971). The Michigan Alcoholism Screening Test: The quest for a new diagnostic instrument. *American Journal of Psychiatry, 127,* 1653–1658.

SEXIAS, J. S., & YOUCHA, G. (1985). *Children of alcoholism: A survivors manual.* New York: Harper & Row.

SHAFFER, H. J., & NEUHAUS, C., JR. (1985). Testing hypotheses: An approach for the assessment of addictive behaviors. In H. B. Milkman & H. J. Shaffer (Eds.), *The addictions: Multidisciplinary perspectives and treatments.* Lexington, MA: D.C. Heath.

SHAVER, P. R., & CLARK, C. L. (1994). The psychodynamics of adult romantic attachment. In J. M. Masling & R. F. Bornstein (Eds.), *Empirical studies of psychoanalytic theories: Vol. 5. Empirical perspectives on object relations theory* (pp. 105–156). Washington, DC: American Psychological Association.

SHEDLER, J., & BLOCK, J. (1990). Adolescent drug use and psychological health. *American Psychologist, 45,* 612–630.

SHER, K. J. (1985). Subjective effects of alcohol: The influence of setting and individual differences in alcohol expectancies. *Journal of Studies on Alcohol, 46*(2), 137–146.

SHER, K. J., & TRULL, T. J. (1994). Personality and disinhibitory psychopathology: Alcoholism and antisocial personality disorder. *Journal of Abnormal Psychology, 103*(1), 92–102.

SHIFFMAN, S. (1982). Relapse following smoking cessation: A situational analysis. *Journal of Consulting and Clinical Psychology, 50,* 71–86.

SHIFFMAN, S. (1984). Coping with temptations to smoke. *Journal of Counseling and Clinical Psychology, 52,* 261–267.

SHIPKO, J. S., & STOUT, C. E. (1992). A comparison of the personality characteristics between the recovering alcoholic and non-alcoholic counselor. *Alcoholism Treatment Quarterly, 9,* 207–214.

SIGAFOOS, A., REISS, D., RICH, J., & DOUGLAS, E. (1985). Pragmatics in the measurement of family functioning: An interpretive framework for methodology. *Family Process, 24,* 189–203.

SINGER, M., & ANGLIN, T. (1986). The identification of adolescent substance abuse by health care professionals. *The International Journal of the Addictions, 21*(2), 247–254.

SIRIS, S. G. (1990). Pharmacological treatment of substance-abusing schizophrenic patients. *Schizophrenia Bulletin, 16,* 111–122.

SKINNER, H. A., STEINHAUER, P. D., & SANTA-BARBARA, J. (1983). The Family Assessment Measure. *Canadian Journal of Mental Health, 2*(2), 91–105.

SMITH, D. E. (1986). Cocaine-alcohol abuse: Epidemiological, diagnostic, and treatment considerations. *Journal of Psychoactive Drugs, 18*(2), 117–129.

SOLOMON, P., & DAVIS, J. M. (1986). The effects of alcohol abuse among the new chronically mentally ill. *Social Work in Health Care, 11*(3), 65–74.

SOMMERS-FLANAGAN, J., & SOMMERS-FLANAGAN, R. (1993). *Foundations of therapeutic interviewing.* Boston: Allyn & Bacon.

SONNE, S. C., BRADY, K. T., MORTON, W. A. (1994). Substance abuse and bipolar affective disorder. *The Journal of Nervous and Mental Disease, 182*(6), 349–352.

SOUTHWICK, L., STEELE, C., MARLATT, A., & LINDELL, M. (1981). Alcohol-related expectancies: Defined by phase of intoxication and drinking experience. *Journal of Consulting and Clinical Psychology, 49*(5), 713–721.

STANTON, M. D., & TODD, T. C. (1981). *The family therapy of drug abuse and addiction.* New York: Guilford.

ST. CLAIR, M. (1986). *Object relations and self psychology: An introduction.* Pacific Grove, CA: Brooks/Cole.

STEELE, C. M., & JOSEPHS, R. A. (1990). Alcohol myopia: Its prized and dangerous effects. *American Psychologist, 45*(8), 921–933.

STEINGLASS, P. (1980). A life history of the alcoholic family. *Journal of the American Medical Association, 254,* 2614–2617.

STEPHEN, T. D., & MARKMAN, H. J. (1983). Assessing the development of relationships: A new measure. *Family Process, 22,* 15–25.

STREISSGUTH, A. P. (1986a). The behavioral teratology of alcohol. In J. R. West (Ed.), *Alcohol and Brain Development* (pp. 3–44). New York: Oxford University Press.

STREISSGUTH, A. P., BARR, H. M., SAMPSON, P. D., DARBY, B. L., & MARTIN, D. C. (1989). IQ at age 4 in relation to maternal alcohol use and smoking during pregnancy. *Developmental Psychology, 25*(1), 3–11.

STREISSGUTH, A. P., SAMPSON, P., BARR, H., CLARREN, S., & MARTIN, D. (1986b). Studying alcohol teratogenesis from the perspective of the fetal alcohol syndrome. In H. Zisniewski & D. A. Snider (Eds.), *Mental retardation and developmental disabilities* (pp. 63–86). New York: New York Academy of Sciences.

SUIN, R. M., & DEFFENBACHER, J. L. (1988). Anxiety management training. *The Counseling Psychologist, 16,* 31–49.

SWEENEY, D. F. (1989). Alcohol versus mnemosyne-blackouts. *Journal of Substance Abuse Treatment, 6,* 159–162.

SWEENEY, D. F. (1990). Alcoholic blackouts: Legal implications. *Journal of Substance Abuse Treatment, 7,* 155–159.

TALBOTT, J. A. (1986, July 1). Chronic mentally ill young adults (18–40) with substance abuse problems: A review of relevant literature and creation of a research agenda. Manuscript submitted by chairman of the University of Maryland Task Force on Chronically Mentally Ill Young Adults with Substance Abuse Problems to the Alcohol, Drug Abuse and Mental Health Administration, U.S. Department of Health and Human Services, and Department of Health and Mental Hygiene, State of Maryland.

TAMERIN, J. S., WEINER, S., POPPEN, R., STEINGLASS, P., & MENDELSON, J. H. (1971). Alcohol and memory: Amnesia and short-term memory function during experimentally induced intoxication. *American Journal of Psychiatry, 127*(12), 1659–1664.

TARTER, R. E. (1976). Blackouts: Relationship with memory capacity and alcoholism history. *Archives of General Psychiatry, 33,* 1492–1496.

TARTER, R. E. (1990). Evaluation and treatment of adolescent substance abuse: A decision tree method. *American Journal of Drug and Alcohol Abuse, 16,* 1–46.

TERENZINI, P. T., LORANG, W. G., & PASCARELLA, E. T. (1981). Predicting freshman persistence and voluntary dropout decisions: A replication. *Research in Higher Education, 15,* 109–126.

TEYBER, E. (1992). *Interpersonal process in psychotherapy: A guide for clinical training.* Pacific Grove, CA: Brooks/Cole.

THACKER, W., & TREMAINE, L. (1989). Systems issues in serving the mentally ill substance abuser: Virginia's experience. *Hospital and Community Psychiatry, 40,* 1046–1049.

THOITS, P. A. (1985). Self-labeling process in mental illness: The role of emotional deviance. *American Journal of Sociology, 91,* 221–249.

THOMPSON, K. E., & RANGE, L. M. (1991). Recent bereavement from suicide and other deaths: Can people imagine it as it really is? *Omega, 22*(4), 249–259.

THORNTON, R., & NARDI, P. M. (1980). The dynamics of role acquisition. *American Journal of Sociology, 80,* 870–885.

THORP, A., & NIKKEL, B. (1983). Alcohol's effect on medications. In Marion County Mental Health Department, *Dual diagnosis resource manual* (1989).

TIEBOUT, H. M. (1946). Psychology and treatment of alcoholism. *Quarterly Journal of Studies on Alcohol, 7*(2), 214–227.

TIEBOUT, H. M. (1949). The act of surrender in the therapeutic process with special reference to alcoholism. *Quarterly Journal of Studies on Alcohol, 10*(1), 48–57.

TIEBOUT, H. M. (1953). Surrender versus compliance in therapy with special reference to alcoholism. *Quarterly Journal of Studies on Alcohol, 14*(1), 58–68.

TOBLER, N. S. (1986). Meta-analysis of 143 adolescent drug prevention programs: Quantitative outcome results of program participants compared to a control or comparison group. *Journal of Drug Issues, 16*(4), 537–567.

TRAD, P. V. (1993). Substance abuse in adolescent mothers: Strategies for diagnosis, treatment, and prevention. *Journal of Substance Abuse Treatment, 10*, 421–431.

TURNER, W. M., & TSUANG, M. T. (1990). Impact of substance abuse on the course and outcome of schizophrenia. *Schizophrenia Bulletin, 16*, 87–95.

TUTTON, C. S., & CRAYTON, J. W. (1993). Current pharmacotherapies for cocaine abuse: A review. *Journal of Addictive Diseases, 12*(2), 109–127.

TYLER, J. D., CLARK, J. A., & WITTENSTROM, R. C. (1989). Mental health values and response to alcoholism treatment. *Counseling and Values, 33*, 204–216.

ULLMAN, A. D., & ORENSTEIN, A. (1994). Why some children of alcoholics become alcoholics: Emulation of the drinker. *Adolescence, 29*, 1–11.

U.S. DEPARTMENT OF HEALTH AND HUMAN SERVICES. (September, 1993). *Eighth special report to the U.S. Congress on alcohol and health* (NIH Publication No. 94-3699). Washington, DC: U.S. Department of Health and Human Services.

VAILLANT, G. E. (1983). *The natural history of alcoholism.* Cambridge, MA: Harvard University Press.

VAILLANT, G. E., & MILOFSKY, E. S. (1982). The etiology of alcoholism: A prospective viewpoint. *American Psychologist, 37*(5), 494–503.

VAN DER VEEN, F. (1965). The parent's concept of the family unit and child adjustment. *Journal of Counseling Psychology, 12*, 196–200.

VAN IJZENDOORN, M. H., JUFFER, F., & DUYVESTEYN, M. G. C. (1995). Breaking the intergenerational cycle of insecure attachment: A review of the effects of attachment-based interventions on maternal sensitivity and infant security. *Journal of Child Psychology and Psychiatry, 36*, 225–248.

VAN WORMER, K. (1987). Group work with alcoholics in recovery: A phase approach. *Social Work with Groups, 10*, 81–97.

VAN WORMER, K. (1989). The male-specific group in alcoholism treatment. *Small Group Behavior, 20*, 228–242.

VANNICELLI, M. (1982). Group psychotherapy with alcoholics: Special techniques. *Journal of Studies on Alcohol, 43*, 17–37.

VANNICELLI, M. (1987). *Group psychotherapy with adult children of alcoholics: Treatment techniques and countertransference considerations.* New York: Guilford.

WALFISH, S., STENMARK, D. E., SHEALY, S. E. & KRONE, A. M. (1992). MMPI profiles of women in codependency treatment. *Journal of Personality Assessment, 58*, 211–214.

WALKER, R. D., HOWARD, M. O., WALKER, P. S., LAMBERT, M. D., & SUCHINSKY, R. (1995). Practice guidelines in the addictions. *Journal of Substance Abuse Treatment, 12*(2), 63–73.

WALLACE, J. (1988). Children of alcoholics: A population at risk. *Alcoholism Treatment Quarterly, 4*, 13–30.

WATSON, L. (1991). Paradigms of recovery: Theoretical implications for relapse prevention in alcoholics. *Journal of Drug Issues, 21*, 839–858.

WAY, N., STAUBER, H. Y., NAKKULA, M. J., & LONDON, P. (1994). Depression and substance use in two divergent high school cultures: A quantitative and qualitative analysis. *Journal of Youth and Adolescence, 23*(3), 331–357.

WEBSTER, D. (1990). Women and depression. *Family and Community Health, 13*, 58–66.

WEGSCHEIDER, S. (1981). *Another chance.* Palo Alto, CA: Science and Behavior Books.

WEGSCHEIDER-CRUSE, S. (1985). *Choice-making for co-dependents, adult children and spirituality seekers.* Pompano Beach, FL: Health Communications.

WEIDEN, P., & HAVENS, L. (1994). Psychotherapeutic management techniques in the treatment of outpatients with schizophrenia. *Hospital and Community Psychiatry, 45*, 549–555.

WEISS, R. D., MIRIN, S. M., & FRANCES, R. J. (1992). The myth of the typical dual diagnosis patient. *Hospital and Community Psychiatry, 43,* 107–108.

WEITZMAN, J. (1985). Engaging the severely dysfunctional family in treatment: Basic considerations. *Family Process, 24,* 473–485.

WELTE, J. W., & BARNES, G. M. (1985). Alcohol: The gateway to other drug use among secondary-school students. *Journal of Youth and Adolescence, 14,* 486–498.

WERNER, E. E. (1986). Resilient offspring of alcoholics. *Journal of Studies on Alcohol, 47,* 34–40.

WEST, J. R. (Ed.). (1986). *Alcohol and brain development.* New York: Oxford University Press.

WEST, J. R., & PIERCE, D. (1986). Perinatal alcohol exposure and neuronal damage. In J. R. West (Ed.), *Alcohol and brain development* (pp. 120–157). New York: Oxford University Press.

WEST, M. O., & PRINZ, R. J. (1987). Parental alcoholism and childhood psychopathology. *Psychological Bulletin, 102,* 204–218.

WHIPPLE, S., PARKER, E. & NOBLE, E. (1988). An atypical neurocognitive profile in alcoholic fathers and their sons. *Journal of Studies on Alcohol, 49*(3), 240–244.

WOLIN, S., BENNETT, L., NOONAN, D., & TEITELBAUM, M. (1980). Disrupted family rituals. *Journal of Studies on Alcohol, 41,* 199–214.

WOODSIDE, M. (1982/1984). *Children of alcoholics.* Children of Alcoholics Foundation. (Original work published 1982 by the New York State Division of Alcoholism and Alcohol Abuse.)

WRIGHT, D. M., & HEPPNER, P. P. (1991). Coping among nonclinical college-age children of alcoholics. *Journal of Counseling Psychology, 38,* 465–472.

YALOM, D. (1995). *The theory and practice of group psychotherapy* (4th ed.). New York: Basic Books.

YESAVAGE, J. A. (1992). Depression in the elderly. *Postgraduate Medicine, 91,* 255–261.

YOCKEY, W. L. (1984). Children of alcoholics: psychometric substantiation of adjustment. Unpublished masters thesis, Cleveland State University, Cleveland, OH.

ZETTERSTROM, R., & NYLANDER, I. (1985). Children in families with alcohol abuse. In U. Rydberg, C. Alling, & J. Engel (Eds.), *Alcohol and the Developing Brain* (pp. 153–160). Stockholm: Raven.

ZILBERG, N. J., WEISS, D. S., & HOROWITZ, M. J. (1982). Impact of event scale: A cross-validation study and some empirical evidence supporting a conceptual model of stress response syndromes. *Journal of Consulting and Clinical Psychology, 50*(3), 407–414.

ZINKER, J. (1977). *Creative process in gestalt therapy.* New York: Vintage.

ZITER, M. L. P. (1989). Treating alcoholic families: The resolution of boundary ambiguity. *Alcoholism Treatment Quarterly, 5*(3/4), 221–233.

ZUCKER, D. K. (1985). Variables associated with alcoholic blackouts in men. *American Journal of Drug and Alcohol Abuse, 47*(2), 156–160.

ZUCKER, R. A., & GOMBERG, E. S. L. (1986). Etiology of alcoholism reconsidered: The case for a biopsychological process. *American Psychologist, 41*(7), 783–793.

ZUROFF, D. C. (1994). Depressive personality styles and the five-factor model of personality. *Journal of Personality Assessment, 63*(3), 453–472.

Name Index

Subject Index